Depression in Kerala

This book examines depression as a widely diagnosed and treated common mental disorder in India and offers a significant ethnographic study of the application of a traditional Indian medical system (Ayurveda) to the very modern problem of depression. Based on over a year of fieldwork, it investigates the Ayurvedic response to the burden of depression in the Indian state of Kerala as one of the key processes of the local appropriation or glocalization of depression. More broadly, Lang considers: What happens with the category of depression when it leaves the West and travels to South Asia? How is depression appropriated in a South Asian society characterized by medical pluralism? She explores on the level of ideas, institutions and materialities how depression interacts with and changes local worlds, clinical practice and knowledge and subjectivities. As depression travels from 'the West' to South India, its ontology, Lang argues, multiplies and thus leads to what she calls 'depression multiple'.

Claudia Lang is an ERC-funded postdoctoral research fellow working on the GLOBHEALTH project at Cermes3 (Center for research in medicine, science, health, mental health and society) in Paris, France.

Routledge Studies in Health and Medical Anthropology

Depression in Kerala
Ayurveda and Mental Health Care in 21st-Century India
Claudia Lang

Diagnosis Narratives and the Healing Ritual in Western Medicine
James P. Meza

For a full list of titles in this series, please visit http://www.routledge.com/Routledge-Studies-in-Health-and-Medical-Anthropology/book-series/RSHMA

Depression in Kerala

Ayurveda and Mental Health Care in 21st-Century India

Claudia Lang

Routledge
Taylor & Francis Group
LONDON AND NEW YORK

First published 2018
by Routledge

2 Park Square, Milton Park, Abingdon, Oxfordshire OX14 4RN
52 Vanderbilt Avenue, New York, NY 10017

Routledge is an imprint of the Taylor & Francis Group, an informa business

First issued in paperback 2020

British Library Cataloguing-in-Publication Data
A catalogue record for this book is available from the British Library

Library of Congress Cataloging-in-Publication Data
A catalog record has been requested for this book

ISBN: 978-1-138-48280-7 (hbk)
ISBN: 978-0-367-58958-5 (pbk)

Typeset in Sabon
by Taylor & Francis Books

Contents

Acknowledgements

Many people have contributed to this book in ways that are more profound and deep than I can express. I first acknowledge my deepest gratitude to the mentors of this project: Frank Heidemann who has been a teacher and friend for many years for helping me sharpen my anthropological perspective and for his unfailing support. William (Bo) Sax for opening up much of the network of mental health scholarship to me and for teaching me a great deal about healing in South Asia, ontologies, and the art of ethnography. He and the workshops he organized in Heidelberg and elsewhere were a constant source of inspiration. Mitchell Weiss for sharpening my thinking on cultural factors and the cultural epidemiology of depression resulting from his long interest in mental health and psychiatry in India and for sharing his knowledge on mental health and psychiatry in Indian films. I appreciate their extensive comments and suggestions for preparing this book.

I also own gratitude to Helene Basu – her vision of cultural and transcultural psychiatry and her work and thinking about psychiatry and ritual healing in India have strongly shaped my own understanding and emphasized the important contribution of anthropology in this field. Murphy Halliburton has been of invaluable help since the start of this project: he introduced me to the field of Ayurvedic psychiatry and into mental health care in Kerala and was a major support and good friend throughout this research.

I extend my warmest gratitude to the doctors and students at the Government Ayurveda Mental Hospital, the P.S. Varier Ayurveda College, Kottakkal, the Ayurveda College Thrippunithura, and the doctors, psychologists, social workers and the students at the three hospitals in Ernakulam and the private clinics whose names I have anonymized in the manuscript. I further thank all those who were either in state of deep despondency or recovered from it as well as those who cared for them for sharing their experiences of suffering with me. My special thanks goes further to my Malayali friends Babu Appat, Bino, Father Binoj, Burton Cleetus, Father John Maria Das, K. Gireesh, Sanat B. John, Anoop Kumar, Dilip Kumar, Father Xavier Manickathan, Rajan Mathai, Sister Miriam, Neela Nair, Rahul Nair, Father Bosco Njaliath, Indu P., Litto Palathingal, M.P Eshwara Sharma, K. Sundaran, Roy Southil, Sister Tessy and Muhammad Mashoor Thangal for their friendship, help, and hospitality and for many inspiring conversations. I am especially indebted to my friends Babu and Ancy and to Tom Paul who taught me a great deal about health, culture and suffering in Kerala and in whose homes I spent many months and was always made welcome. Thanks also to my friend and colleague Eva Jansen with whom I shared the challenges and spirit of the beginning of this project and to Anni Feiler, Janina Geist, Ursula Lang and Maria Wander for helping to take care of my children in India.

I particularly appreciate the support of Hilde Link and Matthias Laubscher during the early phase of this research. My research benefited from the work of other scholars whose challenging intellectual exchange was a source of inspiration, including Ananda Chopra, Hansjörg Dilger, Stefan Ecks, Jean-Paul Gaudillère, Byron Good, Sumeet Jain, Anne Lovell, David Mosse, Harish Naraindas, Heike Oberlin, Johannes Quack, Laurent Pordié, Ursula Read, Brigitte Sébastia, Roman Sieler and Annika Strauss. Thanks also to the participants of: the Oberseminar at the Institute of Social and Cultural Anthropology, Munich; the Medical Anthropology Forum, South Asian Institute, Heidelberg; the Seminar Series Medical Anthropology, Institute of Social and Cultural Anthropology, Berlin; and the Arogyam Network meetings in Heidelberg and Istanbul for comments on earlier iterations and sections of this manuscript. Moreover, the keen interest and often critical remarks of my students in München and Münster have contributed to refining my thinking on mental health in India. Many thanks to Emma Battell Lowman for her invaluable help in editing and commenting on the manuscript.

The research and writing up of this project were made possible by grants from the German Research Foundation (HE 2034/18–1 and LA 3225/1–1) and by grants from the Hochschul- und Wissenschaftsprogramm (HWP) and the Bavarian Gender Equality Grant (BGF) of the Ludwig-Maximilians-University, Munich.

Finally, thanks to my parents Hans and Ursula Lang for their constant support and to my brother Stefan Lang for creating the maps that appear in this manuscript. I am particularly grateful for my children Anand, Georgie, Jonathan and Gita Feiler for bringing the most precious joy and meaning to my life. Their readiness to accompany me on fieldwork, immerse themselves in school life in Kerala, and critically discuss cultural differences expanded my own horizons exponentially. Much more than I can say I owe to the friendship and love of my closest friend Andreas.

Preface

When I began this project in 2009, my main concern was tracing the appropriation, translation and reframing of depression as a mental health category in (re)invented Ayurvedic psychiatry.[1] I started in Kottakkal, a middle sized town in the mainly Muslim Malappuram district in Northern Kerala. Each morning, I travelled three kilometres by auto rickshaw to learn about Ayurvedic psychology and psychiatry in a way similar to that experienced by postgraduate students attending the Medical Doctor (MD Ay) qualifying course *Mano Vigyan avum Mano Rogam* [knowledge of the mind and mental illness]. At the P.S. Varier Ayurveda College and the Government Research Institute for Mental Diseases – popularly known as the Government Ayurveda Mental Hospital – I learned about the theory and practice of Ayurvedic psychiatry and Ayurvedic concepts of mind, mental health and mental disease, and about drugs and procedures to treat people whose thinking, feeling and, most importantly, behaviour deviated from what was considered socially acceptable or was bearable for both the patient and the patient's family. I conducted fieldwork at these two places, and at a third location, the private clinic of Dr Joseph John located in a mostly Christian town in Ernakulam district. I spoke with doctors, patients and caregivers, observed daily routines and sat in on consultations.

Though I have researched Ayurvedic psychiatry intensively for several years, I have done so as a medical anthropologist and not as a practitioner. Ayurvedic training is recognized by the Bachelor of Ayurvedic Medicine and Surgery (BAMS), a graduate degree involving four-and-a-half years of instruction and a one-year rotating internship. My research assistant, Neena, had just finished the taught portion of her training at the Ayurveda College in Kottakkal and was undertaking her internship (called the "house surgency") at the Government Ayurveda Mental Hospital (GAMH) when we met. She was one of the very few students who explicitly planned to specialize in psychology and psychiatry. During one of my stays at GAMH, we were given a separate office next to the consultation rooms of the medical officers. Patients and caregivers interested in talking with us came to share their stories. For many, the opportunity to vent about their problems and experiences of treatment was a welcome relief during their approximately forty-day stay at the hospital.

> It is just weak mind. You can give it any bloody name. I don't like the name the modern science gives, I also don't like the name *dhat*[2] syndrome, but I totally disagree with the name "major depressive disorder". You can call it "the sensitive mind syndrome". And antidepressants are not anti-depressants, they are depressants. They suppress your thoughts and emotions.

Subhash was usually soft-spoken, but this statement was anything but soft. It was a passionately voiced exclamation at the end of his account of all the different diagnoses he had received from the many psychiatrists he had visited before being admitted to GAMH in Kottakkal. Apart from major depressive disorder and *dhat* syndrome [semen loss, a condition psychiatrists and anthropologists have described as a "culture-bound syndrome" resembling depression and anxiety], he had been diagnosed with obsessive-compulsive disorder (OCD), anxiety disorder, somatoform disorder and hypochondriasis. Twenty-six-year-old Subhash and his mother Mallika arrived at GAMH just two days before we first met in February 2014. They were exhausted from the one-day train journey from Thiruvananthapuram to Kottakkal and had put all their hopes into this hospital, the only one of its kind in India. It was Subhash's mother who first unobtrusively peeked her head into the little office Neena and I shared and asked if she could come in. Mallika was a university lecturer in English literature. From a Brahmin family, she was physically delicate and strong-minded. And in that small room, she began to tell us the story of her son.

The problems started when he was fourteen. He was a bright student, a brilliant, ambitious and naughty child, who liked to challenge his teachers. He had a lot of similarly naughty and intelligent friends, liked to play cricket and was the captain of his team. Mallika spoke fondly and fiercely of her son in a way that seemed typical for a proud and loving mother. These were the happy days of childhood – a happiness to which she imagined her son would return when she told us later the good news that her son's appetite had returned. "I have bought four chapattis, two for him, two for myself," she told me excitedly.

> And he finished all the four. That was a happy sign that he is going back to his childhood. If that happens, if he is going back to his childhood days, that would be the luckiest for me. Because that was a time when he used to be very happy; in the company of his friends, admirers, all admirers.

Subhash was a keen and confident student but when the results of his ninth standard examinations did not meet his ambitious expectations, it came as a severe shock. He suffered palpitations. His mother took him to a heart specialist for treatment, but anxiety followed, then depression. He used to say again and again, "how can I show my face to the world?" Mallika told us. Even after the discovery that his teachers had miscalculated his results – which once corrected took his grade from a deplorable 50 per cent to a respectable 80 per cent – things did not improve. On the contrary, the situation worsened when Subhash began planning for postsecondary studies at one of the highly prestigious Indian Institutes of Technology (IIT) despite his concerned mother's advice to take things more gently. At this time the first OCD symptoms manifested: he would complain about small things and forced his mother to change the tables and other furniture in the house because "it was not good enough". "I didn't know that it was something related to his mind," Mallika explained, seemingly embarrassed for having acquiesced so unquestioningly to all of his wishes. "All I wanted was to please him."

When Subhash visited our office one day with his mother, he told a different story. When he was fourteen, he "had a chronic addiction to pornography videos and to masturbation", and believed it was this affliction that ruined his physical and mental health. Apart from causing lower back pain, weakening his body and mind and creating mood swings that impacted those around him, as a "sensitive guy" frequent masturbation had increased his anxiety and driven him into depression. Ayurvedic doctors diagnosed him with dhat and gave him medicines. The allopathic[3] psychiatrists he visited years later found nothing wrong with these habits and diagnosed him instead with depression, OCD and anxiety. He graduated from the IIT and later completed a degree in electrical engineering at a US university, but these accomplishments came at a cost.

> To a certain extent I was able to finish school, do my engineering. But with a lot of daily struggle for years. [...] I was not able to do engineering with good marks. Sometimes I used to sleep for forty-eight hours. Sometimes I didn't sleep for five, six days. Sometimes I didn't eat anything. Sometimes I used to overeat. All these things deteriorated my body and my mind.

With these difficult years in mind, Subhash was determined to stop taking the allopathic medication he had used for several years in the attempt to help him achieve some stability during the time he worked in northern India and Italy for an Italian software company. "After taking the medicines for years", he explained,

> I know that it's not good to be on medicines and going for work. Because I have worked for three years and I was not happy at all. I was getting a very good salary at a good position. But I was suffering so much. Nothing gave me happiness, buying something, watching a movie didn't bring me happiness. So it's not worth it! It was a struggle; it was a torture.

"He used to tell us about listlessness, lack of concentration, sadness," Mallika added. "It's a miracle how he passed the exams; he had to struggle very hard. In spite of all these troubles he managed."

The first psychiatrist he saw was a friend of his father. Many others followed. Their quest for successful treatment took Subhash and Mallika to the most renowned psychiatrists all over India, "keeping on," he stated sarcastically, "switching treatments, switching doctors, switching hopes" and, as he stressed in another context, switching diagnoses. Yet, in hindsight he realised that doctors could offer him neither a satisfying explanation nor a cure. "I was told that this is just the game of serotonin. You take the medicine, then you recover. If required increase the dose, but never stop taking it." "They told us," Mallika added, "that just like diabetes, mental illness is a chronic disease for which he has to continue the antidepressants over a long period". Unlike most other patients I met who smoothly combined a scientific narrative of neurochemical imbalance with other medical and religious explanations, Subhash was sceptical about the neurochemical imbalance explanation. He was well informed from online research, and explained that psychiatrists do not understand the relationship between depression and serotonin:

> First of all they have seen many patients with depression who had good serotonin levels. Second, even if the patient had a low serotonin level, they don't know whether the low serotonin level causes depression or the depression causes low serotonin level. So serotonin is not a help. It's high time that they realign, that they admit they have made a mistake.

Both local and global discourses resonate in Subhash's critique of allopathic pharmacological treatments for depression. In his experience, antidepressants and other psychopharmaceuticals were potent and fast acting but weakened his body and mind, which were both already compromised by the disease. As an extreme example of their damaging effects, he recounted that tricyclic antidepressants made him collapse for fifteen minutes each time he took them. Moreover, he added,

> Antidepressants are in fact depressants, they suppress everything. The mind stops thinking and that too has a deteriorating effect on the body. Your physical capacities get lost. You become emotionless. [...] You become someone else. You don't remain the person you used to be.

Going a step further – following a narrative of decline from a golden past that is characteristic for many practitioners of "ancient Indian sciences" such as Ayurveda – he added: "modern science can maybe kill antibiotics and viruses, but in treating the mind it's a total failure. Those people who went to the mountains, went to the forests, the ones who tried to master their mind, those were the ones who knew the mind." Subhash concluded that none of the many allopathic diagnoses he was given captured the true nature of his problem, namely a weak mind, a lack of mental strength or, if regarded from a more empathetic perspective, a sensitive mind. Both mother and son reflected extensively on this character trait, identifying it in themselves in combination with the intellectual strength they both possessed. For Subhash, his weak mind made him vulnerable to mental illness and accounted for the disproportionate physical and mental stress he experienced compared to others. His sensitivity also made him empathetic, compassionate and intelligent. "People who have a weak immune system," Mallika observed, "get one disease after the other. Similarly, people with a weak mind, they will have their fears, apprehensions, doubts about people." "Yet," Subhash chimed in, "many people with anxiety, depression, they are actually very creative." Following this comforting line of thought, Mallika continued: "They are caring and compassionate also. I don't think he can even think of hurting anybody's feelings." Framing Subhash's problem in terms of a weak or sensitive mind located the issue in an essential and integral part of him in contradiction to religious and psychiatric framings that propose to achieve a cure by eradicating or removing the problem – a foreign intrusion – with rituals or drugs.

Subhash's treatment journey included both religious and allopathic efforts before he came to Kottakkal to try Ayurvedic medicine. Astrologers diagnosed faulty planetary constellations and rituals carried out by malevolent relatives, and recommended various remedies. Brahmin and lower caste priests but also – as he interjected – some quacks prescribed certain remedial religious actions. He stressed the mind-pacifying effects of the ritual actions while at the same standing aloof from the ontologies invoked by them, a stance I found not infrequently among mental health professionals. Still, Subhash remembered that religious cures helped only for a short time before the problems returned. He exclaimed wearily,

> In the beginning when my parents got to know about my problems, we went to a Brahmin who did the mantras. At that time, the effect was good. But after few months when the problems were still there, you think that something is wrong with the astrologer and go to another astrologer. But we spent years!
>
> I have tried ten astrologers, I have tried magnetic therapy, I have tried acupuncture, I have tried acupressure, homeopathy, allopathy, Ayurveda, hypnotism, black magic, witchcraft. All these things I have tried, not only from one place, but from different practitioners, different places. There are so many people in India, everywhere.

Subhash and Mallika's navigation of therapeutic options and management of the attendant etiological and ontological uncertainties had no end in sight. The multiplicity of their experiences and interpretations creates a corresponding potential for multiple readings of their story, and evades a single coherent interpretation (Good 1994, 153). Subhash seemed to recognize the instability of his own narrative, explaining that efforts to locate the cause of his problems in magic poisoning or occult violence[4] sometimes collapsed, and that he then reorganized them into different layers of his mind.

> Yesterday also I was getting negative thoughts. [...] There are small moments of hypochondriasis [or "the doubting disease", as he called it] when I am thinking that some of my friends or relatives [...] that maybe they have done something. Now I am telling my mind, "no, this is your disease, so come back to your original self. This is your disease, your ailment, your thinking. In fact, they have done nothing!"

Diagnoses, root causes, etiologies and treatment efficacies are essential but remain provisional and temporary, ready to give way to other more powerful readings and more effective treatments.

Dr Sarasvati, Subhash's physician at GAMH, later told me that though he had tried many other treatment options, she thought he would improve here because they were doing the *shodana* [purifying] treatment. Although Subhash and his mother found it difficult to adjust to the atmosphere of the hospital, Dr Sarasvati noted, "I told them to complete. With *snehapana* [drinking of large quantities of ghee to lubricate the body] alone they will not get much improvement. They have to do *vasti* [enema], at least vasti." I asked her about Subhash's diagnosis. "He got many diagnoses," Dr Sarasvati replied.

> I think the correct diagnosis will be *vata* [wind, moving principle] and *kapha* [phlegm, stabilizing principle] both symptoms are there. But there is no need to stick upon the diagnosis. Diagnosis is needed but we cannot say that diagnosis is the most important thing.

I asked whether in this case psychotherapy, which is not part of the Ayurvedic treatment at this hospital, might be helpful. The problem was in an "advanced state" and too "deep rooted" for psychotherapy to have a positive effect, she explained. "After shodana it will become flexible, it will become of a fluctuating type. Then only there will be an effect of psychotherapy. Otherwise, I think there is not much relief with psychotherapy."

Even though they had placed great hopes in Ayurvedic treatment, Subhash left GAMH before his forty-day therapy was complete. Unlike many other patients, he was deeply disappointed with what he had experienced. He wrote to me several months later and said of the Ayurvedic treatment he received, "it's sad to say that apart from the de-toxifying part that it played, the rest was of no use to me. For my OCD and depression, it wasn't good and I am sure about it." Though he found the logic behind the treatment "interesting", Subhash believed the changes in mood he experienced were due to withdrawal from allopathically prescribed pharmaceuticals he had been taking. His condition worsened about seven days before he and Mallika left, he wrote, and he "was advised by the Ayurvedic doctors to restart the allopathic treatment and continue it under medical supervision." Although necessary at the time, this return to reliance on a psychopharmaceutical cocktail had immediate and long-term negative effects on his health. "It is difficult to explain how horrifying it was to be dependent on benzos for 1.5 years", he wrote. But the period of alarming withdrawal after going without "SSRI, SNRI, and Benzos (when I came from Kottakal) was worst. I couldn't sleep for so many days. My body weight got reduced by 10 kg. I remember having severe problems with my memory. [...] I used to be afraid of people around me." Subhash has since worked with various doctors to improve his dosages of some drugs and withdraw safely from others. He wrote to me one final time, stating proudly that after struggling for six or seven months after leaving Kottakal, he was much improved. He was off of the benzodiazepines and still taking SSRIs and tricylcic antidepressants. "There is one thing that has helped me," he added, "but I wouldn't be able to mention it till I go with it for some longer period of time, and am able to go strong without SSRIs and tri-cyclics. If it bears some fruit in the future I will reveal it to you." I still hope to hear this secret, and with it that Subhash has achieved some measure of cure he and Mallika have sought for so long.

I tell Subhash and Mallika's story not as representative of the stories and experiences that were shared with me in Kerala but because their narrative combined global and local, medical and critical discourses, and phenomenologies of depression in a singular way. Subhash stood out from the other patients and caregivers I met at GAMH for being constantly involved in self-analysis and introspection. Indeed, a doctor who noticed this told me that Subhash was too intelligent to be treated at the hospital. However, what is quite ordinary in Subhash and Mallika's story is something they have in common with many of the other patients I met: he had tried almost every other treatment available. Ayurvedic psychiatry was his last resort, as allopathic psychiatry was for Nura, who I met in the psychiatric unit of the Syrian Christian Hospital. This private allopathic multi-specialty hospital had a psychiatric unit, and I moved to research there because it was possible to meet many more patients diagnosed with depression there than in Ayurvedic psychiatric settings. It was located in a rural area of the Alapuzha district, a two-hour bus journey from the town where Hamid and Nura lived. We first met in January 2012 in a small office allotted to my research assistant, a Bachelor of Medicine and Bachelor of Surgery (MBBS) student undertaking her obligatory internship in psychiatry, and me in the psychiatric unit by the institution's doctors after the couple agreed to participate in a narrative interview after their regular psychiatric consultation. This was not the first time this lower class Muslim couple sought psychiatric outpatient treatment. Lorry driver Hamid first brought his twenty-seven-year-old wife to the facility eight years ago when she had become "depressed", Nura explained. Her use of that English term stood out to me, and I was keen to hear their story.

Hamid began: The birth of their first child was difficult. In the second half of her pregnancy, Nura felt as if a darkness was entering her mind; as if she was falling unconscious into a tunnel. She was taken to hospital and diagnosed with low blood pressure and a urinary tract infection. After treatment and discharge, doctors at another hospital later discovered a loss of amniotic fluid and opted to deliver by caesarean section. After the procedure, Nura's stitches became badly infected, so she had to stay in hospital for another month. A year later, she began experiencing severe headaches. "We took her to a hospital." Hamid continued, "They told us to take a scan. But no significant complaint or mental problems were seen in the scan." There was also no relief from the headaches, and Nura "used to be mentally disturbed the whole day." The couple then came to Syrian Christian Hospital. A doctor they saw about the headaches suggested they meet the facility's psychiatrist, who then prescribed ten tablets of which Nura took one. "By evening she stopped talking. She was lying flat on her stomach and when we looked she was staring with eyes wide open," Hamid recounted.

> Our neighbours said that some spirit that has entered her body. She was very noisy. But she didn't seem to realize that she was noisy. She acted as if some spirit had entered her body. By evening she came to the level of "Manichitrathazhu" [a popular Malayalam movie in which the heroine is under the influence of the spirit of deceased person].

Hamid paused then, visibly uncomfortable, and said: "When we say we should say the whole thing, isn't it?" Although his narrative moved easily between focusing on the body, the mind and external agents (spirits), he seemed to need to distance himself from any impression of being superstitious or backward – a pattern repeated many times in the course of our conversations.

Hamid went on:

> Every time this happened, we went to an *ustad* [Muslim scholar] who chanted mantras [in the Muslim context reciting chapters of the Qu'ran and Qu'ranic verses]. After our ustads did this she used to be energetic and all right. It went on like this for some time.

It was mainly at the urging of Nura's family, he emphasized, that they sought further treatment from religious healers. This was contrary to his inclination, he stressed, because as a communist he didn't believe in "those things". But Nura's parents preferred religious treatments and rejected psychiatry, fearing the stigma and side effects of psychotropic medications. But when treatments with the ustads failed to result in a cure, Nura and Hamid were on their own when it came to seeking treatment beyond religious options. Hamid took Nura to a psychologist who provided counselling and under whom she practised yoga for some years. "There were no more problems. She was able to do any kind of work," he said. Along with yoga and counselling she was prescribed tablets by a psychiatrist who diagnosed *vishada rogam* [depressive disorder] after Nura first diagnosed herself having learnt that depression can manifest in physical symptoms. "I have seen on TV that my problems of pain could be related to depression", she explained. "If there is depression physical diseases will not get cured. After I took this tablet [...] the backache disappeared." Nura explained the somatization of depression and the efficacy of anti-depressants in her case, however, by switching into the idiom of spirit possession: "After that time, I didn't have the problem of the earlier spirit [*badha*] entering me any more."

Nura became pregnant again shortly after the birth of the couple's second child. This time, Nura remembered, her brother and his wife pressured her to terminate the pregnancy, a rather extreme move, probably in response to Nura's earlier problems. She gave in, although this was contrary to both her and her husband's wishes. In addition to the abortion, Nura underwent sterilization. After this, she remembered, "the diseases started coming. My thoughts were always about these things". Starting with backache, she soon suffered pain all over her body. The couple sought treatment at various hospitals and also from *musliyars* [Muslim priests], *thangals* [Muslim healers] and ustads, never achieving a complete cure. "Different people said different things just like different doctors treat in different ways", Hamid said wearily. "They blew *surats* [chapters of the Qu'ran] over her, asked her to do *namaz* [daily prayers] and recite *ayats* [Qu'ranic verses], give a *vazhipadu* [offering] to a mosque, tied *elassu*[5] and *thakkidu* [protective amulets] on her body", he explained. "They diagnosed *dosham* [fault, affliction] in the family and *peti* [fear] inside me," Nura added. They also diagnosed problems with the couple's house relating to the placement of the toilet and *sarpa dosham* [an affliction related to the serpent deities][6] and carried out remedial actions.

For Nura and Hamid, each new explanation and each suggested remedy gave them a new sense of purpose. Nura was treated by various religious practitioners and Hamid rebuilt some parts of their house. As Hamid noted, "We were searching for any source that could bring some relief." However, he positioned himself firmly within a modernist discourse, saying "But this can be cured by consulting a doctor and doing some counselling". Seeking religious treatment, he said, was a "last resort." However, these treatments did, he stressed, bring change to her *subconscious mind* [Hamid used the English term], and "she felt some relief" after each healer's treatment. I once asked if anybody had diagnosed *kaivisham* or *kudotram* [local forms of occult violence] in her and Hamid answered, "No, nobody has. But does it really exist?" The way he asked reminded me of the suggestive power my questions could hold – that my mentioning kaivisham and kudotram somehow cemented the reality of these vernacular notions of affliction, coming as they did from someone with the cachet accorded a European researcher in this context. My research assistant was quick to explain my question: "Some people here say these things, that's why she asked. She is here to understand the customs and the culture of Kerala." Hamid took issue with the question. "From my experience, if we tell patients like her that something has entered their bodies it is likely to enter into their subconscious mind. I have experienced that with her." Then he told us how a *vastu* specialist they consulted for Nura's feelings of suffocation had diagnosed the spirit of a drowned person, provoking further negative changes in her subconscious mind.[7] "At the moment the specialist had said this she started to act like that drowned person. When we watched this we really got afraid." Hamid returned to his rationalist stance, stating that he did not trust "those people", such as the *vastu* specialist they consulted. Hoping for a psychiatric cure, Hamid took Nura to an elite mental hospital but left the same day after seeing the institution's patients and being afraid "that she might also become a full blown case". Online research turned up a hypnotherapist, "an atheist", Hamid stressed, "famous from magazines and TV shows for solving many court cases." Hypnotherapy improved his wife's condition, but she didn't continue the treatment, Hamid lamented. Nura remembered:

> He made me talk about what was inside my mind. He asked me to take a deep breath and then to exhale it thinking that my will power [*manobalam*]

> will increase day by day. I did it but didn't have the power to do it on a regular basis.

"Whatever was in her *subconscious mind*," her husband explained, "was removed." "Now she has no *mental* problems, now she is only tired, she wants to lie down always", Hamid continued.

> She cannot get up early and do work in a timely and orderly manner. But laying down she cannot sleep. Inside she is sad. She thinks that I will leave her. She says, "you will marry again. You will leave me."

Nura interjected: "I don't feel confident, that's all." "There is no other problem. The reason why we came here today is that she feels darkness in the mind. If it is needed we can do a scan. If there is any other problem we can go for a medical check-up". "This needs a permanent cure," Nura concluded. After emphasizing that hers is not a mental problem any more but merely a somatic and an emotional one the couple focused on the feeling of sadness.

> I feel sadness. In my heart I feel like a weight has been put on my chest, my heartbeat increases. Then I feel very tired and only want to lie down keeping my eyes closed. Tears will flow without me even realizing it. I will not care about anyone.

Hamid added: "She likes to stay in the dark. If we turn on the light she screams. She doesn't like to hear my voice then. She feels it as a very loud voice." "There is fear inside," Nura interrupted,

> I love my husband and my children very much. But in a depressed mood I don't talk to them then. When they come and kiss me I feel distressed and cry inside but I cannot express to them and cannot talk to them then. I talk to them when I am out of that mood. But when I am in a depressed mood I cannot talk to them.

Nura and Hamid's story vividly depicts an experience of dealing with depression in Kerala, and the impact one person's illness can have on those around them. In their narrative, global and local discourses, multiple ontologies of therapeutic practice and patient experience, and multiple contingencies and uncertainties combine and clash. Like so many stories I heard in the course of my fieldwork in Kerala, their narrative is less coherent than ambiguous and fractured, unstable and fragile, and engages, accentuates and merges different – often contradictory – subjectivities and ontologies. It reveals a subjunctive rather than an indicative mood, fluidity rather than stability. As with Subhash and Mallika, Hamid and Nura's story has the potential for multiple readings as well as the identification of ambiguous and fluid ontologies.

As with many other narratives I collected, Subhash and Nura's stories show that depression has not replaced vernacular theories and ontologies of affliction but is added to and sometimes syncretized with them in a creative and hybrid manner. They also show that many patients diagnosed with depression not only follow multiple itineraries and pragmatic modes of seeking help, but also express multiple and complex interpretative and ontological openness, pragmatism and insecurities. This exposes the ways that the category of depression is made multiple, unstable or liquid through multifold therapeutic practices in Kerala.

Depression arises out of a network of conceptual, institutional and material transformations, both global and local. It is these transformations and various ways of stabilizing, doing and experiencing depression in this part of India that *Depression in Kerala* examines. My aim is to explore local engagements with discourses and practices around depression by linking together several levels of analysis. Subhash's and Nura's narratives, along with many others, contributed to the development of this approach and impacted my research experience, demonstrating to me that depression is not one condition but many, not single but multiple.

Notes

1 I use the term (re)invention to denote that inasmuch as Ayurveda has been reconfigured since its encounter with biomedicine (Langford 2002). Ayurvedic psychiatry has been reconfigured as a presumed branch of classical Ayurveda (cf. Chapter 5).

2 For better readability I am not using diacritics and other particularities of the scripts for Sanskrit and Malayalam in transliterating Sanskrit and Malayalam terms.

3 Allopathy (or modern medicine) is the term used throughout India for biomedicine.

4 The term "occult violence" that I use in this manuscript denotes malevolent practices intended to harm others. It does not refer to practices of ritually healing the consequences of occult violence and spirit possession. It is not the healing practices that involve "occult violence" but those practices of "sending sickness" (Farmer 1990).

5 Mantras or Qu'ranic verses written either on a piece of paper or on copper, which are then rolled and inserted into a small round silver or golden case and worn around the neck, waist, or upper arm.

6 Many compounds of houses and temples have a *sarpa kavu*, a piece of land for the snakes, left untouched and wild with one or several snake idols engraved in stone for worshipping and appeasing the serpent deities. A neglect of the serpent deities is said to lead to *sarpa dosam*, an affliction fault brought about by the wrath of the serpents.

7 Vastu shastra is an ancient Indian body of knowledge about sacred and profane architecture and its relationship to inhabitants (Chakrabarty 2013), which has experienced a dramatic revival in recent years through promotion in TV shows and newspaper articles.

1 Introduction

The making of an epidemic

> An upbeat nation hides a terrible secret: the disease of loneliness that hijacks the brain, eats away at personality and snuffs out lives. Money, youth, success, talent, nothing safeguards against its grip. Yet India lives in denial.
>
> *India Today*, 5 March 2015

When one of India's largest English weekly magazines published the exposé "Depression: The Silent Epidemic" in 2015, it brought depression into mainstream public discourse in India and made it impossible to ignore. By framing depression (loneliness) as the opposite of one of the core values of India's collectivist society, *India Today* also emphasized the physical nature of the disease and noted that depression can impact anyone. In fact, the magazine sketched typical sufferers in order to give their readership a better understanding of those likely to be affected by depression. Most strikingly, they described a creative and talented urban woman, with a successful career and marriage, prosperity and active social life. By doing so *India Today* clearly established depression as targeting not the marginalized – those affected by hunger, poverty and economic insecurities – but rather India's prosperous middle class. In the article, a psychiatrist explained, "People from affluent sections of society have a very low threshold. They haven't suffered too much and can't cope when faced with the realities of life." The message is clear: depression is the new epidemic of "India Shining".[1]

India Today's exposé not only raised the spectre of depression as a new epidemic, it also presented it in scientific terms describing it as a brain disease. Chemical imbalance is described as the result of a "neurochemical storm" and in relation to the quantity of neurotransmitters and activity in certain areas of the brain. An insufficiency of the neutrotransmitters serotonin or norepinephrine affects the activity or the size of the prefrontal cortex, amygdala, the parietal lobes and the hippocampus and the outcome is depression, *India Today* explained. It also noted typical psychological symptoms of the disease such as "negative attitude towards everything, feeling of sadness, irritability, sudden lack of interest in everything, emotional behaviour and feeling of loneliness". Beyond the biochemical imbalance narrative, the article also made connections with the socio-economic transformations experienced in India since the 1990s, moving from a Nehruvian socialist to a neoliberal political economy and from a collectivist to an increasingly individualist society. These changes have been accompanied by related shifts in family and residence patterns, education, employment and lifestyle, and increasing loneliness and social disconnection in spite of – or because of – an increasing technological connectivity.[2] With the nation "losing" an estimated one out of every four women and every ten men to depression, "enough to fill a state the size of Maharasthra", the national economic burden is considerable.[3] But who is the real victim of this epidemic and its associated hardships? India Shining.

But there is hope, *India Today* assured. Depression is not the result of a lack of willpower, though this is a prevalent popular assumption in India. It is a disease studied by experts and for which evidence-based treatments are available. Cognitive behavioural therapy, positive lifestyle changes around sleep and exercise, and psychopharmaceuticals are presented as useful therapies. In reality, efforts to design "silver bullet" drugs have failed, and mainstream psychiatry has not moved much beyond the discovery of Valium in the 1970s and Prozac in the 1990s. However, the article assured, new medicines for severe depression could reach the market within the next few years. However, the medicalization of depression was not problematized. On the contrary, the article describes the relief many sufferers experience when told their problem is not their fault or due to a lack of willpower but that it is a disease, and with the latest drugs that are so easy to administer with so few side effects, there is every chance to treat depression before it can develop into a full-blown debilitating disorder.

Celebrity endorsements from those who have recently "come out" to the public with their experiences of depression have improved popular understanding that depression can and does affect anyone, including the prosperous and famous. By mentioning famous actors, poets, filmmakers and others as celebrities known to struggle with depression, *India Today* told us that if depression can happen to them, it can happen to anyone. However, though celebrity endorsement has played an important role in the marketing of treatments for depression (in particular antidepressant drugs) since the 1950s, in the early 2000s, psychiatrists complained that no celebrities were coming out with depression (Ecks 2013). In response, Indian media have recently begun to feature articles and interviews with Bollywood stars about this issue. It was a landmark moment, therefore, when actress Deepika Padukone, one of India's most popular and highest paid celebrities, was interviewed by Barkha Dutt on a popular English-language talk show aired on NDTV about her experience of depression (NDTV 2015). "India is the most depressed country in the world according to the world health organization," Dutt began, citing the prevalence of the disease in India at 36 per cent.[4] However, she went on, there is an "unneeded stigma and a sense of embarrassment when it comes talking about depression". Dutt then praised Padukone for helping to "break through the shroud of silence" of depression with her bravery of "going public with her own struggles". Though the stigma associated with depression could conceivably have damaged her reputation, Padukone emphasized her moral and ethical obligation to "save" the lives of other sufferers by using the platform afforded by her celebrity status to speak out. She began by refuting prevailing assumptions about depression and noting that ignorance about the disease is due to lack of knowledge and stigma that prevent people, and especially their family members, from seeking professional psychiatric help. She described her experience of depression as arising in the midst of a very successful career. She "suddenly woke up" to a feeling of "emptiness", of "a pettish feeling in my stomach", to a "feeling so low that I would just start crying at the drop of the hat. I couldn't understand what was happening to me". This was not just emotional, there were also physical manifestations: "My breathing was different. It was not a deep breath; it was a very shallow, uneven breath, sometimes struggling to breath. [...] It felt like a knot in my stomach." Unlike many Western accounts of depression as an experience of cognitive and emotional emptiness, Padukone identified a physical location for the sensation, and made use not of a psychological, but a somatic idiom. In fact, Padukone also identified the difference between sadness and depression in physical terms, noting that "sadness comes from a different place in my body and in my stomach and having anxiety and going through depression comes from a completely different one and it does something completely different to my body".

Presented alongside her mother, her psychiatrist and her counsellor, Padukone's interview functioned as a carefully staged performance of the increasingly hegemonic mental health discourse on depression and of the imagined power of the psychiatric profession to cure a depressed Indian people. When discussion shifted to the cause of the high rates of depression in India, the psychiatrist made a connection with the country's recent and rapid social transformations. He also noted that the problem was likely to worsen as 70 per cent of the nation's population was under the age of thirty-five and the 15–29 age group was experiencing the highest national suicide rates in the world. "If we continue to face stigma we will have an epidemic", he warned. "If we don't start learning how to prevent and to treat this we are in a huge problem in the coming ten to twelve years." Treatment, however, was not presented as solely curative but also as transformational. As explained in the interview, "the process of taking care of your depression is a voice of self-awareness and self-discovery and optimizing your lifestyle and your mind". Treatment of the disease need not disrupt its creative benefits when through treatment, "You can actually optimize someone's mood and retain, in fact enhance creativity. So, the suffering artist doesn't have to suffer any more." Like *India Today,* this celebrity interview addressed India's English-speaking middle class but this time also provided it with a Renaissance fantasy of depression as a condition of the creative, the artistic, the beautiful and the brilliant, one with the transformative potential for personal achievement and recognition.

Even more recently, on 6 June 2016 Professor Abhik Roy published "Tagore's Triumph over Depression", a powerful and timely piece in *The Statesman*, a prominent Indian English-language newspaper. Roy notes that millions of people in India are affected by depression but still face significant stigma that prevents them speaking about their illness or seeking help. In response, he highlights an important exception: the experiences of the Bengali literary genius and Nobel prize winner, Rabindranath Tagore who in the early twentieth century wrote of his struggles with depression. In letters to confidents, Tagore's descriptions of his suffering are vivid and shocking: "Night and day I think of death and hanker for death. I feel that I have achieved nothing and will achieve nothing, that my life has been a big failure from beginning to end". In another letter he wrote, "My heart is at this moment like a leaky boat, full of water, that can just keep itself afloat, but the least burden of responsibility becomes too much for it". Reflecting on the importance of Tagore's candid discussion of depression and the courage and dignity of his efforts to transcend the pain of this illness, Roy calls Tagore "a source of inspiration for all those who suffer from depression". Roy explains that Tagore's honest descriptions can encourage others to speak of their own struggles, that his example shows the value of engaging with spirituality and nature for sufferers, and that in Tagore's eventual triumph over his depression, other sufferers can find "ultimate hope" (Roy 2016).

Articles and TV broadcasts that aim to bring depression and its sufferers out of the shadows impact the stabilization of depression in India as a common, universal and a largely physiological problem that can affect everyone and, indeed, also affects India Shining and the rich, famous and creative. They place emotional suffering within a mental health discourse for which psychological and pharmacological treatment in line with recent neuroscientific research is available.

Depression multiple: dynamic ontologies

> Diseases of the brain become as much fabricated as sorcerers and spirits.
>
> (Basu 2014)

Depression is a disorder with global significance. According to reports (Murray and Lopez 1996; World Health Organization 2001b), it will be the second largest cause of disability worldwide by the year 2020. As such, not only the search for a cure, but also improved understanding of depression's specific manifestations, causes, experiences, and preventative and therapeutic options is required. The importance of this issue in India is difficult to overstate. As noted in both the high-profile exposé by *India Today* and Deepika Padukone's interview with Barkha Dutt but also the stories of Subhash and Mallika, Nura and Hamid, the impacts are widespread and can be devastating to individuals and their families.

Depression in Kerala explores the appropriation of psychiatric discourse on depression in a South Indian state. More precisely, I analyse the conceptual and ontological movement of depression, in particular how it comes to be rooted, fabricated and translated in Kerala while at the same time attending to the ways depression is integrated into and shaped by various global and local webs of meaning and practice. To trace this journey, it is also necessary to examine depression and its treatment in practice, and the ways related institutions and materialities are appropriated, adapted and reconfigured in response.

By combining qualitative and narrative interviews, participant observation in clinical and religious settings, awareness programs and conferences, and media analysis, it is possible to describe the different actors involved in establishing these at once global *and* local networks of depression in Kerala. Identifying and analysing the nodes and actors involved in these networks allows me to explore the links between mental health politics, clinical and academic institutions, economic interests, access to treatment, ontologies of affliction, the relationship between body and mind, and various subjectivities. I borrow the term "stabilization" from actor-network theory to refer to the ways in which these networks of depression gain coherence and consistence.

My aim is to explore local engagement with discourses and practices around depression by linking together several levels of analysis. By doing so, it is possible to demonstrate that depression is co-constituted on four closely interrelated, parallel levels: materiality or *Dinglichkeit*; institutions; ideologies and ideas; and practices. In other words, *Depression in Kerala* explores the multiple ways of stabilizing, doing and experiencing depression in this part of India. In so doing, it contributes to cross-cultural research on depression and global mental health in anthropology and cross-cultural psychiatry.

In this study I analyse local engagement with depression framed through the key concepts of glocalization and appropriation. The notion of "glocalization" (Robertson 1995) facilitates the exploration of the simultaneous and dual processes of globalization and localization of depression. The lens of glocalization helps to clarify how the global network of depression is locally appropriated and how local realities in turn shape global flows and discourses. First coined by Robertson in 1995, glocalization refers to the ways in which global flows are appropriated and transformed in various local contexts. With regard to what could be called *psychoscapes*, adding to Appadurai's (1996) five scapes namely ethnoscapes, technoscapes, financescapes, mediascapes and ideoscapes, psychoscapes could be flows of experts in the psy-sciences, mental health institutions, psychopharmaceuticals, psychiatric knowledge, mental health policies and disease concepts. And it is not only the concept of depression that has gone global: actors such as psychiatrists and other experts, knowledge about neurochemistry and the brain, broad institutional shifts from the asylum to outpatient and community care, and the imaginary of effective disease-specific drugs all flow literally and intellectually around the globe. Once locally appropriated, particular manifestations then contribute to the growth of depression as a disease and discourse, globally and in specific locations.

My use of the term "appropriation" follows that of anthropologist Hans-Peter Hahn (2004) who uses it to describe the creative processes of reinterpretation and localization of technical artefacts in Africa. Appropriation also provides a valuable conceptual framework for understanding the translation and stabilization of a disease concept.[5] The notion of appropriation is particularly useful as it emphasizes the agency and creativity of the people who adopt, translate, reframe and integrate ideas and ideologies, diagnostic technologies, pharmaceuticals, institutions and practices into different frameworks thereby reconfiguring local institutions. Appropriation runs counter to cultural homogenization and focuses on the persistence of local diversity despite presumed global conformity.

In the way fellow anthropologists follow the "social life of things (Appadurai 1986) or the "social life of pharmaceuticals" (van der Geest, Whyte and Hardon 1996), I follow the conceptual, institutional, material and experiential life and the "multiple reality" (Mol 2002) of depression in Kerala. Key to this project is the notion that globalization of depression does not lead to the "globalization of the American psyche"; that the world is not becoming "crazy like us" (Watters 2010). Local framings of mental illness and vernacular healing knowledge and practices have not simply been washed away by a "tide of modernization" (Taylor 2001), which in the case of mental distress refers to the theory and practice of mainstream psychiatry and Western psychology. Instead I show that depression is locally stabilized in Kerala by various actors and on different levels leading to identifiable regional or local discourses on depression. The intent is not to ignore colonial and postcolonial asymmetries of power and wealth. On the contrary, the hegemony of biomedicine and, for that matter, allopathic psychiatry, as a contested terrain and "a zone of cultural debate" (Appadurai 1988) in defining and treating depression and in dominating mental health care over Ayurveda and other institutionalized and non-institutionalized medical and religious healing practices as well as the hierarchy of knowledge and practice are a central theme of this book. Mainstream psychiatric institutions, ideas and drugs are hegemonic in the "psy disciplines" (Rose 1996) or "psy-ences" (Raikhel and Bemme 2016).[6] The relationships between mainstream psychiatry, psychology, Aryuveda, and religious and ritual healing are deeply asymmetrical. Thus, the question of how depression is appropriated that permeates this book also highlights the contested fields of power, legitimization and exclusion within mental health care in Kerala. It relates the issue of global circulation and local appropriation of psychiatric nosologies and therapeutics to global and local mental health politics and struggles of legitimization, contestation and demarcation, and also to the subjectivities of patients and their caregivers in Kerala. The ethnography of the appropriation of depression is therefore also a depiction of a local medical modernity and of processes of negotiating science, modernity and tradition and of positioning, legitimizing and re-defining therapeutic practices and practitioners within it. Further, it is an ethnography of subjectivities and narratives forming a nexus of discourses from which an illness narrative draws and within which subjects position themselves and thereby expresses different ontologies. The subject of this book is then the constitution of "depression" as a medical and/or religious problem, as an ontological and experiential entity, and as a public health concern and its local translations and reframings. I follow the modern notion of depression as a neurochemical imbalance, initially established in the 1950s as a product and requirement of both the development of antidepressants and the ideology of mental health care de-institutionalization, wherever it is used to diagnose or to self-diagnose, to treat or to understand distress, suffering and despondency, or to create awareness. In other words, I map depression as a glocal ontological entity. Tracing a specific iteration of local appropriation and understanding its multiple realities and reframing of depression, I explore in detail how mental health policies, clinical and academic institutions, economic interests, access and pathways to treatment, ontologies (of affliction, the mind and the body), and subjectivities are linked and interrelated.

Disease categories such as depression are the product of a network of theories, professions, institutions, pharmaceuticals and technologies that stabilize them. This network – or global web – also flows into and intersects with other local networks so that it gradually changes shape in each specific locality. As de Laet and Mol (2000) illustrate, flexibility, portability, fluidity, need and ease of incorporation into a local setting may all influence the uptake and appropriation of items and by extension also of ideas, institutions and practices and thus help to stabilize diseases such as depression. Lakoff's notion of "diagnostic liquidity" (Lakoff 2005) denoting a process of abstraction that brings diverse patient subjectivities and life trajectories into the same classification scheme and thus renders psychiatric concepts malleable, and Latour's concept of the "immutable mobile" indicating objects that associate the features of "being mobile but also immutable, presentable, readable and combinable with one another" (Latour 1986) are both useful for understanding how symptoms and experiences are rendered compatible or commensurable. The mobility, portability and fluidity of depression and its diagnostic liquidity facilitate the global flows of depression. Since the early 1980s,[7] depression and other psychiatric diagnoses have lost their specificity and locality and can more easily be incorporated into diverse local contexts. This loss of specificity and singular focus on a symptomatic approach may be partly responsible for a general avoidance of the exploration of deeper existential meanings that facilitate local appropriation and the creation of new stabilizing global-local networks. Beyond merely medicalizing distress and social suffering, depression then provides an idiom for articulating locally relevant experiences of distress and social suffering for mental health professionals and laypeople alike. I argue that it is the ontological instability, fluidity or malleability of depression and its associated practices that stabilizes depression in Kerala.

Depression in Kerala arises out of a network of conceptual, institutional and material transformations both global and local. It is stabilized through clinical, research and pedagogic practice and experienced locally in multiple ways. It is these transformations and the multiple ways of stabilizing, doing and experiencing depression in this part of India that give rise to depression multiple. Various ways of appropriating, translating, enacting and doing depression not only stabilize its ontology but also make it fragile, fluid and multiple. Because of the fact that numerous actors appropriate and translate depression into different contexts and spaces depression is stabilized not as one, but as many. As depression moves through different worlds, people navigate different ontologies. In Kerala, then, ontologies of depression are not stable but dynamic, flexible and pragmatic.

Though they often appear in medical talk and practice as such, diseases are not independent entities. They are the products of specific historic and cultural discourses and configurations. However, disease entities are not mere interpretations or perspectives (of the body, the mind, suffering). As objects, diseases are always enacted. The first assumption is now conventional knowledge in anthropology, but the latter is the result of the so-called "ontological turn" and the influence of Science and Technology Studies (STS). My argument that depression is multiple draws from STS and from this recent ontological debate in anthropology. One of the theoretical approaches that informs my approach comes from the philosopher Ian Hacking who, in his historical works on psychiatric disease entities that he describes as "dynamic nominalism", explores the relationship between ontology and epistemology; or in other words, "the interactions between what there is (and what comes into being) and our conceptions of it" (Hacking 2002). Following Hacking I will investigate the "looping effects" of the disease entity depression and knowledge about it, the people classified as being of a depressive kind, experts or professionals who generate or legitimate knowledge about depression, and institutions that guarantee their status as experts (Hacking 2007). People diagnosed with depression (as well as depression itself) are

> moving targets because our investigations interact with the targets themselves, and change them. And since they are changed, they are not quite the same kind of people as before. The target has moved. That is the looping effect. Sometimes our sciences create kinds of people that in a certain sense did not exist before.
>
> (Hacking 2007)

The focus of Hacking's historical ontology is "objects or their effects which do not exist in any recognizable form until they are objects of scientific study" (Hacking 2002, 11). In line with Hacking, I suggest that depression offers not only a new sense of who others are but also produces a new sense of who one is and why one is a certain way. Prominent examples of the process in which new categories of diseases are related to the reconfiguring of persons include trauma (or post-traumatic stress disorder) (Young 1995) and multiple personality disorder (Hacking 1995). But we can also observe this process in the case of depression. Depressive disorder came into being as a disease category in the 1950s – and changed in the 1980s with pharmaceutically influenced neurochemical ideas. Thus emerged a new kind of patient: individuals suffering from depression. Along with it – whether as its precursor or its effect is disputed – came the drugs and therapies to treat depressive disorder, the institutions in which these new kinds of patients could be treated, the experts who generated and used specific knowledge of the disease category, and a body of expert knowledge that also trickles down into popular knowledge. These different realms reinforce and transform each other, thereby constantly moving their target, again feeding back into the other domains. The stronger the loops, the more stable, natural and taken for granted depression as a medical ontology becomes. Depression then becomes a new way of talking and thinking about distress, marginalization and social (in)equality and enables the "biomedical reshaping of global citizenship" (Mills 2014).

What happens when this looping effect stabilizing depression travels around the globe and lands in a place such as Kerala? Does it hold? As I will show in *Depression in Kerala*, it does. But there is more to it. In the local context of Kerala, the looping effect is expanded, assembling elements that at first seem unrelated, such as the Ayurvedic *doshas* and *gunas*, blocked body channels, spirits, occult violence or exorcists. Moreover, it involves people and patients navigating the actors and the ontologies created by therapeutic practice. Furthermore, in adapting to patients' worlds, medical and religious practitioners are often highly pragmatic in creating different ontologies through the same therapeutic practices. Global and local loopings interact and help to stabilize and locally appropriate depression in Kerala.

To better understand how this works in practice, it is useful to draw on another body of work that has had a strong influence on this book: science and technology studies focusing on actors and networks. Actor-network theory is not a single, coherent concept, but rather a suite of theoretical frameworks that help to reveal or interpret diverse relationships across space and time, and as such I take only what is most useful from ANT for the work at hand (per Mol 2010). My approach has also been influenced by the work of Annemarie Mol who investigates the process of practising ontologies, or doing diseases. To focus on the multiple ways diseases are "done in practice", Mol argues, reveals the object of manipulations as many through which reality multiplies. This leads to complex relations between these objects in practice. For Mol, a "praxiography" (Mol 2002, 33) is a turn away from perspectivism that explores what a disease means to different actors towards the disease "itself" that includes both the way doctors and scientists do a disease through clinical, research, and pedagogic practice and the way patients live a disease. This is a move away from epistemology and representation towards ontology that manifests in practice and therefore can be studied with ethnographic methods. Objects are not out there in the world waiting to be interpreted or represented but they are enacted in practice. "Reality is secreted" not only in the laboratory as a "set of productive forces", as Latour and Woolgar (1979, 243) argue, but also, I suggest, in a multiple set of clinical, research and pedagogic practices. This is not only true for medical but also for religious practices that deal with spirits, possession and sorcery. Basu (2014, 176) argues: "The shrine provides a setting that Bruno Latour might compare to a laboratory, where – instead of 'natural facts' – 'divine facts' are fabricated by means of actions of human and nonhuman actors or 'existential forms' (Latour 2010)." Langwick (2011) has shown that ontologies are created through therapeutic practice and are orchestrated through ontological politics.

How are the objects of multiple practices related? How is depression as the object of mainstream psychiatric intervention, of Ayurvedic treatment and of practices that address spirits and sorcery assembled? I suggest that it is an "ontological choreography" and the practical work of alignment that creates a commensurate world (Cussins 1996) or "coordination work" (Mol 2002, 66) that assembles the enacted depressions multiple whose ontologies are no longer stable but fragile and which differ between sites (Cussins 1996; Mol 2002). In this process of assembling, translations "draw together and establish difference at the same time" (Mol 2002, 83). These works of alignment link diverse entities and agents together into a network (Latour and Callon, 1981) "to the extent that they come to understand their situation according to a certain language and logic, to construe their goals and their fate as in some way inextricable" (Rose 1999). It is through these works of alignment that depression enacted in Ayurveda or ritual healing practice may be considered the same as depression enacted in clinical encounters and practice of mainstream psychiatrists and again as depression enacted by neuroscientific research as well as depression experienced by sufferers in multiple ways. Ontologies are often rendered commensurable, but they regularly also stand parallel to each other instead of speaking "on behalf of" (Latour and Callon 1981, 279) each other. In the latter case, depression ontologies of neurochemicals, DSM and ICD categories, of doshas, of spirit affliction or occult violence may also remain resolutely distinct. These alternative figurations sometimes meet – for instance in patients' narratives or in the treatment practice of various practitioners – but they do not necessarily fit together. They may also "rub against each other" (Brives 2013) with the frictions and dilemmas that such contact entails.

In the same way that divination "brings novel entities forth into existence" (Holbraad 2009), diseases are enacted (Mol 2002) and "ontologies are created through therapeutic practice" (Langwick 2011, 12), depression multiple is brought forth and created not only through clinical but also through teaching and research practices. These again create and stabilize depression and the "kinds of people" that are classified and perceive themselves as suffering from depression as "moving targets" (Hacking 2007). Multiple therapeutic practices produce multiple, often frictious and interfering interpretations, representations, meanings and etiologies of depression that are, as Rhodes (1980) has shown, linked by the itinerary of patients and their families though different systems that constitute mental health pluralism in a South Asian local reality. These, in turn, are not conflictual but cumulative in their effect on their perspectives and experiences of their illness (Good 1985; Callan 2012). They are also linked by the itinerary of medical and ritual healing agents and by the framing of similar practices as acting on neurochemicals, doshas, spirits or occult violence. More importantly, therapeutic practices produce multiple materialities and ontologies of depression as moving targets that, again, lead to different kinds of depressive people, different phenonomenological experiences and understandings of depression, and different therapeutic agents and methods for treating depression.

Multiple glocal (global and local) assemblages and looping effects of concepts, institutions, drugs and therapeutic practice produce depression as neurochemical imbalance in the brain, as doshic imbalance, as mental and moral weakness, as heat and anger, as spirit affliction, or as occult violence. Depression then flows through these multiple spaces and simultaneously transforms and is transformed by them. As *Depression in Kerala* shows, neurochemical imbalance can then, for example, be at once an underlying physiological cause to be addressed by psychopharmaceuticals, a doshic imbalance to be addressed by purifying, pacifying and mind strengthening treatment, and/or a symptom and physiological manifestation of spirit affliction or occult violence. Mental and moral weakness can be both cause and symptom of neurochemical imbalance, doshic imbalance, spirit affliction or occult violence. Likewise, one and the same therapeutic practice may create or stabilize different ontologies. Ayurvedic therapeutic vomiting may then be a therapy to treat vitiated *kapha dosha*, neurochemicals and *kaivisham*. Fumigation may address both doshas and spirits. Psychopharmaceuticals may correct a neurochemical imbalance as well as acting as a protection against occult influences. Psychopharmaceutical and Ayurvedic pills may become antidotes for occult violence. Similarly, an increasing number of ritual healers prescribe psychopharmaceuticals or Ayurvedic medicine. Deliverance prayers, exorcism or kaivisham treatment may remove not only spirits or occult violence but also correct neurochemical imbalance or balance vitiated doshas. These treatments target a multiple ontology of depression.

Multiple ontologies of depression are also experienced differently and may become part of diverse local phenomenologies of depression. Such translations and assemblages further

> demand that people move back and forth between healing settings, that they take a variety of kinds of medication, and that they subject themselves to different therapeutic tools and procedures. They also open up the possible emergence of bodies and disease entities that are enacted through the coordination of a variety of biomedical procedures and a variety of non-biomedical therapies.
>
> (Langwick 2007)

Depression multiple that is produced through different practices is not free from power asymmetries. "Ontological politics" (Langwick 2011, 9) defines which bodies and threats are allowed to exist and which ones are marginalized or excised in postcolonial time and space. On the other hand the narratives in this book illustrate often other layers of occult power that attributes healing agency to deities or God rather than to medical substances or procedures as it attributes illness causing agency to spirits, malevolent occult actions or nocuous passions and thus turn hierarchies of finance, knowledge or legitimacy on their head. In most of the cases, however, these different layers of epistemological and ontological power and agency get entangled and are fugacious, ephemeral, unstable and pragmatic, ready to transform into other framings of affliction and always adapted to and shaped by different healing contexts.

As it grows, the network of depression can take various forms, create new connections and discard others, be approached and construed through various entryways, and break off and begin again along new lines. Through the dynamic creation of new networks and dynamic ontologies, depression is not one unitary pathological reality but many. Depression becomes multiple as new conceptual and therapeutic networks are created. Following Deleuze and Guattari's (1987) rhizomatic approach I capture the meanings and ontologies created through new connections and assemblages and decentre psychiatric origins.

The global dynamic network of depression is then expanded and stabilized by a local network of depression created not only by practitioners of mainstream psychiatry and (re)invented Ayurvedic psychiatry, but also by other actors such as religious practitioners, agents of occult violence and remedies of all varieties. All of this happens in spite of efforts of the "worldwide web of doctors, hospitals, universities, clinics, journals, experiments, and professional associations" (Sax 2009) to purify their own established network of social and historical context on the one hand and of assemblages with other "non-modern", "backward", superstitious networks on the other. I have argued that in spite of or rather because of all these efforts of growing depression – and mental health literacy – the neurochemical imbalance narrative of depression has not neatly replaced other ideas and practices around causes and treatment of mental affliction. Rather, it has become meaningfully entangled with them. This is why, as Nura's and Subhash's narratives at the outset of *Depression in Kerala* and so many others like them exemplify, the ontologies of depression thus produced and engaged by sufferers and caregivers are fugacious and unstable, often highly pragmatic, and tend to reflect rhetorical moves rather than deep convictions. Further, they are mixed, if necessary, with other narratives of spirits and occult violence and weak-mindedness. Depression often becomes, in the narratives of doctors, healers and patients, "not an endpoint, a stable signified, but only another touchstone, another sign" (Langford 2002, 258) mixed with other narratives of doshas, spirits and sorcery. It is frequently more of a "rhetorical moment" (ibid.) used to emphasize affiliation to a scientific medical discourse or citizenship (Ecks 2005) and employed as a statement to emphasize a desirable and modern "scientific temper" and to demarcate oneself from backwardness and superstition.

By moving through the mental health pluralism of Kerala, patients find multiple options of treatment and care for their suffering. They are thus able to experiment in order to find a therapy that works for them (Halliburton 2004) and this also prevents sufferers from becoming locked into a single diagnosis (Rhodes 1980). Through mental health pluralism, meanings, worlds and experiences multiply. Suffering and distress transform and are transformed by these multiple worlds that both produce and heal depression multiple. My own understanding of depression as a fugacious research target was shaped by my movement through the network that makes up depression, its treatment and its experience in Kerala, and through the multiple worlds of those in distress. Like many of those who shared their stories with me, I moved through multiple worlds, meanings and transformative experiences that stabilized and challenged notions of depression as a biomedical category, or Ayurvedic psychiatry as a single regime. The implication of the observably shifting ontologies of those who seek treatment for depression in Kerala is evidence of my contention that depression is not one, but many. This is critical because, as statistics and narratives agree, depression is an increasingly common experience, and thus treatment for depression involves a necessarily ongoing and open-ended discourse. We need sustained and critical attention to the specificities of experience and ontology in order to create robust strategies to deal with an illness stabilized by various processes that seems to be constitutive of our modernity.

Critical and cross-cultural research on depression

Depressive disorder is a medical condition that is the product of a long history that stretches back to Hippocrates. Then, the disorder was understood through humoral theory as arising from an excess of black bile with symptoms including despondency, irritability and sleeplessness. Christian theological ideas of acedia (a sinful state of the soul characterized by listlessness, feelings of spiritual futility and despondency) attributed to the interference of demons were revived in seventeenth and eighteenth century descriptions (Jackson 1986) that then gave way to narratives of melancholy as madness. Melancholy was constructed as a condition associated with genius and cultural distinction in the late Renaissance when Greek melancholia as character trait or mark of genius (not as disease) was rehabilitated and later developed into the romantic melancholia of the nineteenth century related to ennui and *weltschmerz* (Jackson 1986; Jadhav 2000). Acedia was treated by priests, melancholia by doctors. This divergence in their diagnosis and treatment was a part of a wider shift around the growing importance of medicine over religion in issues related to the mind and the associated transition from regarding emotional distress and different perceptions of reality as a problem of morality or possession towards understanding them as a medical problem and a disease (Good, Good and Moradi 1985).

Depressive disorder as we know it today is a relatively recent phenomenon. Despair and hopelessness were the core symptoms of melancholia but somatic symptoms were not recognized. Medically unexplained aches and pains were diagnosed as hysteria and as having little in common with depression, as melancholia increasingly came to be called. In the nineteenth century – the age of neurasthenia – a broad range of psychological and somatic diagnostic criteria soon became coterminous with depression. It was with the advent of the opium cure for depression in the 1860s that depression began to appear as a diagnostic category. It was further stabilized with the introduction of electroconvulsive therapy in 1938 that contributed to the idea that depression was a treatable disease. But the major breakthrough occurred in 1958 with the launch of the first antidepressant that made depression pharmacologically treatable. The 1950s marked a major shift in the treatment of mental disorders. The advent of new active ingredients that were regarded as disease-specific, such as chlorpromazine and imipramine (Moncrieff 2008), changed the main location of psychiatric treatment from the asylum into the community (Ecks 2011; Shorter 1997). This development not only stabilized depression as a disease entity but also cemented the status of psychiatry as a scientific medical discipline. Yet, it was not until the 1980s that SSRIs were introduced and the prevalence rates of depression skyrocketed. Depression went mainstream: psychiatrists diagnosed with increasing frequency, and people increasingly framed their dysphoria or unhappiness in terms of depression. Before SSRIs, benzodiazepines were routinely prescribed for anxiety, and anxiety, not depression, was the most diagnosed psychiatric condition. The problem of benzodiazine dependency, in particular Valium or "mother's little helper", combined with the new availability of pharmacological treatment options in the 1980s provoked a rapid rise in SSRI use as they became known as safe drugs for the treatment of depression *and* anxiety as well as for a range of other conditions. Cases that would have been treated with "benzos" were now being treated with SSRIs, and anxiety was slowly transformed into depression (Healy 2006). By the mid-1990s, sales of antidepressants had overtaken those of tranquilizers (Rose 2003). SSRIs, epitomized in Prozac, were hailed as wonder drugs and achieved cult status. Though there is as yet no evidence confirming a causative link between lowered serotonin levels and depression (Healy 2006), the model of depression as a lack or insufficiency of certain neurotransmitters (mainly serotonin though later also norepinephrine) through which the subjectivity of insufficiency was transformed into a neurochemical insufficiency, has become the prevailing narrative. As a result, in the 1990s the American Psychiatric Association and the British College of Psychiatrists launched "defeat depression" campaigns supported by pharmaceutical companies that stressed recognition of the condition as key to effective (pharmacological) treatment (Jadhav and Littlewood 1995).

In the second half of the twentieth century depression was invented and stabilized in a complex interplay of disease mongering, drug marketing and scientific research through collaborations between the pharmaceutical industry and the psychiatric profession. Healy (2006) addresses the role of the pharmaceutical industry in structuring expert and popular understandings of mental illness in North America and Great Britain in the late twentieth century, including marketing disorders through "celebrity endorsements and the sponsoring of disease awareness campaigns, clinical trials and ghostwritten scientific articles". This transformation is reflected in advertisements. From the 1960s to the 1980s, depression was depicted as a rare disorder targeting middle-aged or older people, but in the 1990s advertisements for SSRI antidepressants featured progressively younger women (Healy 2006, 65). With the medicalization of states otherwise regarded as normal parts of everyday life, depression as a psychiatric category (not only its treatment) was what was being sold to the public. But not only were pharmaceutical companies and psychiatry selling depression, they were selling a specific model of depression as neurochemical imbalance related to a lack of certain neurotransmitters. Conveniently, they also sold the cure – drugs intended (or at least reputed) to correct that chemical imbalance.

Psychiatrist Joanna Moncrieff (2008) debunks the very concept of an antidepressant as merging the interests of the psychiatric profession and those of the pharmaceutical industry to present psychiatric interventions as disease-specific treatments since the launch of *Miltown* and other tranquilizers in the 1950s. When it was suggested that imipramine was effective in the treatment of depression in the 1950s, it was presented as acting solely on a specific disease. The idea that some drugs have a specific action on the underlying basis of depression caught on rapidly and was well established by the 1960s – before evidence was available to support this understanding. Forces that could have driven the adoption of this view include the psychiatric profession's desire to integrate with general medicine to improve its status and to escape the confines of the asylum. Underlying the idea of a specificity of antidepressants is what Moncrieff calls the "disease-centered" theory of drug action that is closely related to the "rise of specificity" (Lakoff 2005) that arrived with the third edition of the Diagnostic and Statistic Manual (DSM-III). This suggests that the drugs produce their effects by reversing the particular brain abnormalities that give rise to symptoms or, in more colloquial terms, by rectifying a biochemical imbalance. This model is in contrast to earlier drug-centred theories of drug action where psychiatric drugs were perceived as psychoactive substances which were helpful not because they rectified an imbalance in the brain but because the psychoactive state might suppress or mask the symptoms. This shift was based on the localization of diseases in body parts and physicians becoming specialists in them instead of in humours or the body as a single fully integrated entity that arose in the early nineteenth century (Foucault 1973). In developing disease-specific models of the action of psychopharmaceuticals and in locating psychological problems in the brain, psychiatry also aimed for recognition as a scientific discipline.

The growth of depression as a category is also related to the growing importance of the psy disciplines over the course of the twentieth century where psy experts became the "technicians of subjectivity" (Rose 1996). Through these psy disciplines people came to understand themselves as fundamentally psychological beings, as creatures inhabiting a deep interior psychological space, which is the locus of our personhood, emotions, beliefs and personality.[8] The emergence and growing importance of the psy disciplines were again closely linked to new forms of governance and self-governance (Rose 1996). Similarly the rise in psychopharmaceuticals and especially antidepressants in many countries led to new technologies of the self and the emergence of neurochemical or pharmaceutical selves (Jenkins 2011; Rose 2003).

The shift from anxiety and tranquilizers to depression and SSRIs was also the product of developments in psychiatry in the 1980s. Until the 1970s, psychoanalysis dominated the models and treatment of depression and other conditions. The launch of DSM-III marked a turning point in the history of psychiatry from psychoanalysis to biopsychiatry from the 1980s onward. Now hegemonic, biopsychiatry considers psychiatric disorders as similar to physical disorders and having underlying organic causes and disease-specific pharmaceutical treatments. Biopsychiatry owes its allegiance not to Freud but to Emil Kraepelin, which is why this approach is often called neo-Kraepelinian. Born in the same year as Freud (1856), he is often seen as the precursor of biological psychiatry, in opposition to Freud who stands for a biodynamic approach to psychiatric disorders. It is important to note that in this ideological shift from psychoanalysis to neo-Kraepelinian biological psychiatry, economics exerted significant influence: pharmacological treatment was simply cheaper than psychoanalytic or psychodynamic psychotherapy (Luhrmann 2000). The psychophysiological narrative of depression as a brain disease due to imbalanced neurochemicals replaced the notion of depression as a profoundly social and psychological disorder (Good, Good and Moradi 1985).

Drug companies and psychiatrists are involved in medicalizing depression but so are awareness campaigns that proclaim mental illness to be an organic disease, a brain disorder treatable with medication just as Type 1 diabetes is treated with insulin. Awareness campaigns in India and beyond do just this but also proclaim a treatment gap of depression and antidepressants as the first line of treatment. The growing influence of psychiatrists might be taken as a sign of scientific progress, but in North America and Europe critics have voiced concern about the close relationship between the rise of depression and the development of new antidepressants (SSRIs and SNRIs). Problems that are deeply social or socio-economic are redefined as individual and relocated in neurochemical imbalance of the brain. Antidepressants, they argue, silence dissent and diminish people's capacity to reflect upon the social and political roots of their affliction (Illich 1975). The consequence is a pharmaceutical kind of self-surveillance, a de-politicization and decreased autonomy. Moreover the medicalization of sadness and despair leads to a "loss of sadness" whereby people lose the capacity for tolerance, patience, suffering and grief and also the resources for dealing with the hardships of life (Horwitz and Wakefield 2007). Some critics (Horwitz and Wakefield 2007) argue that medicalization of sadness and other "natural states" primarily serves the interests of the pharmaceutical industry. They see a conspiracy behind the worldwide rise of depression rates, the global export of Western psychiatric diagnostic categories and sales rates of antidepressants. This kind of global medicalization and pharmaceuticalization is often equated with "globalization of the American psyche", as a tool of "top-down biomedical domination and homogenization" (Watters 2010). Psychiatry "imposes certain categories on the world that may not fit equally well everywhere and that never completely capture the illness experience and concerns of patients" (Watters 2010, 197). This critique also holds for the Movement of Global Mental Health. Although it tries to address structural issues, the Movement's focus on discrete psychiatric disorders and their treatments tends to decontextualize diseases and undermine structural, political and economic solutions which are more difficult to implement. The transformation of social problems into inadequacy of delivery of mental health services might also serve political and economic interests and help stabilize inequalities (Jain and Jadhav 2009; Kirmayer and Pedersen 2014; Mills 2014).

Since the publication of DSM-III practitioners and researchers have criticized the over-diagnosis of depression (Horwitz and Wakefield 2007; Frances 2013). The ascendance of depressive disorder as a major social trend becomes obvious in the ubiquity of depression manifested in various ways: in the amount of depression in the community, the number of patients in treatment, frequency of prescription of antidepressant medication, the social cost calculated for depression in relation to the Global Burden of Disease modelled by the World Bank and media attention to depression. This exorbitant rise of putative depressive disorder does not stem primarily from a real rise. Rather, it is a product of the convergence of two categories: normal sadness and depressive disorder. The classification of many instances of normal sadness as mental disorder became possible with the focus on symptoms rather than on causes and contexts in what is called the "phenomenological approach" of DSM-III and its later editions. The current epidemic of depression has been made possible by these changed definitions of depressive disorder that allow the diagnosis of sadness as pathology even when it is not (Horwitz and Wakefield 2007).

The medicalization critique of depression was reinforced after the publication of DSM-5, and roundly critiqued by the Chair of the Task Force that published DSM-IV in 1994. Psychiatrist Allan Frances (2013) criticizes the DSM's impact on mental health practice and research, and revolts against "out-of-control psychiatric diagnosis" and the "medicalization of everyday life" in DSM-5. Frances targets the influence of Big Pharma but also the designers of the new edition for being blinded by their own over-valued ideas and not understanding the distortions brought about translating DSM-5 into clinical practice – in particular that the ever-widening diagnostic criteria for depression leads to over-diagnosis. For example, the "bereavement exclusion" for depressive disorder in DSM-IV was repealed, and in DSM-5, two weeks of symptoms like sadness, loss of interest, appetite or energy, insomnia and difficulty following bereavement qualify for a diagnosis of Major Depressive Disorder. The resultant medicalization trivialises common and necessary emotional reactions to death and loss, substituting pills and superficial medical rituals for the deep consolations of family, friends and religion.

It is this narrative of depression as a neurochemical imbalance and epidemic – along with the network that constitutes and stabilizes it – that is being globalized. Further, this is the model being glocalized and stabilized on local levels. However, new networks of depression are also being created in local contexts. Here, Deleuze and Guittari's (1987) rhizome model is useful: the network of depression as it grows can take up various forms, create new connections and discard others, be approached and construed through various entryways, and be broken off and start again along new lines. Depression is therefore not one unitary pathological reality but many. For this reason, I explore the multiple ontologies of depression while new conceptual and therapeutic networks are being created. A rhizomatic approach to the local appropriation of depression is able to capture the different meanings and ontologies created through different new connections and decentres its meaning from its psychiatric origin.

But isn't depression a Western import, a product of psychiatric imperialism and the globalization of the American Psyche? Watters (2010) asked whether the world was becoming "crazy like us", and until at least the late 1970s and

1980s, psychiatry and epidemiology assumed a cross-cultural validity or universality of depression, regardless of differences in cultural, social, educational or economic background. This changed, but slowly, following anthropologist and psychiatrist Arthur Kleinman's (1977) announcement of what he called the "new cross-cultural psychiatry". Kleinman observed that Chinese patients in Taiwan diagnosed with depression mainly showed somatic symptoms such as headache, body pain, back pain, fatigue or sleeplessness instead of psychological ones such as guilt, sadness (dysphoria), despair, hopelessness or low self-esteem. On this basis he argues that "depressive disorder" with its psychological core symptoms was a Western construct, grounded in a long Western intellectual and medical tradition and deeply rooted in particular and specific Western understandings of body and self that could not be found cross-culturally. The "old cross-cultural psychiatry", Kleinman contends, focused on identifying universals in psychiatric disorders, minimizing cultural differences and ethnocentrically superimposing cultural-derived categories on to other cultural contexts. The new "cross-cultural psychiatry" is primarily interested in "the ways culture influences the perception, classification, process of labeling, explanation, experience of symptoms, course, decisions regarding and treatment of sickness" (Kleinman 1977, 5). Kleinman is less clear, however, on the nature of psychiatric disease entities and whether universal psychiatric diseases actually exist but with different cultural manifestations or whether there are different medical ontologies. In other words, Kleinman (1977) is not clear if illness was only a psychosocial experience of a perceived disease or whether disease exists as an objective universal entity. As such, his "new cross-cultural psychiatry" represents a shift to focusing on differences rather than on similarities in the manifestation or symptoms of depression and other psychiatric categories, instead of a fundamental reframing.

Similar arguments had been made from the 1950s onwards by psychiatrists from postcolonial countries such as Nigeria and India, but they received neither the recognition nor notice accorded to Kleinman. In arguing against ethnopsychiatric assumptions of the non-prevalence of depression in colonized peoples (once believed incapable of depression because of their mental and emotional inferiority) these psychiatrists argued that mental disorders such as depression are universal and differ only in their manifestation, which in turn is related to specific cultural contexts. As Heaton (2013) argues, psychiatrists from postcolonial countries such as Nigeria or India contributed more to the development of transcultural psychiatry than has yet been acknowledged.[9] In an effort to move from ethnopsychiatry towards transcultural psychiatry, they identified the emphasis of cultural and racial differences in psychopathology as a colonial enterprise, depriving colonial subjects of the same civilized status as the colonizers (Heaton 2013). In contrast to arguments that critique the universalization and export of psychiatric categories around the globe as a colonizing endeavour (Watters 2010; Mills 2014), for these psychiatrists it was precisely the universality of psychiatric categories that led to the decolonization of psychiatry.

The question of whether mainstream psychiatric categories as laid out in the American Psychiatric Society's DSM and the World Health Organization's International Classifications of Diseases (ICD) are truly universal is still widely discussed, with some criticizing cross-cultural psychiatrists for reifying and universalizing psychiatric categories that are in fact cultural and historical (Kirmayer 2000; Summerfield 2008; Fernando 1991). They questioned the universality of Western diagnostic categories and therefore the validity of the knowledge base of global mental health. Today, this debate seems somewhat obsolete because neuroscience research increasingly discards disease categories as laid out in the DSM and ICD (including depression and bipolar disorder). Even the prestigious American National Institute of Mental Health (NIMH) that previously only approved research based on DSM categories has reoriented research away from these to focus instead of what the director of the US National Institute of Mental Health (NIMH) Thomas Insel (2014) calls Research Domain Criteria (RDoC) that can be studied "across multiple units of analysis, from genes to neural circuits to behaviors cutting across disorders as traditionally defined". Further, the globalization of psychiatry has meant that these categories have been taken up in local contexts and are increasingly used not only by experts but also by laypeople to classify and describe problems.

The scientific categories of mainstream psychiatry have become part of local meaning and local meaning is imbued in scientific categories such as psychiatry. My approach in *Depression in Kerala* is thus to ask how the network of the globalized disease category depression is appropriated and stabilized in the local reality of Kerala. Following more recent research on depression, I challenge the dichotomy of the West and the rest that lurks behind debates on somatization and psychologization and the dichotomy of global and local framings of depression. Where psychiatrists have criticized global medicalization of depression as a form of top-down biomedical domination and homogenization leading to "globalization of the American psyche" (Watters 2010) or colonization of the mind (Mills 2014), anthropologists have begun to explore the process of glocalization of psychiatric diagnostic categories as grounded in social, historical and political contexts. In her ethnography of suicide in Kerala's capital Thiruvananthapuram, Chua (2009) argues against the disjuncture between Western psychiatric discourse and culturally embedded idioms of distress and healing, but without denying the importance of historizing and de-centring Western psychiatric paradigms. As Chua (2009) argues with regard to the vernacularized psychiatric category "adjustment disorder" that is included in DSM-5 and ICD-10), I suggest that depression as a chemical imbalance also does not in itself stand in opposition to local idioms of suffering. Rather it lends itself to other expressions and elaborations that go beyond and are sometimes in opposition to the formal criteria of these diagnostic categories. Depression is thus integrated, I argue, not only into a local "web of significance" (Good 1994, 57) but also into a local network of ontologies. The interpretive and ontological instability (and resultant flexibility) of psychiatric terminology has a double effect: it enables vernacular forms of meaning making and agency, facilitates pathologization (and stigmatization) and extends the reach of psychiatry into the everyday. As I will show throughout this book, beyond the binary of Western psychiatry/Indian culture it is, in the words of anthropologist Sarah Pinto, "different layers of experience, explanation, and practice that make diseases less objects than dialogues" (Pinto 2014, 15).

Anthropologists of late have described how the local forms of disease appropriation and medicalization can be generative for the articulation of political dissent, contrary to the assumption that medicalization of depression leads automatically to depolitization (Kleinman 1986; Young 1995; Kitanaka 2012; Chua 2014). For example, work in the Japanese context has shown that the medicalizing psychiatric language of depression might indeed be liberating and lead to a diversified expression of distress and individual suffering (Kitanaka 2012). Kitanaka argues that the new psychiatric language of depression also becomes a "socializing" language in that it reappropriates a Japanese cultural discourse about the social nature of depression and thus psychiatrists have become "unlikely agents of liberation" (Kitanaka 2012, 5). Anthropologists have started to address asymmetrical power relationships as well as the agency involved in translating between medical languages. This is an important issue that is taken up in this book.

With his stress on somatic modes of experiencing and expressing depression in Chinese patients, Kleinman (1977) focus on "somatization", which means that depression is primarily experienced as perceived physical or somatic complaints such as pain as opposed to psychological symptoms such as despondency or guilt. This notion is now widely used by psychiatrists (and anthropologists) around the globe to describe the experience of depression in societies other than those of North America and Northwest Europe or, crudely speaking, in "the rest" as opposed to "the West". The theory of somatization of depression in "non-Western patients" soon became shared knowledge among psychiatrists all over the world, and somatization rapidly became associated with disempowered groups or those regarded as somehow inferior, especially people of the global South, ethnic minorities, migrants, those belonging to lower social classes or with low educational attainment, children and, of course, women. In India, psychiatrists often frame the experience of depression in binary opposition to "the West" and relate somatization to lower classes, lower education, rural areas, women or, in the case of psychiatrists from Kerala, to Northern Indian states. Psychologization is regarded as more sophisticated, somatization as more primitive. Though certainly not intended by Kleinman and others, somatization theory shares some continuity with the racism of colonial ethnopsychiatry. For instance, well into the twentieth century and before the presumed worldwide rise of depression, British psychiatrists working in Kenya assumed that Africans were not able to experience depression because of their assumed ethnic incapacity to feel guilt due to the underdevelopment of the frontal lobes of their brains (Heaton 2013). The psychological symptoms of depression (dysphoria, sense of guilt and self-blame) were regarded as signs of maturity and adult selfhood (Jadhav 2000). Even if not associated with differences in brain structures or with racism, it has been widely assumed that people from non-Western backgrounds cannot experience depression in psychological form since they do not possess reflexive and autonomous selves and the capacity for the introspection required to perceive and express depression in a mature way (Ernst 2007; Kakar 1982, Littlewood and Dein 2000).

Criticizing this binary model of somatization versus psychologization, cross-cultural psychiatrists have set out growing evidence that somatic symptoms are commonly presenting features of depression throughout the world, including "Western" cultures as becomes evident from Bhugra and Mastrogianni's (2004) review. Moreover, somatization theory has been criticized for creating a split between the imaginary illness (somatic complaints) and the "real" disease (psychological complaints) (Kirmayer 1988; Langford 2002). From a slightly different theoretical perspective, social historian of medicine Edward Shorter recently criticized the psychologization that accompanied the diagnostic shift from nervous disorder (neurasthenia)[10] to depression (Shorter 2013). Most people diagnosed with major depression today, he argues, do not actually have it. The symptoms they experience – anxiety, fatigue, sleep problems and obsession with their symptoms – are those which in the nineteenth century led to a diagnosis of nervous disorder which was regarded as a problem of the entire body involving the mind. Its symptoms were diverse and involved fatigue, mild depression (non-melancholic), mild anxiety (non-psychotic), somatic symptoms such as pain, insomnia and disordered bowel function, and some kind of obsessive thinking (Shorter 2013, 11). Under the influence of Freud, nervous illness shifted from neurology to psychiatry, focusing on the mind and ignoring the rest of the body. The result has been "a scientific disaster, resulting in the misdiagnosis and inappropriate treatment of millions" (Shorter 2013, 198). This has given rise to "the paradox of depression without depression" (Hamilton 1989). The notion of nervous disorder has survived in Japan as neurasthenia (Kitanaka 2012), and is manifest in the Latin American folk illness *nervios* (Baer et al. 2003), and as nerves [*nara*] in India. Accounts of patients experiencing nara at the National Institute of Mental Health and Neurosciences (NIMHANS) in Bangalore, India suggest that patients have an illness of the entire body (Raguram et al. 2001) in contrast to the notion of depression that locates a mood disorder in the mind and in the brain. It is exactly the idea of an illness that affects the entire body and not just the mood that Shorter aims to push forward when he argues for a reintroduction of an illness called nerves, nervous breakdown or neurasthenia (weakness of the nerves). I argue that the present understanding of depression in Kerala resembles neurasthenia as it is understood in Japan (Kitanaka 2012) or China (Kleinman 1982) today or as it was understood in Europe and North America in the nineteenth century before the advent of psychoanalysis. It is a term designating distress, tension, mental and physical weakness, and often anger avoiding the stigmatizing connotations of mental illness. Talking to psychiatrists and other physicians, to patients and their caretakers, and analysing media reports on depression, I suggest that depression in Kerala is conceptualized as a form of brain distress that manifests through both psychological and physical symptoms and not a mental illness. Leaving the psychoanalytical history of the concept of depression and all the psychodynamic connotations many people in contemporary Europe and North America still connect with it aside and, after a short flirtation with psychoanalysis, jumping directly into the somatic, neo-humoral and organic notion of depression as a brain disorder with psychopharmacology as the treatment of choice, psychiatrists in India are able to capture depression simultaneously as somatic *and* epidemic. Just as nervous disorder was seen as a product of modernity at the end of the nineteenth century in the US and Europe, in India depression is now seen as related to the pathological effect of socio-economic transformations associated with modernity.

In North America and Western Europe the symptoms of depression are construed as inner states with the source assumed to lie primarily in the individual mind and brain as opposed to the social, spiritual or ecological world. In cultural contexts where happiness, pleasure and self-confidence are highly valued, these symptoms are particularly stressful and disturbing. There is a certain paradox in the normative phenomenology of depression as a psychological rather than somatic crisis. Although scientific efforts to understand depression have become more and more focused on neurophysiological processes, a psychological phenomenology testifying to the rise of global mental health literacy is normative for subjective experience of depression. In other words, while the professional somatization of depression on the *conceptual* level is promoted as more scientific than a conceptualization couched in terms of psychodynamics and the mind, the somatization of the depressive *experience* is discarded and seen as inferior and a sign of poor mental health literacy.

From a different vantage point, the theory of somatization of depression and the trend of including more and more somatic symptoms under the diagnosis of depression are also part of a strategy for expanding the market for antidepressants into the treatment of unspecific somatic symptoms. Gaudillière (2015) analyses how the advent of scientific marketing and the close collaboration of pharmaceutical companies with psychiatrists and general physicians in Switzerland and Germany since the 1960s has impacted the stabilization of depression and the expansion of its boundaries, especially through the introduction of the category "masked depression". When almost any not otherwise explicable somatic complaint can be regarded as a symptom of (masked) depression, antidepressants are the means by which to solve it. Including somatic symptoms under depression acknowledges non-psychological forms of expressing depression, but it also facilitates an ever-expanding medicalization of diverse forms of (experiencing and expressing) suffering.

Not only the symptoms of depression, but also the ways emotions such as sadness and despair are culturally framed and evaluated vary dramatically. For example: Obeyesekere (1985) points out that Sinhalese Buddhists value suffering or dysphoria positively as an esteemed feature of the human path to salvation; Good, Good and Morani (1985) demonstrate that for Shi'ite Muslims in Iran suffering and grief are highly elaborated religious elements associated with martyrdom, and the capacity to experience dysphoria is a characteristic of the personal depth; and Tousignant (1984) and Jenkins (1988) show that in Latin American societies suffering is associated with a culturally profound sense of tragedy. These valuations of suffering provide a sharp contrast to Anglo-American attitudes in which suffering is neither expected or acceptable and as such should be overcome through effort and willpower. As Kleinman and Good (1985, 3) identify, "describing how it feels to be grieved or melancholy in another society leads straightforward into analysis into different ways of being a person in radically different worlds". This is an issue that I will take up in Chapter 4.

It might even be suggested that the psychological conceptualization of depression with core symptoms including low mood, loss of pleasure, loss of self-esteem, guilt, loss of a feeling of social connectivity are rather "peculiar in the context of the worlds' cultures", as the anthropologist Clifford Geertz once put it so aptly with regard to the Euro-American concept of the person (Geertz 1974). It is the sharp distinction between pathologies of the body and those of the mind, and between the disciplines designated to understand and to treat them in the age before neuroscience, that do not allow for easy concourse between them. As it stands, "contemporary psychiatric discourse on depression reproduces conventional knowledge in American society" and "postulates an abstract, desocialized individual, whose symptoms are seen to reflect an inner psychophysiological state rather than aspects of social interaction or local power relationships" (Good, Good and Moradi 1985, 374). Further, the "correspondence of the disease category to a natural phenomenon is seldom challenged" (Good, Good and Moradi 1985, 370). Though this holds true for anthropological and social science research on physical diseases, "[d]iseases of the mind have quite a different history in anthropological theory" and have been understood as behavioural abnormalities and deviancies, and "analytic attention has been on the cultural production and societal response to such behavior, rather than on the cultural interpretation of an underlying disorder" (Good, Good and Moradi 1985, 370). Illness categories are therefore "not merely a reflection of symptoms linked with each other in a natural reality but a set of experiences associated through networks of meaning and social interaction" (Good 1977, 27).

For a long time, disease was the realm of medicine just as the physical body was the realm of the sciences while culture was the dominion of the social sciences. The disease-illness distinction, developed by Leon Eisenberg (1977) in the first issue of *Culture, Medicine and Psychiatry*, goes back to Parsons who in the 1950s argued that social scientists should study the role of sickness and everything a disease means for a patient while medicine should focus on the study of the disease. Social scientists did not intrude into "body-talk" (Mol 2002, 7) and were satisfied focusing on the role of sickness and the meaning of disease for patients and later, doctors. This interpretative slant did not intrude into the study of the physical or physiological body (Mol 2002). This is in part why the physiological processes of neurochemical changes involved in a disease such as depression were not questioned by anthropologists though they were under investigation by neuroscientists. The brain has been left untouched (with some notable exceptions such as Choudhury and Kirmayer 2009; Choudhury and Slaby 2012; Röttger-Rössler and Markovitsch 2009; Seligman and Brown 2009; Slaby 2010) and not subjected to research in the social sciences and the humanities. My approach in this book is not so much to critically analyse neurobiology or neuroscience except in my critique of the construction of the neurochemical or brain narrative of depression. For many neuroscientists and neurobiologists, even culture has to "pass through the brain" (Rose 2003). In a practical ontographic approach (Latour and Woolgar 1979; Mol 2002) the brain would have to pass through culture. But my cultural ontographic approach to depression focuses rather on practices of stabilizing depression, on the question of how depression manifests in the local context of Kerala. The fabricated fact of depression as a brain disorder or a chemical imbalance has gone global. It is time to explore their local appropriations and new rhizomatic connections with local epistemologies, ontologies and experiences. It is the ontology of depression that is at stake, not only its interpretation and subjective experience. I argue that the ontology of depression, established, stabilized and grown on institutional, material, cognitive and practical levels by a host of actors, is a fabricated fact that creates embodied or psychologized subjectivities.

Methods, personal orientations and the mental health pluralism of Kerala

I explore the appropriation of psychiatric discourse on depression in Kerala and chart the conceptual and ontological movement of depression, in particular how it came to be rooted, fabricated and translated in Kerala, while at the same time attending to the ways depression is integrated into and shaped by various global and local webs of meaning and action. To trace this journey, it is necessary to examine depression and its treatment in practice, and the ways related institutions and materialities are appropriated, adapted and reconfigured. I explore these conceptual, institutional and material shifts in the context of mainstream psychiatry, Ayurvedic psychiatry and ritual healing. Kerala not only has a large proportion of psychiatric facilities, mental health personnel, and responsive public and private health care compared to other Indian states, but also has experienced significant media coverage and multiple awareness programmes on mental health issues that contribute to a high mental health literacy in the state. Moreover, Kerala not only has a long and unique history of Ayurveda but also boasts the only Ayurvedic psychiatric hospital in the country and a postgraduate specialization in psychiatry for Ayurveda students. I use Ayurveda in Kerala as a case to explore how an indigenous medical system responds to the epidemic of depression and how depression is conceptualized, translated and dealt with in pedagogic and clinical practice. Finally, many people seek Hindu, Muslim or Christian ritual healing for depression, emotional suffering and behavioural problems, spirit possession or occult violence, and the significance of these traditions existing alongside and overlapping with mainstream and Ayurvedic treatments of depression is high.

The state of Kerala was formed in 1956 when the two princely states of Tranvancore and Cochin were merged with the formerly British-administered Malabar in the North, nine years after these regions became part of the newly-founded nation-state of India. Kerala today is a densely populated state with over thirty million people inhabiting a small area of 38,664 square kilometres, which amounts to around 800 people per square kilometre. The three main cities – Thiruvananthapuram and Kochi/Ernakulam are the former capitals of the two princely states of Tranvancore and Kozhikode was the former capital of British administered Malabar. Thiruvananthapuram is the administrative capital, Kochi/Ernakulam the economic centre and Kozhikode is notable as the source of many migrant workers who leave the city for the Persian Gulf region.

The state is bounded on the east by the Ghat Mountains separating Kerala from Tamil Nadu, and on the west by the Arabian Sea. Its location has led to various historical contacts with West and East Asia, Europe and other parts of the globe. The state boundary was determined according to the spatial distribution of a particular linguistic community. Most of Kerala's inhabitants speak Malayalam, a Dravidian language into which many Sanskrit terms were introduced by the Namboodiri Brahamin elite who came from North India in the first centuries CE. Additionally the educated middle class is often quite skilled in English, especially individuals educated in the private English-language schools, colleges and universities. The majority of the people who live in Kerala refer to themselves as Malayalis. They consist mostly of descendants of Dravidians, North Indians or Arab people and of less than half a million *Adivasi* [tribal people] who mostly live in the Western Ghats. Kerala is known for its high literacy rate that reached 100 per cent in the 1990s. The reasons for this rise are manifold, and range from the matrilineal history of the dominant Nair and some other communities, to the large proportion of Christian private education facilities, to good climatic conditions that enabled a large proportion of the population the leisure to become literate.

The majority of the population of Kerala (around 60 per cent) regard themselves as Hindus consisting of a small elite of Namboodiri Brahmins, the dominant matrilineal Nayar identified in part by their former specific *sambandham* [sexual relations] relationships with Namboodiri men (Gough 1959; Fuller 1976b) and the Izhavas or Tiyyas, a formerly untouchable caste before the reform movement led by Narayana Guru that largely impacted their upward mobility (Osella and Osella, 2000), as well as several other, smaller communities. Kerala, once characterized by an extremely rigid and unequal caste system and an unequal distribution of wealth, has seen several anti-caste social reform movements leading to increased social mobility in the region.

But Kerala has also a large proportion of Muslims (around 20 per cent) and Christians (around 20 per cent). Muslims in Kerala differ from North Indian Muslims mainly with regard to the strong Arabic influence in the former. Islam spread to Malabar earlier than to the North through trading relationships beginning in the seventh century and, later, through travelling Hadrami saints. The influence of Arabian culture and language continues today through the migration of Malayalam-speaking Muslims seeking work in the Gulf region, a trend that began in the 1970s. Mappilas are the largest Muslim community in Malabar, settled mainly in the inner Malabar area (Osella and Osella 2008).

Kerala Christians are divided into at least three groups: Syrian Christians, Latin Christians and New Christians. Syrian Christians regard themselves as descendants of Namboodiri Brahmins who converted to Christianity in the first centuries CE after the missionary activity of apostle Thomas who is said to have arrived in Kerala in the first century CE. Missionary activity in the sixteenth century by the Portuguese led to the conversion of mainly fisher castes that later came to be known as Latin Christians. Finally, the New Christians are the descendants of those converted in a missionary wave in the end of the nineteenth century led mainly by European Protestants (Fuller 1976b; Visvanathan 1993). There is evidence that Christians and Muslims practice caste in a similar manner to the caste practices of Hindus in Kerala (Fuller 1976a, Osella and Osella 2008).

Kerala is famous in part because it was one of the first governments worldwide to democratically elect a communist government when the state was founded in 1957, and communism has persistently remained an important political movement in Kerala, along with the Congress party and several religious- or caste-based parties. Today, the communist parties take turns with the Congress party in every alternate election. Kerala is also well known for what is called the Kerala model of development, a model based on the state's achievement of significant improvements in material conditions of living, and social development indices such as low birth and mortality rates, high life expectancy, literacy and provision of social services in spite of its relatively low per capita income, low gross domestic product (GDP) and a lack of local employment opportunities (though this model is increasingly challenged from various sides – cf. Chapter 2). The social emphasis on the importance of education, which can be traced to historical forces of colonial and postcolonial modernity, has led to a highly competitive education system. Together with the low employment rates due to low investment in industrialization and other factors, this creates an immense pressure on young adults that often results in stress, mental distress and suicide. Gulf migration largely leads Malayalis into construction and other manual work which contributes to the GDP and general wealth in Kerala, though not all migration stories are success stories and migrants often fail to find prosperity abroad.

I began my fieldwork in the mainly Muslim Malappuram district of Northern Kerala, in the town of Kottakkal at the P.S. Varier Ayurveda College and the Government Ayurveda Mental Hospital (GAMH). The hospital's newer and official name is the Government Research Institute for Mental Diseases, but the institution is popularly known by the older name.[11] There, I learned about the theories and practice of Ayurvedic psychiatry and Ayurvedic concepts of mind, mental health and mental disease. I was taught by college teachers, students and doctors at GAMH about Ayurvedic psychiatry, what it is and what it is not – an important issue in the legitimization process of Ayurvedic psychiatry. Unlike the students I spent time with, I had not completed the four-and-a-half-year BAMS (Bachelor of Ayurvedic Medicine and Surgery) and as such lacked the depth and breadth of their formal training.[12] Most of these students decided to become doctors during their "plus one" (eleventh class), had attended Sunday tuition during their "plus two" (twelfth class)[13] and had taken extra tuition following their final exam in preparation for writing the several entrance exams required to gain admission into one of the many medical colleges in Kerala or beyond. When they failed to achieve results that would qualify them for a place on a biomedical course, they slipped into Ayurveda more by coincidence than by design. Similarly, most of the postgraduate students of Ayurvedic psychiatry enrolled in the Ayurvedic MD (Medical Doctor) course that I met would have preferred a more prestigious subfield of Ayurveda like general medicine, *panchakarma* [the famous purifying procedures] or at least gynaecology or otolaryngology. My exposure to Ayurveda was a sort of crash course, beginning with an introduction to Ayurvedic theory by way of anthropological, historical and medical material I was able to access in Germany before my fieldwork, and then after, spending valuable time with Dr Rahul, to whom I was referred by one of his former teachers.

Dr Rahul had just finished his BAMS and as he was free for a few weeks before starting his MD course, he was able to spend time teaching me about Ayurvedic theory in the way it is taught at the approximately fifteen public and private Ayurveda colleges in Kerala. He introduced me not only to the teachers and students of different departments of the college but also to the medical officers at GAMH. Dr Rahul was engaged in translating Ayurvedic ideas into "modern" ones[14] during our daily teaching sessions, in part due to my unfamiliarity with many Ayurvedic terms and ideas. To a much larger extent, these translations are part and parcel of Ayurvedic training and the result of a pedagogics of teaching students who had been trained up to plus two in Western biology, anatomy and physiology and were themselves unfamiliar with Sanskrit and Ayurvedic concepts. More importantly, the translations of (for example) the *tridosha* [three humours or principles] into modern physiology and chemistry (including neurochemistry), of *agni* [digestive fire] into metabolism, of *kapha unmada* [a despondent phlegmatic state] into depression testify to asymmetrical power relations and the hegemony of biomedicine in India. The appropriation of depression in Ayurvedic psychiatry is an important part of the story of the appropriation of depression in Kerala.

I also learned from many of the small group of specialists in Ayurvedic psychiatry in Kerala, and Ayurvedic general practitioners – both college- and *parampara-* [hereditary] trained – in institutions and private practice. I observed Ayurvedic psychiatry in practice in three different Ayurvedic settings in Kerala and conducted narrative interviews ranging from twenty minutes to two hours with patients suffering from depression and other mental health problems and their caregivers with a focus on subjectivities, experiences and pragmatics of relief. As an anthropologist with a special interest in psychiatry, the aim of my engagement with Ayurvedic psychiatry was never to treat patients but to conduct ethnographic research in Ayurvedic contexts. On several occasions during my fieldwork, I experienced doubts about purpose and meaning of an anthropological study whose theoretical research into the permeation of the concept of depression into Ayurvedic pedagogics and treatments, but also into public health politics and planning and the experiences of patients and caregivers, did nothing to ameliorate the problems and pain of the sufferers and their families. Often my research was understood as a kind of study of the efficacy of Ayurvedic treatment.

Another point of dissonance is that my theoretical frame of reference was not based in classical Ayurvedic texts, modern medical textbooks or even general "medical knowledge", but rather the books and articles written by anthropologists. This accords with the debates I seek to engage and contribute to that are taking place in the social sciences (and more specifically within psychiatric or medical anthropology) instead of the advancement of treatment options for patients. This difference between applicability and social scientific research came into sharp focus when, unlike most of the Ayurveda students I met, I moved from Ayurveda into mainstream psychiatry – and sometimes back to Ayurveda again. I was constantly confronted with and expected to take a position on the question of which treatment was better and which was most effective because I was presumed to speak from an independent, scientific and objective perspective. I avoided responding mainly by noting that as an anthropologist I was neither trained for nor capable of making a pronouncement one way or the other, but was much more interested in the answer of the people who asked me the question. Some of the Ayurvedic psychiatrists I worked with pushed me, a foreign scholar with an obviously strong interest in Ayurveda, into the role of advocacy for Ayurveda and a bit of action anthropology at two press conferences of Ayurvedic psychiatrists advocating for this (re)invented discipline, one in 2013 in Kottayam, the other in 2014 in Thrissur.

Many patient narratives reveal the difficulties of accessing "thick descriptions" of patient subjectivities in the context of psychiatric inpatient treatment in Kerala. Difficulties conducting interviews with individuals diagnosed with depression arise not so much in terms of reliability of the narrative (cf. Pinto 2014) but because most patients in a severe state of depression do not speak much or easily. Further, in the psychiatric contexts in which I conducted my fieldwork, family members and caregivers did most of the talking – both in medical consultations and in interviews with me.

I conducted fieldwork in three different Ayurvedic settings. At GAMH, I spoke with doctors, sat in on outpatient consultations, participated in doctors' rounds in the inpatient department, and chatted with patients and those accompanying them. During one stay, I was given a small room to use as an office where I could talk privately with patients and caregivers. At the Department of Kaya Chikitsa of the P.S. Varier Ayurveda College, I participated in outpatient and inpatient consultations, classroom teaching and debates, interviewed and had long discussions with psychiatric and general doctors, teachers, students, and patients and their family members using qualitative and narrative interview techniques. I analysed patient files and observed and attended political demonstrations of students and faculty of Ayurvedic psychiatry, focus group discussions and press conferences of Ayurvedic psychiatrists and followed up with several former students of Ayurvedic psychiatry. In the private clinic of Dr Joseph John in a mostly Christian town in Kottayam district I observed the daily routine of doctor and patients, and had long discussions with the doctor in his office, in the car, and during visits to his relatives and friends, church meetings, and meetings of several Ayurvedic associations of which he was a member. I also had the opportunity to accompany some of his patients to additional religious therapies outside his clinic. At Dr Joseph John's two private clinics, which he named (in English) the Centre for Ayurvedic Treatment, Counselling and Psychotherapy especially for Psychosomatic Diseases and the Arogya Manovikas Kendra [centre for health and mental development], I was able to observe the workings of two of the very few private clinics specializing in Ayurvedic mental health care in Kerala. Although most of his patients were Christian, Dr John also treated Hindu and Muslim individuals (mostly middle class), from around twenty to fifty years of age, the small majority of which were women. At his clinics, I was integrated into clinical encounters, and presented to patients as a doctor from Germany who wanted to learn about Ayurveda. Although not a clinician, I was sometimes given a medical device – such as a stethoscope – by the attending doctor to make me appear like a medical professional. In other cases, I was asked for my opinion on cases or thrown into a situation in which I was expected to counsel patients. Many of the explanations Dr Joseph John gave, and the discussions we had regarding depression, were included in discussions he had had with his patients and their caregivers, as part of the clinical encounter. Moreover, I was able to talk with inpatients, outpatients and family members. Apart from my main Ayurvedic psychiatry field sites, I also visited other government and private Ayurvedic colleges and hospitals in Thrippunithura and Thrissur (see Figure 1.1), had extensive conversations with around thirty institutionally and traditionally trained Ayurvedic practitioners and teachers all over Kerala specialising in psychiatry, general medicine and other fields, and with several dozen students.

I had several reasons for following depression from the Ayurvedic to the allopathic context. First, it was analytically useful to access another perspective on depression (and on Ayurvedic psychiatry itself) in Kerala. More importantly, Ayurvedic psychiatry is somewhat marginal and still largely unknown in mental health care in Kerala so the bulk of those diagnosed with depression will at some point seek the help of an allopathic practitioner (a psychiatrist or a non-psychiatrist). Approximately one-tenth to one-fifth of the patients of general practitioners come in to discuss somatic or psychological symptoms of depression, depression-anxiety or other common mental disorders, so it might have been useful to conduct participant observation in that context. Another useful possibility would have been to conduct fieldwork with a psychologist or in one of the many counselling centres mushrooming in Kerala's three larger cities.

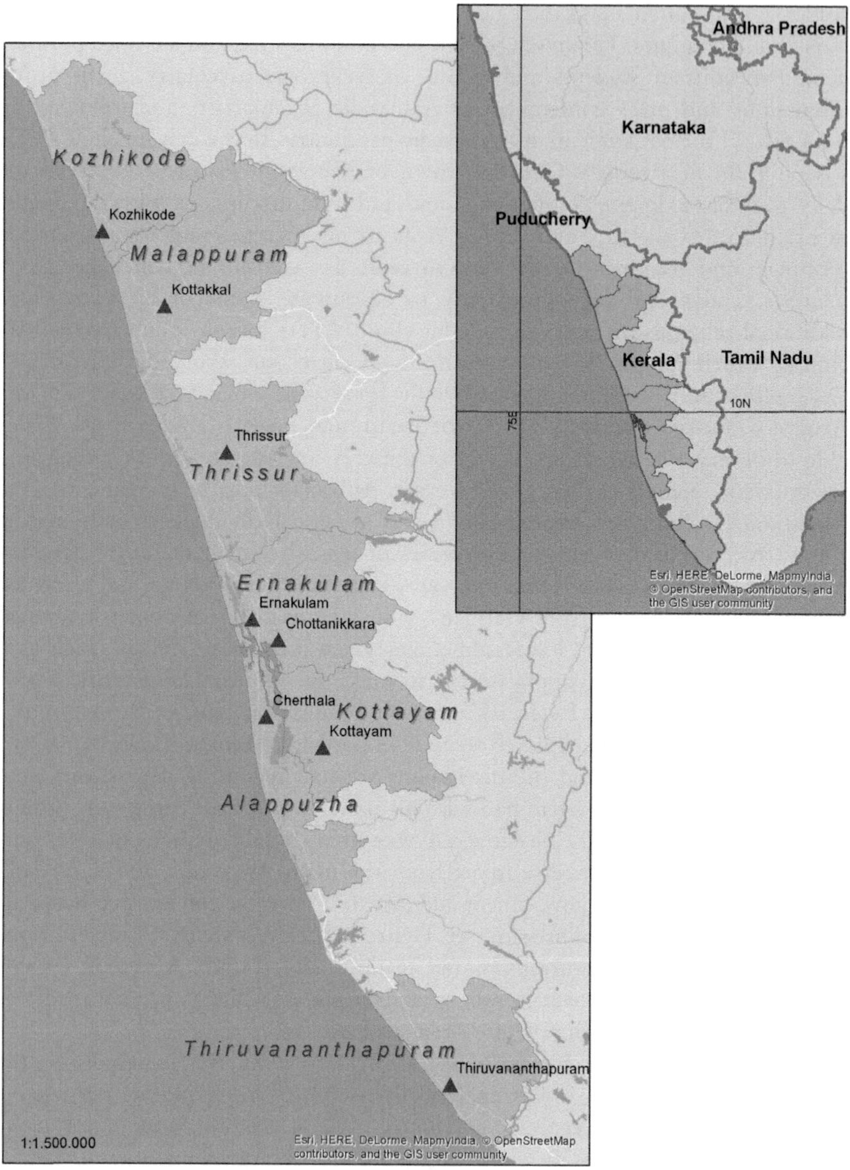

Figure 1.1 Map of the state of Kerala, India

However, the psychologists and counsellors that I met who talked with me about Western methods, the difficulties they experienced adapting them to their Malayali patients, "Indian psychology" and the social changes that led to the rise of depression would not allow me to sit in their consultations (with rare exceptions). The reason was that psychological consultations were regarded as much more intimate and confidential than psychiatric ones. Interestingly, at the Little Flower Mental Health Centre (a private mental hospital) it was the other way around. There, psychiatric doctors allowed me to shadow them during their daily rounds, together with the other students, residents, social workers and nurses, and to speak with inpatients and their caregivers. However, they did not want me to sit in on their outpatient consultations for reasons of confidentiality and sent me instead to the psychologist, which was regarded by the hospital *and* the psychologist as unproblematic. I chose to conduct research first in the Little Flower Mental Health Centre and then in the psychiatric departments of two multi specialty hospitals because psychiatrists are the opinion leaders that largely shape discourse on mental health through defining diagnoses and identifying and endorsing treatments which then trickle down to non-psychiatrists through "floating prescriptions" (Ecks and Basu 2009) and media presence. Equally important to my decision was that I expected to see many more patients diagnosed with depression in these specialized care institutions than in general practice. I was right *and* wrong.

The Little Flower Mental Health Centre was established and run by Christian nuns, specialised in autism and had an attached rehabilitation centre for female patients. I conducted research there for a month, and it turned out to be one of the most important and well-known psychiatric institutions in the state. But after some time I found that apart from some very rare exceptions almost no patients were diagnosed with depression – not in the inpatient ward, the private rooms or in the outpatient department. However, this was not a peculiarity limited to this institution. In an overview of the three big "mental health centres" (as the former asylums are now called) in Kozhikode, Thrissur and Thiruvanathapuram, I found that only a very small percentage of those seeking treatment as inpatients or outpatients were diagnosed with depression. The vast majority were diagnosed with bipolar disorder (in the state of mania) that has replaced schizophrenia as the most common diagnosis, followed by schizophrenia. Similarly, a very small number of patients were diagnosed with bipolar disorder in a depressive state. Seeking reasons, I learned that the stigma of the mental hospital prevents families from bringing patients whose condition is not so severe and disruptive to the social order as is mania and schizophrenia. There is a related fear that the mental distress of a sufferer might be reinforced by seeing and socializing with other patients. Finally depression is not widely regarded as a mental illness in Kerala, so many do not consider seeking treatment at a mental hospital.

Later, I moved to work in two private multi-specialty hospitals with psychiatric units (one in and one near a major city) and the situation was markedly different. Both at the Syrian Christian Hospital and in the Guruji Institute of Medical Sciences, a much larger percentage of patients were diagnosed with mild, moderate or severe depressive disorder, anxiety disorder and other common mental disorders. In the more rural private hospital, patients came from the surrounding area and were predominantly lower middle class and were less affluent than those attracted by the urban institution. Outpatients waited in long lines in front of the consultation rooms, and doctors saw up to fifty patients a morning. Wards, especially the general free ward, were full. In both hospitals, I had the opportunity to sit in on outpatient consultations, accompany staff on their rounds, and talk to inpatients and outpatients and their family members. Moreover, I participated in three conferences of the Indian Psychiatric Society (IPS), at regional and national levels. Though I had maintained contact with Ayurvedic doctors over the months I spent in allopathic psychiatry (between 2012 and 2013), my fieldwork in mainstream psychiatry entailed not only a spatial move but also a shift in perspective and perception, both about depression and Ayurvedic psychiatry. Equipped with multiple perspectives and their attendant blind spots, I returned to Ayurvedic psychiatry for another two months in 2014.

By following depression and the therapeutic itineraries of people diagnosed or self-diagnosed with depression, I further expanded and shifted my spatial and cognitive perspective to vernacular diagnosticians and to what is often referred to as ritual healing, or in India as religious healing or faith healing. Mental health care in Kerala consists of various formalized and non-formalized medical and religious practices. Mainstream psychiatry and psychology exert strong influence on professional and lay discourses on mental illness. Patients and their families in Kerala use Ayurveda, Homeopathy and Naturopathy in their institutionalized and non-institutionalized configurations, and seek additional help from astrological diagnostics and religious healing (Muslim, Hindu or Christian) and do so before, after, alongside or instead of medical treatment. Most Hindu and Muslim sufferers come to Hindu religious healers referred by a *jyotishi* [astrologer], and most are members of the Panikkar or Kaniyan castes who traditionally work as astrologers (though they might also be Namboodiri Brahmin or other persons informally trained or self-trained as astrologers). Depending on the astrologer's background, his clients' preferences and the kind of affliction diagnosed in the *prashnam* [problem-oriented horoscope], those seeking help are referred either to a Namboodiri Brahmin, a lower caste *mantravadi* [a specialist who performs what is usually referred to as black magic or sorcery in Kerala], or a Hindu temple or treatment centre. Another kind of vernacular Hindu diagnostician of mental affliction in Northern Kerala, frequented by Hindus and Muslims, are *velichappadus* [oracles] who, apart from their function in Hindu temple festivals, routinely act as a medium for Bhagavati or other goddesses who diagnose not only the source of mental affliction and recommend the best treatment – be it psychiatric or religious – but also problems related to families, learning, loss and any other kind of issue. Some others seek the diagnosis of a vastu specialist.

There are several Namboodiri houses well known for the treatment of mental illness and cosmological afflictions; the most famous are Poonkudil Mana that combines Ayurvedic treatment and *mantravadam* [magic, sorcery][15] (Sax and Bhaskaran Nair 2014) and Kattumadam Mana that offers religious treatment (Smith 2006; Tarabout 1999), both located in Northern Kerala. If *kaivisham* [magic poisoning or sorcery] is diagnosed as the cause, an astrologer might also refer sufferers to a kaivisham treatment centre – either to the Shiva temple in Cherthala, Alapuzha district, or to one of the smaller centres in Kerala. If possession or spirit affliction is considered before, alongside or after psychiatric treatment, people also try the Chottanikkara temple near Ernakulam or Beemapalli mosque in Thiruvananthapuram for shorter or even long-term treatment (Halliburton 2009). Beemapalli mosque and Chottanikkara temple also offer shelter for mentally ill or destitute people (often widows or abandoned women), for months, years or sometimes the rest of their lives. In the largely Muslim Malappuram and Kozhikode districts of Malabar, Northern Kerala, it is thangals to whom many Muslims with mental distress or mental illness turn (Lang 2014). When discussing the type of Muslim people who seek the help of thangal healers, a historian working as a teacher in a Muslim college quipped: "Uneducated people visit thangals during the day. Educated people go at night." This succinctly illustrates the fact that not only Sunnis but even those Muslims who identify as *mujahid* [post-1950s Islamic reformers and proponents of rationality, science, education and progress] who publicly criticize the thangals' treatments as superstitious, financially exploitative and even dangerous secretly visit them in times of serious personal crisis. This is likewise also true in the case of seeking help from astrologers, velichappadus, mantravadis and in part from Christian exorcists.[16] This attitude shows "that the overt rejection of ritual healing was not so much a statement of disbelief in its efficacy as it was an assertion of one's social position: modern, educated, and scientific" (Sax 2009). In order to avoid jeopardizing this position, educated people seek help from these sources under cover of night. Christians – and sometimes Hindus and Muslims, too – also seek the help of Christian priests (often though not always a priest-psychologist), nuns or one of the many religious counsellors in Charismatic retreat centres and beyond. People also participate in one of the weekly *dyanam* [one-week retreats] in large centres such as Divine Retreat Centre in Muringur (Jansen and Lang 2012) or Potta, or in smaller retreats of shorter duration operating in a similar way. Similarly, the increasing importance of the Charismatic and Pentecostal movements in Kerala, the growing number of churches holding deliverance prayers, and some priests offering Christian exorcism sanctioned by the Catholic Church, encourage many Christians turn to weekly prayers either collectively or in separate individual or family sessions with one priest. Situated somewhere between the formal and informal sectors, religious or secular counselling centres are mushrooming everywhere in Kerala, especially in the major towns. Counsellors range from formally trained clinical psychologists to self-made laypersons, retired schoolteachers or college professors, Christian priests or nuns, or any other person regarding themselves as sufficiently experienced. Like religious healing, counselling centres do not carry the stigma of psychiatric (and psychological) treatment. Whereas Hindu and Muslim religious healing often carries the connotation of superstition and backwardness, Christian counselling centres do not. Moreover they are less associated with stigmatized mental illness than with positive enhancement, personal development and other forms of counselling not associated with illness or disorders such as career counselling or the widely obligatory marital counselling. Most clinical psychologists in private clinics and in hospitals practise a form of cognitive behavioural therapy and therefore provide another option for people suffering from depression and seeking help. Although still not as popular as in North America or Europe, the number of clinical psychologists in Kerala is rising, especially in the larger towns. Psychology is probably more influential in Kerala than in other places in India: it is represented and promoted on television, in print media and in awareness programs (Halliburton 2005; Chua 2014) and is highly influential not only for how people express their distress (Halliburton 2005) but also for perception and self perception of religious healing (Tarabout 1999; Lang 2014).

Psychiatric and psychological healing on one hand and ritual healing on the other have become increasingly important in recent decades. As psychiatric and psychological knowledge increasingly pervade public discourse in Kerala and mental health professionals see a rising number of patients that they diagnose with depression and other common mental disorders, religious healers are also seeing an increasing numbers of patients (Osella and Osella 2000). In other words, despite or perhaps because of the increasing psychiatrization and psychologization of mental distress and suffering, ritual healing has gained in importance. This is true in spite of efforts of the Indian government to discredit ritual healing not only as superstitious but also as potentially violent and exploitive and to spread what is regarded as a rational and scientific understanding of mental illness and mental health literacy. Since the accident in Erwadi, a Muslim shrine in Tamil Nadu, in 2001 when twenty-eight people died in a fire because they were chained or tethered, ritual healing centres have come under heavy criticism (Quack 2013; Basu 2014). Mental health policies in India have since then been characterized by an intensification of existing medicine policy agendas of the Indian state with their ideology of the centrality of science. This involves the rejection of practices that are regarded not only as superstitious and backward but also as violent and inhumane. In some places, this led to efforts to integrate psychiatric services into the spaces of religious healing and thus to bring these centres under the purview of psychiatry and therewith the Indian state (Basu 2014; for a critique see Sax 2014). It was this science-centredness of Indian medical policy that has been blamed for leading to neglect and antipathy towards recognized Indian systems of medicine. It can be speculated that it is the increasing power of global and national health policy stakeholders that has now led to extensive efforts to implement an otherwise unimplemented policy.

Because of their importance in the treatment of depression, I visited many of these religious healing centres and spoke to ritual practitioners, participated in consultations and healing sessions, and talked with the sufferers seeking help there. Although main field sites during the seventeen months of ethnographic fieldwork conducted between 2009 and 2014 were institutions of mainstream and Ayurvedic psychiatry, I also included a heterogeneous field of other, non-psychiatric practitioners and approaches and opposite views. This multi-sited research (Marcus 1995) was complemented by the analysis of media reports on depression in the print media, in TV programmes and in online reports. Finally I learned how mental health awareness and public mental health programs are organized in Kerala. Mental health is increasingly pushing for integration into primary health care, but it was also important to understand the specific roles of mental health NGOs, the function of rehabilitation centres and how psychiatric discourse on depression (and other mental disorders) is transported and translated to laypeople. My own literal and metaphoric itinerary of following depression was not unlike the way sufferers seeking help navigated different framings, epistemologies and ontologies of depression. The cognitive map that I present here, I would note, is not exhaustive. My story of the appropriation of depression in Kerala in relation to wider health political, institutional and economic processes is necessarily fragmentary and partial, in much the same way as are the stories and narratives told by patients, their caregivers, and by medical and religious practitioners. Whatever the spatial field of my research, it was defined and demarcated by the theoretical approach of following the conceptualization of depression and its treatment.

In the course of my fieldwork, I employed research assistants who helped me in different contexts. When I visited Hindu or Muslim ritual healers in Northern Kerala, Babu Appat was always by my side. As an economics graduate, and employee in the automotive and pharmaceutical industries, Babu was a student of psychology and a freelancer who had jobs ranging from newsreader, to college teacher and coach, to *chenda* [drum] player with a music ensemble at festivals. With this background and hailing from the Izhava community, a numerically large former untouchable caste that had succeeded in upward social mobility in recent decades, he was not only an excellent English speaker and an open-minded person, but also knew many people in various communities and was able to communicate easily and befriend people from all religious and socio-economic backgrounds. His assistance was invaluable in helping me to understand the culture, society, politics and history of Kerala. Before I got to know Babu, it was Sanat B. John, a tourism graduate and son of Dr John Baby, a famous naturopathic doctor and professor of psychology, who accompanied me to Hindu ritual healers, psychiatrists and psychologists.

At GAMH, I had the assistance of several students. Apart from Dr Rahul from the Nair community, who introduced me to Ayurvedic theory and practice in institutional Ayurveda, my main research assistant in Ayurvedic psychiatry was Neena. A student of Ayurveda likewise from the Nair community, Neena, had just finished the taught portion of her training at the Ayurveda College in Kottakkal and was undertaking her internship at GAMH. She was one of the very few students who explicitly planned to specialize in psychology and psychiatry. In allopathic psychiatric institutions, I had the help of several MBBS students undertaking their obligatory internship in psychiatry, and several MD students who specialized in psychiatry. For transcriptions of my recorded interview material, I was greatly assisted by Indu P, an Izhava graduate of English literature of the University of Calicut who worked at a college as an English teacher, and mainly from Roy Southil, a Syrian Christian and retired editor of a Malayalam nursing journal, with whom I had many long discussions and whose linguistic explanations contributed much to my understanding of many areas of religious, social and economic life in Kerala and who accompanied me to several trips to Chottanikkara.

My positioning and role as a social scientist conducting research in the field of depression produced certain expectations among those I met. As a foreign scientist, I was expected to be able to determine objectively which treatment for depression was most effective and to make suggestions of how to improve mental health care in Kerala. Some expected me to be able to detect and analyse the social causes of depression of Kerala, as a sort of social diagnostician. Our aims, then, were at odds: mine was to identify and examine the local (or glocal) fabric of depression; theirs was to obtain an objective, scientific analysis. Faced with such questions and the pressure to respond, my solution was to escape pronouncements and instead explain my anthropological approach or, setting my academic endeavour aside, to quote the usual set of answers that I heard so often (see Chapter 2). Others expected me (alone or with my research assistant) to act as a medical expert and though their motivation for talking with us was a chance to vent about their problems and difficulties, their narration mirrored their quest for a diagnosis. My research, they thought, should contribute to helping them find the truth and accordingly the best treatment for their problem. Families' expectations from my research (and from me) then opened a window on to what they were struggling to find. A major element in recent work on medical anthropology in South Asia stresses the importance of pragmatics in help-seeking behaviour rather than previously postulated models of congruence and explanation. However, the narratives I collected show that the quest for meaning is as important for those who seek help as the search for a cure. Those I interviewed in a medical context (allopathic and Ayurvedic) felt comfortable talking to me about their treatment itineraries and medications – most of them regarded me as just another member of hospital staff. They did not mention mantravadam, kaivisham or spirits without being prompted, but when I asked if they ever sought the help of religious healing for their problem, many had their own story to tell. In some cases it happened that my questioning cemented ontologies when some patients or family members answered by asking back "But does it exist?" or "So it is true?" as in Nura and Hamid's narrative. My mere asking effectively established an ontological reality that sufferers knew doctors doubted but also often took into consideration without being fully sure. What medical anthropologists used to call explanatory models (and later explanatory webs) that are less often used as a framework for ethnographic research but continue to be widely regarded as useful for bridging interests of medical anthropology and clinical practice as in the "Cultural Formulation Interview" in the DSM-5, to be elicited in questions such as "What can be a cause for your problem?" or "Which other factors might be involved?" are in fact much more of an explanatory option, a discursive or ontological possibility, negotiated in "ontological politics" and emerging through therapeutic practice (Langwick 2011), to be elicited in certain institutional contexts, buried in others and yet never fully denied. What we as anthropologists then describe is thus not so much what people believe or hold to be true – what psychologists often gloss as "belief systems" – conveniently packaged in a single chapter or section and discerned from other contexts. It is rather the discursive and ontological spaces through which families move (or do not move) in finding relief and finding sense, embracing some framings of their problems at times and rejecting them at others, with power relations endowing some framings with more authority than others. Ontologies as perceived causalities, then, are created and absorbed not only through therapeutic and popular encounters and practices but also through constant negotiations of what constitutes truth. That means that in the end, patients and their families navigating the mental health pluralism shared an uncertainty and incomprehensibility with those treating them and with anthropologists writing about them.

I use pseudonyms for persons and places as far as possible. For the Government Ayurveda Mental Hospital this was not possible since this is the only one of its kind. Similarly the P.S. Varier Ayurveda College is the only one in Kerala to offer a postgraduate specialization. For the allopathic hospitals I worked in and the private clinic of an Ayurvedic psychiatrist I use pseudonyms. I anonymized all my interlocutors except for one who also appears in the work of another researcher.

The book in a nutshell

Depression multiple arises out of a network of conceptual, institutional and material transformations both global and local. It is these transformations and the multiple ways of experiencing depression in this part of India that *Depression in Kerala* explores. To trace this journey, it is also necessary to examine depression and its treatment in practice, and the ways related institutions and materialities are appropriated, adapted and reconfigured in response. This book explores the multiple ways of stabilizing, doing and experiencing depression in the state of Kerala, India. In delineating the rhizoid network that constitutes depression as pathology in a local reality, it contributes to cross-cultural anthropological and research on depression and global mental health.

Depression is one of the most prevalent health problems worldwide. At the same time, figures on depression in Kerala are reportedly the highest in India. Further, popular imaginary in Kerala – fuelled by health statistics and media reports – shows depression on the rise. This is linked to larger socio-cultural transformations in recent decades, usually formulated as a narrative of cultural decline or crisis. In Chapter 2, "Kerala: A Society in Distress", I elucidate the causes for the presumed rise of depression as described by mental health experts, religious practitioners, laypeople and the media. In so doing, I provide an introduction to the ethnographic context of Kerala through the lens of crisis and social critique in an historical moment of accelerated social transformation. The arguments brought forward to account for the rise of depression in Kerala point to a larger context of critique in that they resonate with discontent around modern transformations and the flipside of what is called (today with increasing sarcasm) the "Kerala model of development". Kerala sees itself as a society in distress, suffering from unprecedented rates of depression. For this reason, my particular focus in this chapter is unpicking the ways distress, suffering and emotional breakdown came to be reconfigured and pathologized as depression in Kerala.

Chapter 3, "Glocalizing Depression and Its Treatment in Kerala", focuses on the looping effects of institutions, drugs and concepts within mainstream psychiatry that stabilize depression as a mental health category and a public health concern. These go hand in hand with a shift in the illnesses and complaints that are understood to be the purview of psychiatry and an associated change in the scope of competency of psychiatrists encompassing what are now called common mental disorders. The chapter begins with an exploration of the institutional shifts that enabled psychiatry to expand its scope of competency to encompass – and lay claim to – depression. The relocation of psychiatry from the abandoned spaces of the asylum into the spaces of somatic medicine and the community was, I argue, a prerequisite for bringing depression into the mainstream and the construction of depression as an epidemic. Indeed, psychiatry and depression entered the Indian mainstream hand-in-hand. Since the production and dissemination of expert knowledge further contributes to the construction of depression as a complex moving target in Kerala, I investigate the representation of depression in Indian media and the expansion of psychiatry's increasing influence in everyday life, and explore how psy discourse on depression is vernacularized in Kerala. In the ways and means that professional knowledge is disseminated to the population of Kerala, it is clear that the expansion of the symptomatology of depression and identification of the vulnerable not only produces psychiatric authority but also stabilizes depression as a localized health category. In medicalizing behaviours that deviate (even slightly) from local norms and expectations, psychiatrists and psychologists increasingly bring new population groups under the purview of the psy disciplines, particularly through the widely disseminated notion of masked depression. Taking a material focus, I then turn to another key element of the stabilization of depression: antidepressants. Connecting the pharmaceutical industry to psychiatry, antidepressants as disease-specific agents and their wide availability give rise to a strong focus on pharmacological treatment for depression in Kerala and even for suicide attempts. The chapter concludes with a closer investigation of the cognitive level of the local appropriation of depression in Kerala and the ways doctors explain depression diagnoses to their patients. I show that depression is negotiated between doctors, patients and family members and that, though psychiatrists in Kerala think with global notions of depression as a neurochemical imbalance in the brain, they adapt these to local notions of self, body and mind and to local forms of stigmatization and marginalization. Although psychosocial factors are taken into account, the main pathology is conceptualized as a somatic dysfunction that transforms social suffering, conflict and structural violence into individual somatic pathology which also increases the status of psychiatry within the medical disciplines by conceptualizing depression as a somatic disease and thus psychiatrists as physical doctors.

Chapter 4, "Appropriating Depression in Ayurvedic Psychiatry", follows depression into the context of an indigenous medical system. The translation and reframing of depression and its underlying theories, psychiatric framings and mind/body distinctions in Ayurveda can best be described in conjunction with the (re)invention of institutionalized Ayurvedic psychiatry as an emergent field of specialization. How, I ask, are mainstream psychiatric categories and their etiologies translated into Ayurvedic theory? How is the hegemony of modern psychiatry negotiated, mimicked or contested? How do the institutional regimes of depression come under the purview of, or become mirrored in Ayurveda and how is depression treated in Ayurveda? The (re)invention of Ayurvedic psychiatry as a separate theory, practice and academic discipline in Kerala demonstrates the ontological power of mainstream psychiatry, as does investigating the ways Ayurveda reproduces and partly resists its categories and associated logics. Faced with resistance from biopsychiatric *and* Ayurvedic practitioners and authorities, Ayurvedic psychiatrists are busy not only inventing, defining and professionalizing this field, but they are also involved in a politics of recognition with regards to Kerala's public mental health. This chapter traces the establishment and gate keeping of Ayurvedic psychiatry as a separate discipline, and considers the processes involved in its legitimization as scientific and authentic. I show that the asymmetrical translations of mainstream psychiatric nosologies in general, and depression in specific give rise to important strategies for establishing and legitimizing this discipline not only as scientific and rational but also as a credible actor in the network of depression and mental health care in Kerala. The reconfiguration of bhutavidya into Ayurvedic psychiatry, the translation of depression into Ayurvedic categories in training, research and treatment, and the development and marketing of specific Ayurveda products that address depression not only help to legitimize and stabilize this (re)invented branch of Ayurveda as an actor in public and private mental health care of Kerala but also as an emergent actor in the glocal network of depression.

Finally, Chapter 5, "Possession to Depression and Back: Ayurvedic Psychiatry from the Margin", provides an analysis from the margins of institutionalized Ayurvedic psychiatric health professionalism based on the practice of an Ayurvedic psychiatrist who reinterpreted and reclaimed spiritual therapy as an important component of Ayurvedic psychiatry. This analysis of this figure "from the margins" highlights negotiations in everyday healing practice that are obfuscated by homogenizing narratives of the "scientization" of institutionalized Ayurveda. This is not a story of borrowing scientific authority from biomedicine alone but also the reconfiguration of Christian healing into a scientific endeavour. I analyse how Dr Joseph John understands, translates and treats depression and how depression becomes multiple in his treatment regime.

Before delving into *Depression in Kerala*, in the next chapter I provide an introduction to the ethnographic context of Kerala through the lens of crisis and social critique in an historical moment of accelerated social transformation.

Notes

1 This slogan was coined to refer to economic optimism and popularized by the Bharatiya Janata Party in the elections of 2004 to promote India as the future global superpower. Since then, this slogan has largely shaped the imagination of the new upper middle classes, both those remaining in India and those moving overseas (Brosius 2010).
2 In her book *Alone Together* Sherry Turkle (2011) argues that the relentless connection through the new media and social networks leads to a new solitude.
3 The language speaking of a "burden of depression" or a "global burden of disease" is based on an economic perspective and the economic cost of disease which is closely linked to Global Health and the new influence of the World Bank in defining disease impact. Bemme and d'Souza (2014) argue that it was through the introduction of a new form of metrics – the global burden of disease based on the disability adjusted life years (DALYs) that measure not only years lost through mortality but also years lost through disability – that mental health (especially depression) was thrust into the first ranks and with it into a central position within global and national health policies. Along with this came a public health approach to mental health or what Nunley (1996) has called an "epidemic view" of mental illness. Ominous statistics showing India having the highest rate of depression worldwide (without ever quoting references) appear frequently in media reports. The only study I am aware of that ever published these statistics was a cross-national epidemiological study on major depressive episode (Bromet et al. 2011) that reports the highest prevalence for depression as occurring in India. Data for India were taken in Puducherry, South India.
4 See note 9.
5 For the appropriation of malaria in Cote d'Ivoire, see Granado et al. (2011).
6 The concepts of "psy disciplines" (Rose 1996) or "psy-ences" (Raikhel and Bemme 2016) refer to the emergence and social influence of the disciplines of psychiatry, psychology, psychoanalysis and psychopharmacology and the specific assemblage of scientific expertise, subjectivity and modernity. These notions refer to an argument that psychological and neuroscientific knowledge has become unquestioned and constitutes a specific notion of the self as an object of knowledge and site for intervention.
7 In 1980 the third edition of the American Psychiatric Association's Diagnostic and Statistical Manual of Mental Disorders was published. Since DSM-III, depression and other psychiatric diagnoses have lost their specificity.
8 This assumption has given way to a shift from the psy-ences to the brain sciences and many aspects of our conduct and thought which were explained in psychological terms during the twentieth century are now in the twenty-first century being explained in terms of the brain (Rose 2016)
9 Indian psychiatrists were influential in global mental health in questioning the DSM (Wig 1983), in emphasizing the cultural dimension of mental disorders (Jadhav 2000; Raguram et al. 2001); and in developing community psychiatry (Isaac et al 1982; Murthy and Wig 1983). The current director of the WHO Department of Mental Health and Substance Abuse, Shekhar Saxena, was trained in India.
10 The idea still reflects the differentiation between neurotic and psychotic disorders, the latter involving breaks with reality while the former are regarded as affective or cognitive and therefore milder. The term neurotic refers to the nerves as being the main culprits.
11 Renaming of GAMH mirrors the reconfiguration of large allopathic psychiatric institutions from mental asylums into mental hospitals and later mental health centres and research institutes.
12 As an anthropologist, my focus was not on becoming an Ayurvedic clinician, but rather learning about Ayurveda in order to better study the intersections between depression and Ayurveda. As such, in addition to not completing the Bachelor of

Ayurvedic Medicine and Surgery, I did not undertake the many years of study required to learn Sanskrit, and to study and learn by heart the *Asthanga Hrdayam* and other classic texts. Nor was I examined on basic principles and different elements of Ayurvedic theory, Ayurvedic drugs and treatment practices, and allopathic physiology and anatomy in the systematic manner of the BAMS syllabus designed by the Central Council of Indian Medicine (CCIM).

13 Students are usually between seventeen and eighteen years when they complete their twelfth class and start college or university.

14 "Modern medicine" was the term that Ayurvedic students, teachers and practitioners used for biomedicine or allopathy, as biomedicine is called in India, and "moderns" or "modern doctors" referred to the MBBS-trained biomedical practitioners.

15 It is difficult to translate mantravadam into an English term. Literally it denotes the knowledge of mantras for a specific purpose which may be good or bad according to context. Malayalis differentiate between *satmantravadam* [benevolent mantravadam] and *durmantravadam* [malevolent mantravadam].

16 Christian exorcism and deliverance prayers as part of Charismatic healing practices are often perceived to be more in concordance with modernity and science than are Hindu and Muslim religious healing. Having said this, it should be noted that there are also Christian exorcisms that are publicly debated as violent and violating human rights.

2 Kerala: a society in distress

In Kerala, worry has replaced dysentery.

(John 2009)

The World Health Organization's 2001 *World Health Report* states that depression will be the world's second most prevalent health problem by the year 2020 if calculated by disability adjusted life years (cf. Desjarlais et al. 1995; Murray and Lopez 1996). Another study, the *Cross-national Epidemiology of DSM-IV Major Depressive Episode* (Bromet et al. 2011) reports that the highest worldwide prevalence of depression exists in India. In the South Indian state of Kerala, the number of people suffering from depression is reported in the media as significantly above the national average. If cases of "masked depression" are taken into account in addition to instances of depression as laid out in the International Classification of Diseases 10th edition (ICD-10), the number of people suffering from depression in the state rises to between 30 and 35 per cent of the total population. In 2011, *The Economic Times* quoted the former president of the Kerala branch of the Indian Psychiatric Society, A.J. John, noting that about 35 per cent of all Keralites suffer from depression.[1] Whatever the source of these figures, the numbers used in media reports disseminate the imaginary of depression as a public health crisis erupting in Kerala. Although high numbers are also reported in the rest of India, Kerala is usually identified as the state with the highest rates of depression. Journalist R. Krishnakumar offered an explanation for this situation:

> Kerala has become very materialistic. Increasingly, alien values replaced traditional ones and nuclear families took the place of a once-predominant joint family system. It is today a very individualistic society, caught in a state of imperfect modernisation. Imperfect education and easy Gulf money had led to the creation of a society which has great expectations but not enough resources and other means to bring them to reality. Rapid changes have taken place in the material culture, but there has been no change at all in the State's non-material culture. Kerala society is caught in a cultural lag.
>
> (Krishnakumar 2000)

High rates of depression and suicide are attributed to Kerala's consumerism, "imperfect modernization" and a "cultural lag". Krishnakumar also notes that, in earlier times, there were "popular release mechanisms" built into Kerala society, including "faith healing, hysterical dances in temples or exorcism". These provided emotional outlets, but in the context of modernization they have come to be ridiculed and devalued. However, instead of the development of a positive alternative, it became fashionable to be depressed (Krishnakumar 2000).

Depression is seen to be so common that it is often regarded as a normal condition. From one vantage point, sadness and suffering have always been seen as an existential condition of life, and religions such as Buddhism or to a certain extent Christianity represent a way to deal with life as suffering. In Kerala, women especially are said to be predestined to suffer, at least when considering Malayalam sayings such as "If you are born a woman you must drink tears" or "Women should suffer everything like the earth" (quoted by the psychiatrist C.J. John in an article in the Malayalam magazine *Arogya Masika* in April 2014). The status of women in Kerala is characterized by ambiguity. Some scholars describe women in Kerala as empowered by a matrilineal past, high female literacy and wide employment rates – especially in the spheres of education, health and the social services (Hapke 2013; Jeffrey 2004) – while others describe them as marginalized in public politics (Jeffrey 1992; Lindberg 2005; Mathew 1997), disempowered from domestic decision making and subject to some of the most conservative gender roles in India (Mukhopadhyay 2007). From another vantage point, misery is often said to be a condition that has replaced the once proud character of the Malayalis (Chua 2014). "Is Kerala a workshop of depressed minds? Are Malayalis so ignorant as to invite depression into their lives by being imprudent?" asks psychiatrist Dr C.J. John in a special issue on depressive disorder in the health magazine *Arogya Masika* (John 2010). Along with issues such as low employment rates and lonely elders whose adult children are forced to work abroad or elsewhere in India, Dr John lists what he considers to be "typical characteristics" of the Malayalis that he regards as responsible for their depressed minds: Malayalis "do not have the habit of recording in their minds happy moments of life so that they can think about them and feel good" and generally speaking, the dominating character trait of a Malayali is negativity (John 2010). He further cites wide use of the use of English terms "depression" and "tension" in Kerala (cf. Halliburton 2005) as a sign of Malayalis' "depressed mind" and that "worry" is the main health problem of Malayalis today (John 2010). He goes on to state that child-rearing practices in Kerala play a key role in creating depressed personalities as from a very early age they cultivate good habits by discouraging childishness and through the use of negative and derogatory correction.

Many people I spoke with told me that in every family I would find at least one family member with depression, a term often used as synonymous with mental diseases in general. The debate about the rise of mental health problems in Kerala is often focused on depression and psychotic disorders such as mania or schizophrenia are sometimes perceived to be advanced stages of depression.

Figures citing one-third or more of the population as suffering from depression might be exaggerated, but they accurately depict the imaginary of Kerala as a state in distress. If – as part of the *conditio humana* or as a feature of the contemporary Malayali – sadness, suffering and misery have long been an integral part of normal life in Kerala, then one of the central questions of this book is how depression is now being stabilized as a disease in need of medical management.

There is a discourse linking depression to socio-economic changes experienced in Kerala in recent decades. As has been documented in other local contexts (Kitanaka 2012; Ecks 2013), debates on the rise of depression in Kerala are often tied to narratives of social decline. In this chapter I elucidate the causes for the presumed rise of depression as described by mental health experts, religious practitioners, laypeople and the media. In so doing, I provide an introduction to the ethnographic context of Kerala through the lens of crisis and social critique in a historical moment of accelerated social transformation. The arguments brought forward to account for the rise of depression in Kerala point to a larger context of critique in that they resonate with the discontent around modern transformations and the flipside of the "Kerala model of development". *The Hindu* reported on 11 September 2012 that Kerala rates highly on developmental indices but lags behind other states on mental health indices. Psychiatrists, psychologists, counsellors and social workers are portrayed as solutions for many of the crises Kerala is facing. If Kerala is depicted as a "society in distress" produced by a variety of socio-cultural changes in recent decades, then solutions are sought in the form of psychosocial engineering or governmentality capable of producing mentally resilient subjects able to face the multiple crises of Kerala's increasingly neoliberal society. In this sense, mental health care is often seen as producing enhanced subjects able to achieve their highest potential or, in other words, subjects capable of meeting neoliberal requirements without falling into dysfunction. The non-depressed subject is not only supposed to be productive and highly functional but also happy. This is what Kirmayer has called a "global monoculture of happiness", which demands that everyone be "pain free, completely comfortable, and ready and able to acquire and consume the greatest quantity and variety of the newest goods and fashions" (Kirmayer 2002).

The first social shift is the transformation in residence patterns "from the joint to the nuclear family". The disruption of the joint family[2] is often described in terms of a decline and related to modernization or Westernization. Kerala was once characterized by diverse matrilineal and patrilineal joint family residence patterns, most notably *marumakkattayam* [the matrilineal joint family practices of residence, descent and inheritance] among the Nair and some other castes.[3] The shift from the joint to the nuclear family is often mentioned as one of the reasons for the high rates of depression due to its isolating impact on children and the elderly. Together with the inflow of commodities and technologies since the economic liberalization of the 1990s, these transformations are perceived as a cause of the disruption of earlier systems of social security. Regarding the causes for the high rates of depression in Kerala, clinical psychologist Anand Kutty observed:

> There is a big gap between the newer generation and the just preceding generation. Earlier there was no need of parenting techniques or skills in this country because we had a joint family system. One or the other person would always look after the child. Now it's like papa, mama and both of them go for work, children are at home, computer is there, Internet is there. The whole world is there at their fingertips. And you don't know how to guard your children. So they go to a lot of places, in the virtual world as well as in the real world. And they learn things that they should not learn at that age. The cultural fabric is not able to hold the kind of learning that is happening. So the cultural fabric is broken. Good time for psychologists![4]

Apart from the fact that there was always somebody to look after and listen to the children, in these previous – often glorified – times, elder adults were present to imbue values and morals in children and teach them basic social skills like adjustment, listening to others or how to air their problems. As today more and more nuclear families live "separate" from their relatives, with both parents often working, many children are left to spend time home alone with electronic media as their sole companion. A related problem is one perceived as bad parenting practice: while in times past, children had to cope with their wishes for consumer goods being denied, the "spoilt children" of today are much less likely to learn how to wait for fulfilment of their consumer desires or to be able to cope with denial, and turn to suicide as an emotional reaction if refused. "Nowadays parents are over-protective. They don't expose these children to any type of stress. So the stress-bearing capacity of children has come down. That's why we have so many suicides during the adolescence," said Father Jijo, a priest, clinical psychologist and college teacher in Ernakulam.[5] This inability to cope with denial of desires which leads to depression or suicide once aspirations are not fulfilled is often related to a lack of *manobalam* [will power or mental power] which is perceived by many people I spoke with as closely related to depression (see Chapter 4). In this social scenario, moral education is increasingly institutionalized. Schools offer life skill training programmes, children are sent to summer camps to develop these skills and for personality development, parents are offered "courses for good parenting to produce anti-suicidal children" (Chua 2011), and many communities have established marital courses where couples complete an obligatory course of marital counselling before marriage. Hassan Ahamed, a social worker in Thiruvananthapuram who strongly promoted what he called "mental health literacy" – engaging Global Mental Health and WHO terminology – in schools and other institutions, noted:

> The scarcity or inadequacy of life-skills or social skills is the major problem and it will precipitate in depression and other mental disorders. People have to know how to cope with emotions, cope with stress. People are less and less able. We have to inculcate these life-skills at lower ages, at school education. We have to include them into the curriculum: How to

> speak, what is empathy, how to address the problems of friends, how to face a stressful situation.[6]

The breakdown of the joint family has also consequences for the elderly. The changed status of the elderly related to shifting residence patterns, migration, education and the rise of old-age homes has led to depression in this group being perceived as an important public health and social concern in Kerala. The children of these individuals live in nuclear families, often abroad, so the elderly are increasingly forced to reside either alone or in care homes. In Kerala as in the rest of India where long-term reciprocity and interdependence between parents and their children is still regarded as constitutive of intergenerational social life and care (Vatuk 1990; Cohen 1998; Lamb 2000), the perception of old-age homes is largely negative and they are considered "forms of noncare" (Lamb 2000, 53). Often, they are regarded as the negative outcomes of Westernization, of the loss of the joint family, of urbanization and individualization. Not surprisingly, depression is one of the largest health problems among residents in these institutions and the suicide rate in the population over sixty is rising (Pilania et al. 2013; Rajan and Zachariah 2010).

Closely related is the change in the social status of the elderly. When we talked about depression in Kerala, clinical psychologist Sonia Thomas pointed to the shifts experienced by elder women in the state. In the West, she said, women often become depressed around the age of forty because their social value decreases as they experience the bodily effects of aging and "don't feel attractive any more". In Kerala, the status of women used to increase with age as they assumed more responsibility and became more involved in the decision-making processes of the family they married into. "But now," she said, "this is changing and elder women have started feeling not attractive any more, not competent enough for the demands of the professional world, and often the young daughter-in-law is more educated than her."[7]

Divorce is another problem that often features in debates on the social origins of depression in Kerala in addition to occurring as a consequence of a depression diagnosis. In Kerala, divorce is highly problematic for a woman's status and can often almost be equated with her social death. A divorced woman has to go back to her natal home, sometimes with her children, but more often leaving her children with her in-laws. It can drive women into situations in which they are utterly dependant on their parents or brothers, are branded with the stigma of divorce and have little prospect of remarriage. This issue was raised in an article in *The Times of India* from 27 June 2012 that provocatively observed, "Looks like God's Own Country [the label for Kerala in touristic marketing] is fast metamorphosing into the haven of two ominous Ds – depression and divorce". The piece went on to closely link divorce, depression and suicide. In particular, indebted farmers, students failing their exams, unemployed but highly educated youth, people with high levels of debt incurred for the purchase of consumer goods, young women dishonoured by allegations of indecency or sexual transgression, and youth whose consumer demands are not met are the groups described as particularly vulnerable to depression and suicide. These failures and hardships and their attendant risks run counter to the narrative Kerala has told the world about its bright prospects and success, and for that reason are all the more troubling to many.

Explanations offered for the rise of the two big Ds largely overlap with other explanations I heard for the rise in divorce rates. In the media and in other public and professional discourses, the reasons for divorce and depression are seen in a transformation of the modern self and of subjectivities related to Westernization. Egotism, individualism, ego clash and maladjustment are identified as the most important factors. The English term "adjustment" was frequently used to refer to a quality associated with marriage, employment, migration – so much so that I was tempted to locate it as the key gendered attribute in middle class women and a core quality of young brides. The school psychologist Susan Abraham explained it to me: "Whatever will be the circumstances, it's your responsibility to stay with your in-laws. I may not even utter these difficulties to my parent. I will suffer and be part and parcel of my in-laws."[8] Ego clash is closely related to a failure in adjustment, often also gendered and related to the economic independence of employed women. Ego clashes are seen as responsible for divorce and for depression resulting out of conjugal conflicts. This is how Dr Fatimah, a young female psychiatrist working at the Syrian Christian Hospital expressed it:

> Husbands and wives are working. In Kerala, this is something new. Both of them are working and both are earning money and naturally *ego problems* arise. *Ego problems* means the feeling of "I am getting paid, so why should I obey?" Previously, there was a little difference between husband and wife which contributed to conjugal harmony.[9]

Without resident family elders to act as mediators or counsellors in the household, the couple is left on their own in conflict and discord, in many cases this leads at least one member of the couple into depression.

In a state well known for its high development indicators such as economic growth, social welfare and equitable redistribution of resources, high literacy rates, low birth rates, and access to health care, the current prevalence of depression is a challenge. Like suicide, the high rates of depression expose the flipside of the "Kerala model of development" (Halliburton 1998) and index the disappointment of unfulfilled political and social promises. Kerala's international status rests on a citizenry notable for good health and, as such, depression represents a particularly pernicious threat to the reputation on which the state trades and to the powerful and overwhelmingly positive narrative of development and progress (Chua 2014). In a state where doctors as engineers of the body (and the mind) are seen as able to fix anything, depression represents an accusation that the model is unsuccessful and that the quest for and achievement of development comes at the cost of the mental health of the people. Contradictions have been identified between high physical health indicators and the high incidence of mental distress (Eapen 2002; Chua 2014). In the same way that the state is proud to have successfully combated communicable physical diseases through a comprehensive health care system, the state and mental health NGOs promote a comprehensive technical solution for depression and other mental health problems consisting of early detection and intervention. Neoliberal mental health governmentality now aims to produce docile and resilient bodies, minds and subjects. Despite the many achievements of the Kerala model, problems such as unemployment, political stagnation, environmental concerns and the exclusion of lower castes and tribes have lead many to speak of the "paradox" of the Kerala development model (Chua 2014). Educational attainment has outstripped the availability of skilled jobs. Today, many highly educated young Malayalis are unable to find employment in jobs that match their education. This is especially relevant for men who spend years completing more and more qualifying certificates or experience long stagnant periods waiting for opportunities to arise (Jeffrey 2010) which postpones the process of entering into a locally defined state of male maturity (Osella and Osella 2006). For women, unemployment is regarded as less problematic because middle class norms direct them to invest their education in their own children rather than contributing to the family income by working "outside".

As in many other parts of the world, depression rates in Kerala are reported to be higher for women than men (Eapen 2002; Mukhopadyay, Basu and Rajan 2007). Many of the people I spoke with mentioned female physiology, but emphasized gender role expectations and gender-related inequalities. These "traps set by society", as expressed by Dr C.J. John in an article in the Malayalam magazine *Arogya Masika* in April (John 2014), include the character traits expected from women in Kerala such as adjustment capacity, modesty and the ability "to accept suffering without complaining" as psychiatrist Smitha Ramdas and gynaecologist P.P. Rameshkumar (2014) mention in the same issue. Moreover, competing priorities, such as the burdens of employment and housework, and gender-specific factors such as discrimination, violence and sexual abuse, spousal alcoholism and the exponential rise of dowries are cited as further factors that lead women into depression (ibid.). Indeed, a flipside of the Kerala model is what is called the "gender paradox" of Malayali women. Some have emphasized the high status of women as a historical heritage of the former matrilineality of many groups in Kerala resulting in high rates of women's literacy and educational attainments (Jeffrey 2004). Others, especially feminist scholars, question the dominant imaginary of Malayali women's empowerment and argue that patriarchal inequality is a foundational element of Kerala's modernity and that socio-political reforms were based in "the dichotomization of the male breadwinner and the female housewife" (Sreekumar 2007; Chua 2014). This was reinforced by middle class values based in the Brahmanic ideal that locates women's labour inside the home and equates working women with lower classes and castes (Gulati and Rajan 1991; Eapen and Kodoth 2003; Mitra and Singh 2007). Many middle-class families perceive the shift of women into the private sphere of the household as a rise in female status; feminist scholars interpret this as a decline in the status women held until the disruption of the matrilineal practices of residence, descent and inheritance (Devika 2007; Sreekumar 2007). These transformations in family structure, inheritance practices, gender ideology and economy, together with the discrepancy between high educational achievement and limited agency, make women in Kerala vulnerable not only to domestic violence, dowry abuse and suicide (Kodoth and Eapen 2005; Mitra and Singh 2007; Mukhopadhyay et al. 2007; Chua 2014) but also to depression.

If they work outside the home, women face an enormous double burden: full-time employment and responsibility for the household and the family. Dr Geetha (2009) writes in an article in *Arogya Masika* published in June "It is the nonstop race between home and work without any rest that plunges them into mental stress. [...] With the emergence of nuclear families working women who are under stress have no way to share their stressful problems." In the home of the middle class Christian family where I lived while conducting fieldwork in Kottakkal, both parents worked as teachers. Maria got up by 4 a.m. to have a short walk, cook breakfast and lunch for their two school-aged daughters, clean the house, eat a bit of breakfast in the kitchen, and ready herself for work and her daughters for school. She left the house at 7:30 a.m., caught the first bus to the provincial capital an hour away, then caught a second bus for an hour-long journey that took her to the town where she worked in a government-aided school. On the bus, she might find the time to relax and sleep. After a day's teaching, she started her journey home by 4 p.m., arriving around 6 p.m. Her husband Antony worked as a teacher in a school near their home and commuted by motorbike. He would return home at about 4:30 p.m., and proceeded to relax, watch TV with his daughters and help them with their studies, or read the newspaper. Antony did the shopping, so when Maria arrived home she could immediately begin her remaining household work, wash the clothes and start cooking dinner. Antony was responsible for supervising the children's homework, completed half in the afternoon after school and half in the morning. Dinner was at 8:30 or 9 p.m., and afterward the family would pray together and watch a bit of TV. When the children went to sleep, Maria went to her bed where she corrected her students' work, prepared her lessons for the next day and, in my last months there, studied for an additional postgraduate course. She finally fell asleep around midnight. I further heard of women residing in the capital, Thiruvananthapuram, and commuting each day to the Kochi – a journey of several hours. Situations like this have led to the appearance of a new niche of vendors selling vegetables and other foodstuff on the train from Ernakulam to Thiruvananthapuram so that women are able to complete their shopping on the train, eliminating the need for a separate shopping trip before being able to return home. Employment, then, is often an enormous burden for women because they are still expected to do all the work required of a good housewife and, in the absence of practical and emotional support from the joint family, to do it all on their own.

The term "Gulf depression" refers to the distress of "Gulf wives",[10] left home without their husbands and often shouldering the sole responsibility for bringing up their children and residing either with their in-laws or as a single-parent family.[11] Most – nearly all – families in Kerala have at least one male member working in the Gulf countries. Opportunities for well-paid employment in the Arab states bordering the Persian Gulf (most prominent are the United Arab Emirates, Oman, Quatar, Saudi Arabia and Kuwait) attract individuals who send their wages home to Kerala. Gulf labour migration has substantial sociocultural implications (Gulati and Rajan 1993; Osella and Osella 2006). It helps Kerala's growing middle class achieve a lifestyle comparable to a European middle class lifestyle with families improving their social status through imported consumer goods and large new houses. It also fuels the state's economy. Poor prospects at home and lucrative job availability in the Gulf since the oil boom in the 1970s created a significant shift in Kerala's economy. Gulf remittances "make a substantial contribution to the annual income of the households in Kerala" and constitute around one-third of the net state domestic product (Rajan and Zachariah 2010). Furthermore, labour migrants to the Gulf bring home not only consumer goods but also reformist Islam ideologies and practices that shape religious practice and lifestyle in Kerala (Osella and Osella 2008; Osella 2012).

There is a close relationship between consumption and distress in Kerala (Balachandran 1998). Men and women are affected, and greed sows *adhi* [mental stress] and harvests *vyadhi* [disease], writes Dr Geetha (*Arogya Masika*, June 2009). The consumerism underwritten by migratory labour remittances and media depictions of "consumer citizenship" (Lukose 2009) and national economic liberalization are seen as a double-edged sword. There is the risk of the "disease of consumerism" (Chua 2014: 32), which is often framed as a generational or class conflict between Nehruvian socialist ideas on the one hand and a culture of pleasure and happiness on the other. Hierarchies of moral and social status are being formulated between a more mature consumerism focused around permanent consumer goods such as houses, land and education, versus a pleasure-based short-term kind of consumerism based around transient consumer goods such as clothes, motorbikes, fashion or dining out (Osella and Osella 1999; Lukose 2009). Leftist critics identify consumerism as a manifestation of the growing reach of multinational corporations leading to political passivity, while those on the Hindutva right are primarily concerned with the threats it poses to Indian traditions and values (Chua 2014). Consumerism, especially in combination with "over-ambition",[12] is often mentioned as contributing to dissatisfaction, jealousy and envy. This can lead to depression, as several mental health workers in Kerala explained to me. Father Jijo saw the high rate of depression as related to what he called "relative deprivation".[13] People are not deprived of their basic needs, he explained, but they compare their own situation with others who have more money, more savings and larger houses. To obtain desirable consumer goods, people take out loans that they are often not able to repay. People are prepared to go into debt to obtain prestigious consumer goods and access private education for their children.

Others connected heightened material aspirations with high literacy rates, including Dr Narayanan, an Ayurvedic physician from one of the Asthavaidya families in Thrissur. "Education of the people is very good," he told me, but qualified this by asserting that

> education also creates a great desire in many people to have a better quality of life. Well and good. But what happens is that if you have a desire and you are not able to achieve that target, you slip into a depression.[14]

Psychologist Mohan Menon[15] similarly explained that, surrounded by luxury homes, some people might feel worse living in a smaller house than they would if all the houses were small. With neighbours showing off the newest electronic devices from the Gulf every time they return home, those who cannot afford them feel deprived. The presence and prevalence of English-language private educational institutions means that those unable to afford entry for their children feel cut off from being able to achieve modern middle class ideals, he contended.

Growing consumption, aspirations and increasing economic differentiation have made Kerala a highly competitive and envious society. This manifests also in increasing suspicion of mantravadam, kaivisham and other forms of occult violence being used against neighbours or relatives out of jealousy. As a result, ritual practices of manipulating wealth, dealing with bad luck or occult violence on the one hand and protecting fortunes that left other family members behind on the other are gaining importance in Kerala (Osella and Osella, 2000). There is little hesitation to call on the gods to satisfy consumer desires and achieve wealth. "Nowadays, people are even bribing the gods," my host Antony[16] told me. As the consumerist gap between aspiration and reality drives people into ritual ways of manipulating destiny, increasing consumerism leads to an augmentation of reinvented rituals with which religious practitioners treat not only economic disadvantage and bad luck, but also depression, tension and other pathologies related to consumerism, mobility and modern life.

Alcoholism is described as one of the masks worn by depression in Malayali men. Kerala has been identified as having the heaviest drinkers in India and the highest rates of alcohol consumption (BBC News 2010). Even more recently, Kerala was called "the booziest state" in India, with an annual per capita alcohol consumption of 8.3 litres (The Economist 2013). It is a popular joke in Malayalam that alcohol stalls and toddy bars are the only places in Kerala where people queue in orderly lines, and the Kerala affinity for alcohol and issue of alcoholism are also reflected in popular Malayalam movies.[17] Men in particular, psychiatrists told me, do not express depression in psychological or somatic terms: instead of seeking help, they take refuge in liquor. The heavy consumption of alcohol in Kerala can thus be seen as an idiom of distress for men that, according to mental health professionals, masks underlying depression in need of therapeutic attention. Addiction and rehabilitation programmes in general hospitals offering these services – often free of charge and supported by government schemes – are always over-full, and invariably have long waiting lists. Husbands and fathers with drinking problems featured in the narratives of many of my interlocutors, and this affects whole families, not just the men dealing with depression through overuse of alcohol. They also arise in discussions with medical and religious mental health practitioners, and in media reports on depression in the state. Divorce is often not an option, so women are left to bear the burden of their husband's alcohol abuse, including domestic violence but also his care both in the clinic and the home.

Youth and children in Kerala, too, are not exempt from the state's high rates of depression (Krishnakumar 2010; The Hindu 2012). The pressure on and competition between students is frequently cited as a cause of depression in the young. Behavioural problems and *vishada rogam* [depressive disorder] are seen to be spreading among children in Kerala, and some experts warn that a whole generation would be lost to the disease if timely treatment was not made available. A flipside of high literacy and educational attainment rates in Kerala is the bifurcation and commercialization of higher education into public Malayalam schools and private English schools. The pressure exerted on children due to the high expectations of parents is also in many cases related to the high financial investment – and sacrifice – required to gain entrance to private schools. Beyond this, depression in children has been linked to recent and widespread lifestyle changes in Kerala. In particular, as work patterns have changed so too have food habits. A growing dependence on processed and preprepared packaged foods has been identified as having a negative impact on the bodies of children, drastically reducing "the chance for exercise and lack of proper exercise causes a lot of mental and physical problems" (Krishnakumar 2010). These physiological factors combined with the pressures of a highly competitive educational system and the loss of childhood pleasures further contribute to depression in children. Changing family configurations are also identified as a key factor in depression in the young. The shift from the joint to the nuclear family as the unit of primary social interaction and residence has narrowed children's options for expressing and learning to deal with strong emotions. Further, divorce and the rupture of family relations are said to create a lack of strong positive role models for children with a decidedly negative impact on their mental health. Such familial problems affect children of all classes, but the impacts are particularly marked in communities and families seeking upward social mobility.[18] As part of an awareness session on the importance of befriending and listening skills for improving mental health at a local college, lawyer and activist Matthew Kurian[19] told the following story:

> One boy I know, he got a good rank in the 10th standard SSLC[20] examination. After that, plus two. Then he got admission for medicine and completed the degree. After that, he got admission to the postgraduate course and completed his MD. Very good career. During the examination for the MD, there was an examiner who talked to him in a very arrogant manner. He felt that he would not achieve the right marks. He committed suicide. Was his life successful?

He continued: "They have achieved everything, they are qualified, may have postgraduate, very good employment. But they don't know how to talk to their wives, to their children. How to make good relations with their neighbour. Many parents," he concluded, "consider their children as machines: more productivity, more production, more profit". They are considered to be socially ill equipped as a result of a dehumanizing achievement orientation.

Parental pressure and high expectations are important factors in depression in the young but also lead to a rise in suicide, both reflected in the increasing use of telephone hotline services such as Childline or Maithri. More and more, parents are seeking the help of a psychiatrist, counsellor or religious healer for their children especially during the annual SSLC final exams. Vasudeva Namboodiri,[21] a practitioner at a Hindu religious healing centre, explained,

> This time I have some teenager patients, plus two and 10th standard. These students have lots of depression. Parents and teachers put a lot of pressure on them. We try to comfort them and increase their *manobalam* [mental strength]. I tell the parents, don't put this pressure on the children. It will lead to tension and tension will lead to *vishadam* [depression].

Recognition of the power and prevalence of this pressure and the resulting mental health problems for students have led to the mandatory establishment of a counsellor post in every school to monitor student mental health. However, the daily routines for many of these children allows for little downtime, or time for play. They study in the morning, then go to school until 4 p.m., attend additional tuition until 7 p.m., then return home to eat and study again, often until late at night. While I was in Kerala, the seventeen-year-old daughter of one of my research assistants was preparing for the plus two final exams. At the same time, she spent Sundays at a tuition centre preparing for the entrance exam to study medicine. She had no day of rest in her week, and always studied until late at night. Once, when I returned from their home quite late, I was surprised to see her mother wake her at midnight in order to study until 2 a.m., as a matter of routine.

Competition at school has further consequences for the experience, social behaviour and mental health of children. Psychologist Sonia Thomas related this transformation to a shift in selves and psyches:

> In the Indian system, even at the age of twenty-five years, we do not consider ourselves as an individual. We are only part of a larger group. That kind of dependent psyche was there. But now, because of these family changes, even in school situations, there is so much competition. So even children cannot relate to each other as their intimates. When I was a child of ten years, it was very different from the experience that a child of ten years now. We have become more achievement-oriented. Even school children are competing with each other. So they cannot fully share. Earlier, children in India, we used to share everything. It was so transparent. Even in

> adolescence we used to be very transparent, used to have very close friendly relationships. There were no secrets. But nowadays it is not like that. Actually we are getting more isolated, nobody at home or even outside to fully share and get support from. These are my observations. Probably these are the reasons now even our children have started developing this problem of depression.[22]

The pressure on children through a competitive school system is especially prominent in Kerala where an emphasis on education stems from historical forces of colonial and postcolonial modernity (Jeffrey 2004; Lukose 2009). The rulers of the princely states of Travancore and Kochi (two of the three regions brought together to form the state of Kerala in 1956) were particularly concerned with expanding educational opportunities for all castes and communities. The influence of the previously matrilineal system of the Nair, a high caste in Kerala, is also cited as playing an important role in attitudes and expectations of education in the state. This group accorded women relative freedom including access to literacy (Jeffrey 2004). The influence of the Christian community in establishing and creating an educational infrastructure from the British colonial period onwards is also identified as a factor. Finally, high literacy rates and the importance of education are causally linked to caste-based social reform movements in Kerala since the nineteenth century and to the strong communist influence in Kerala since the middle of the twentieth century (Lukose 2009).

In addition to educational pressures, depression (and suicide) in adolescents is also related to "love failures". Love affairs indicate a disruption of the social order and normative gendered behaviour, and they interfere with what youth are supposed to be mostly concerned with – studying. In a state where the majority of marriages are arranged, love affairs are regarded as highly problematic and the mental state of "being in love" is pathologized. Love affairs are negotiated in relation to new technology, such as mobile phones and social media, which enable adolescents to freely communicate with potential partners without the oversight of the usual forms of cultural control. Love failure features in many stories about suicides or suicide attempts. Young adults may also fall into depression after being forced by their parents into an arranged marriage. The debate around romantic love is often formulated in terms of a conflict between modern and traditional values. Students regard it prestigious in the eyes of their peers to have a love affair, usually consisting of nothing more than chatting on social media, exchanging glances in the classroom or talking in class while others stand nearby.

It should be noted that close interaction between adolescents of the opposite sex is still taboo. While I was in Kottakkal I heard about a girl who hanged herself after her neighbours came to know she had a love affair and that the boy had picked her up from school on his motorbike and taken her home on several occasions. At a private Christian (English) school, teachers told me that they got suspicious and intervened if a boy and a girl became too intimate, that is, if a pair was seen to speak regularly outside the classroom. Clinical psychologist

Jacob Matthew[23] told me that these love affairs are not culturally appropriate. "We are becoming more liberal" he continued, "How good this is, I don't know." Many eighteen-year-olds confessed to him that they had had intimate physical contact. "They say, 'we have taken precautions, so what?'" Overhearing this, a student of psychology who had just finished her MSc thesis under his guidance laughed and said, "Oh my god!" The psychologist remarked, "Their grandparents would commit suicide if they listened to that." He mentioned similar cases and explained me that as a psychologist he could only guide an adolescent in a way that was culturally appropriate, one that corresponded to accepted moral norms. "If a boy and girl are holding hands with each other," Susan Abraham,[24] the school counsellor at a Christian (English) school, told me, "the girl is said to have a loose character or the boy is too much of a freak." When children came to her for help, it was usually because the situation had gotten out of hand. What might be an innocent, friendly relationship can quickly be blown out of proportion if peers start making up stories.

> To a certain extent, the girl may handle it. But after some time, the girl may feel guilty or maybe feels the pressure from the parents. She is not in a position to handle it by herself. Then I have to give courage to her. Basically I have to boost up her morals. She has to know the system. She has to survive in the society. So what the society is I have to make her aware.

Caught in a double bind, adolescents then navigate two opposite standards: those of the older generation and those of their peers. And they do so in the context of a global youth culture endlessly disseminated through mass and social media.

The rise of "depression", usually referred to by its English name, but also by the Malayalam terms vishadam or vishada rogam, is linked to larger socio-cultural transformations in recent decades, usually formulated in a narrative of cultural decline or crisis. This chapter has described the ways local mental health practitioners, religious healers and scholars account for the rise of depression in Kerala by relating it to a social critique and the flipside of the "Kerala model of development". The shift in family patterns from joint to nuclear families, a rise in divorce rates, unemployment, gender inequalities, economic migration to the Gulf and its impact on the Gulf wives left behind, an increase in consumption, pressure on students, alcoholism, love affairs and the tensions in the perceived shift from tradition to modernity are the problems that feature most prominently when Malayalis try to account for the rise of depression in their state. If Kerala is depicted as a "society in distress" produced by a host of socio-cultural changes in recent decades, then solutions are sought in a form of psychosocial engineering or governance intended to produce mentally resilient subjects able to withstand the many challenges of Kerala's increasingly neoliberal society. In this sense, mental health care is often seen as producing enhanced subjects able to achieve their highest potential or, in other words, subjects fitting neoliberal requirements without falling prey to depression or other malfunction. The non-depressed subject is not only supposed to be productive and highly functional but also happy (Kirmayer 2002). This global trend has also led to a "happiness turn" (Ahmed 2007) in policy and governance, a happiness induced, if needed, by the consumption of antidepressants as "happy pills". There is an evident neoliberal mental health governmentality producing docile, productive, happy non-depressive subjects. Yet it is not only mental health professionals, but also religious practitioners that are sought out to address aspects of depression, and provide relief to sufferers. Girish Menon,[25] a member of a foundation that promotes individual transformation as a path to social change through what he calls "harmony counselling", commented: "There is a huge market for mental health. Peace of mind has become a much sought after good. Mental health problems, especially tension, are on the rise, because of the *rat race*."

Mental health professionals have argued that the reason why psychiatry, psychology and counselling have only recently gained in importance is because the need for these services is new. This explanation implies that the current situation is the result of a recent shift in the prevalence and experience of depression. A second understanding identifies the rise in depression rates as tied to changes in the evaluation of what constitutes abnormal behaviour and its social impact. In a joint family with many members in one house, an individual who did not function properly did not have a strong negative impact on the family, I was told. So long as they did not become violent, the family did not consider such individuals as a problem and saw no need to seek treatment. A related view holds that symptoms that are today medicalized as depression were previously understood as existential, moral or religious exigencies and treated mainly by religious or spiritual means. An explanation for the depression crisis in Kerala certainly involves a shifting combination of all three explanations. But what is clear is that Kerala sees itself as a society in distress, suffering from unprecedented rates of depression. For this reason, my particular focus is unpicking the ways distress, suffering and emotional breakdown came to be reconfigured and pathologized as depression in Kerala.

Notes

1 *The Economic Times,* 11 August 2011.

2 The joint family or extended family is a common form of residence in India in which more than one nuclear family of more than one generation live together on the basis of consanguine and affinal relational ties.

3 Social and legislative reform movements beginning in the nineteenth century gradually "modernized" or "civilized" the marumakkattayam system and introduced "patrifocal" (Mukhopadhyay 1994) residence, patrilineal descent, and patrilineal inheritance and succession. Reforms were guided by a moralist and modernist discourse of liberating women from immoral practices by striving for a growing paternal influence and a tax system under which it is difficult to hold properties jointly. New legislation put the conjugal or nuclear family at the centre and redefined relations of protection and dependence (Arunima 2003; Devika 2007; Eapen and Kodoth 2003; Saradamoni 1999). Marumakkattayam was officially abolished by the Kerala Joint Hindu Family (Abolition) Act, although matrilineal thinking and practice continue today.

However, as legislative changes and economic transformations made matrilineal practices less viable, the nuclear conjugal patrifocal family emerged as the accepted economical – and therefore most desirable – option (Chua 2014). In the matrilineal family form, decision-making authority was in the hands of the male manager or guardian but women had property rights and greater agency, authority, and power over decision making (Jeffrey 2004).

4 Anand Kutty, Kozhikode, 15 February 2010.
5 Father Jijo, Ernakulam, 26 September 2010.
6 Hassan Ahamed, Thiruvananthapuram, 10 October 2012.
7 Sonia Thomas, Kozhikode, 13 September 2012.
8 Susan Abraham, Ernakulam, 14 January 2012.
9 Dr Fatimah, Ernakulam, 16 January 2012
10 In rare cases, women migrate alone to the Gulf to work mainly as nurses or doctors, but this is not common.
11 Although the "Gulfans" (male Gulf migrants) themselves often fall into depression, Gulf depression does not generally refer to their mental suffering. For a popular representation of Gulfan struggles, see the novel *Goat Days* (2008) by the Malayalam author Benyamin.
12 Ambition or over-ambition is often pathologized in popular mental health discourse in Kerala (cf. also Chua 2009). Some psychologists and Ayurvedic psychiatrists traced negative connotations of ambition to the Bhagavad Gita in which Arjuna is admonished by Krishna not to let his actions be led by the expectations of the results.
13 Father Jijo, Ernakulam, 26 September 2010.
14 Dr Narayanan, Thrissur, 3 September 2009.
15 Mohan Menon, Kozhikode, 13 September 2012.
16 Antony, Kottakkal, 10 February 2015.
17 Examples are the blockbuster *Spirit* (2012) directed by Ranjith in which Mohan Lal plays the lead role, or *Pavada* [skirt] (2016) directed by G. Marthandan.
18 For an excellent description of the ex-untouchable Izhava caste, see Osella & Osella 2000.
19 Matthew Kurian, Ernakulam, 26 September 2012.
20 The Secondary School Leaving Certificate, a qualification of students after leaving the 10th class.
21 Vasudeva Namboodiri, Manjeri, 15 March 2010.
22 Sonia Thomas, Kozhikode, 13 September 2012.
23 Jacob Matthew, Ernakulam, 13 October 2012.
24 Susan Abraham, Ernakulam, 14 January 2013
25 Girish Menon, Thrissur, 31 March 2010.

3 Glocalizing depression and its treatment in Kerala

It is one of the basic premises of this book that transformations on institutional, material and cognitive levels contributed to the medicalization and expansion of depression in India. This in turn is closely tied to the increasing creation and acceptance of institutions of treatment and education, drugs intended to cure or manage, clinicians, expert and public knowledge, and a concomitant enlargement of the number and types of people diagnosed with depression. This chapter focuses on these looping effects (Hacking 2007) that constitute depression as a mental disorder. These go hand in hand with a shift in the diseases that are understood as the purview of psychiatry and an associated change in the scope of competency of psychiatrists encompassing what are now called common mental disorders. The age of the asylum was also the age of severe mental disorders: that is, psychoses in psychiatry. The "age of Prozac" (Shorter 1997) is also the age of depression, and the disorder is predicted to be the second most prevalent disease worldwide by 2020 (Desjarlais et al. 1995; Murray and Lopez 1996; World Health Organization 2001b). Although depression first became a WHO priority in the mid-1980s, the impact of mental health programmes in India remains questionable, not only because of a lack of resources but also due to their social and cultural inadequacy in Indian contexts. The common imaginary of psychiatry is slowly shifting from dealing with relatively rare and severely debilitating conditions to milder and more common forms of distress. This corresponds to the image psychiatrists in India are constructing for their profession as not only the home for treatment of severe psychopathology but also of specialization in common mental disorders and in what is sometimes called "cosmetic psychiatry" – individual enhancement and treating the neoliberal and consumerist collateral damage to India's new middle class to improve their ability to cope with modern lifestyles thereby creating a new technology of the neoliberal self. In this chapter, I draw on fieldwork in the psychiatric units of two multi-specialty hospitals and a larger private psychiatric hospital in and near a major city where I had discussions with psychiatrists, psychologists and psychiatric social workers in clinical settings as well as participant observation in clinical encounters with patients diagnosed with depression. This allows both observation of mental health professionals and their self reflection regarding current practice in order to focus on the institutional shifts that enabled psychiatry to expand its scope of competency to encompass – and lay claim to – depression.

From the asylum towards community psychiatry: institutional shifts

I knew from my first visits to Kuthiravathom Mental Health Centre in Kozhikode, one of the three large governmental mental hospitals in Kerala, that with some rare exceptions these former asylums did not admit and treat patients for depression. Rather, it was the psychotic, violent and difficult to manage patients whose deviant behaviour disrupted the social order and family life who were committed there, often for months, sometimes years. Some were "dumped" by family members who left a false address so that the patient could not be sent back to them on release. In Kuthiravathom, doctors told me, the majority of patients were diagnosed with bipolar disorder (maniac state) or schizophrenia.[1] Patients with depression, both mild and severe, were rarely admitted either as inpatients or outpatients to these large institutions.[2] Too strong are the memories of the asylum, too close the architectural, spatial and residential resemblances to these infamous institutions that they are chosen for treatment only in the case of emergencies.

The imaginary of the asylum weighed heavily on Kuthiravathom and the other two government-run institutions. It was the key reason why people suffering from mental illness and their families hesitated to seek treatment there except when management at home became absolutely impossible. The Kuthiravathom mental health centre was established in 1872 on the outskirts of Kozhikode as a "lunatic asylum" widely known as *branthan jail* [prison for the mad] offering custody rather than treatment for British lunatics while they were waiting to be sent back to Britain. Unlike the situation in Europe and other former colonies, the aim of psychiatry in India was not social control of the "natives" – they were understood by British colonial authorities as the responsibility of Indian communities, families and Indian-run asylums (Ernst 2007). The renaming that occurred in the 1920s from "lunatic asylum" to "mental hospital" [*manasikarogyasupathri*] and later to "mental health centre" [*manasikarogyakendram*] accompanied a shift from custody to treatment, and from treating British to treating Indian people. Along with other mental hospitals in India, treatment in Kerala developed along the same lines as in European and North American psychiatry, moving from moral therapies to pharmacological treatment of mental disorder in the mid-twentieth century, with increasing importance accorded to vocational training and rehabilitation from the 1990s. It was only with the 1983 foundation of the Institute of Mental Health and Neurosciences (IMHANS) in Kozikode that Kuthiravathom (then renamed an Institute of Mental Health Science) developed into a research institute.

Although armed with the expectation that patients suffering from depression would not frequent the larger mental health institutions in Kerala, I was nonetheless surprised to find that even in the smaller private mental hospitals – which are far less stigmatized than the large institutions – depression patients were rare. Those few who did seek treatment at these smaller hospitals mostly accessed outpatient services. There were almost no inpatients diagnosed with depression, either at the Little Flower Mental Health Centre[3] or in the other private mental hospitals I visited, most of which were managed either by Christian nuns or by individual psychiatrists. Analysis of past patient files confirmed that only rarely were patients diagnosed with depression at the outpatient department (OPD) and referred to one of the three psychiatrists or the psychologist there. On an average day, out of approximately fifty patients, one or two were diagnosed with severe depression; the majority of diagnoses were for bipolar disorder, psychosis or, more rarely, schizophrenia. Additionally some few patients suffering from depression showed up at the office of the clinical psychologist. Singular emergency cases also included patients who had attempted suicide. Here, there was no trace of the depression epidemic so widely discussed in newspapers, on television and in conversations with mental health professionals (Chapter 2).

It was when I moved into two private general hospital psychiatric units, one in and one near a major city, that depression appeared in mainstream psychiatric practice, though still not in the numbers one might expect given the public and professional discourse. In these private psychiatric units, a much larger percentage of patients was diagnosed with depressive disorder, anxiety disorder and other common mental disorders although bipolar disorder, psychoses and alcohol dependency amounted to around half of the diagnoses. It seems that a large number of depression patients in Kerala are treated by a doctor who is not a psychiatrist. Approximately one-fifth of patients seen in general practice and a significant proportion of patients treated by gynaecologists, neurologists, cardiologists and others came in with symptoms such as body pain, headache, lower back pain, burning or tingling in the hands or feet, fatigue or sleeplessness and, often without exchanging a single word about depression or mental illness, general practitioners prescribed antidepressants for these and other complaints. In these situations, depression is "hidden" – as physicians and psychiatrists put it – behind the somatic symptoms of the patient and behind the somatic medicines of the physician. From another angle, depression is thus fabricated as a somatic disease (neurotransmitters gone awry), experienced and dealt with in clinical encounters as a physical problem.

The scenario I encountered was the result of profound institutional and policy shifts in psychiatry in India in the decades since Independence. Since the days of the asylum, psychiatry has continuously expanded its scope to encompass milder kinds of distress that would not have been associated with the field some decades ago. The rise of depression increasingly makes psychiatrists specialists in dealing with the perceived side effects of modernity. With depression reportedly on the rise and numbers in Kerala reckoned to be the highest in India, psychiatry is increasingly thought of and presented as the branch of medicine most suited to addressing the problem. Moving from the age of the asylum to the "age of depression" (Horwitz 2010), psychiatry is expected not only to fill an enormous treatment gap but also to treat the collateral damage of modern social and cultural transformations (Chapter 2). The shift from asylum psychiatry to outpatient psychiatry and to the outreach of psychiatrists towards the public sphere is one part of the vernacularization of the psy disciplines in Kerala (cf. Chua 2013).

The development of psychiatric wings in general hospitals was part of a wider development of de-centralized, community mental health care in India (Jain and Jadhav 2008). Though attempted by pioneers in the 1950s, it was in the 1970s and 1980s, in an effort to shift the treatment of patients with mental illness from asylums to the community, that psychiatric wings in general hospitals (public and private) were created to involve the families in treatment, counter stigma and master the heavy patient load (Wig and Awasthi 2005). Following the World Health Organization's seminal 1975 report *Organization of Mental Health Services in Developing Countries*, Indian psychiatrists made systematic attempts in integrating psychiatric services into primary health care by training general physicians and community health workers. The pilot projects in community psychiatry at Sakalwara near Bangalore by the National Institution of Mental Health and Neurosciences (NIMHANS) in 1976 and Raipur Rani near Chandigarh by psychiatrists at the Postgraduate Institute of Medical Education and Research (PGIMER) in 1975 were part of an international WHO Project "Strategies For Extending Mental Health Care". While Raipur Rani was externally funded and time bound Sakalwara, primarily on domestic and government initiative, continues to date. The District Mental Health Programme at Bellary district that was initiated in 1984 as a pilot model programme has been up-scaled to many other districts in the country (Weiss et al. 2001; Kapur 2004; Jain and Jadhav 2008).

The General Hospital Psychiatry Unit (GHPU) movement further expanded after it was promoted by the 1982 National Mental Health Programme (NMHP) and later the restructuring of mental health care in the country that followed the tragic fire in the Muslim shrine of Erwadi in Tamil Nadu in 2001 and the deaths of twenty-eight mental health patients there. The fallout from Erwadi brought religious healing centres under the purview of the state. It also precipitated closer scrutiny for mental hospitals that were criticized for not implementing the 1987 Mental Health Act. The 2014 launch of India's Mental Health Policy *New Pathways, New Hopes* (Ministry of Health & Family Welfare 2014) pushed the de-centralization of mental health care, especially community care.

National developments were important to this policy shift, but it was intensified by wider global developments promoted by the World Health Organization including the 2001 publication of an influential report on the global burden of mental diseases. The prognosis in *Mental Health: New Understanding, New Hope* was that depression would be the second greatest cause of disability by 2020. It suggests that mental health be included in primary health care. The new policy favoured the distribution of psychotropic medication over community participation and psycho-social interventions and led to a situation where pills "swallowed policy" (Jain and Jadhav 2009). Along with the focus on psychotropic medicines as cheap and effective treatments, changes in mental health policy in 2002 involved a shift towards investment in hospitals, public education, training and research (Jain and Jadhav 2009). The context and driving forces behind the GHPU movement involved several interrelated developments. As in the US and Europe, the advent of psychiatric drugs in the 1950s encouraged movement away from the already discredited mental asylum towards the deinstitutionalization of psychiatry and community-based mental health care in what has been called the shift from "the era of the asylum to the age of Prozac" (Shorter 1997). Within India and similar to other countries of the global South, economic constraints and a shortage of trained psychiatrists were countered by creating training facilities in colleges and general hospitals. In India, the epidemic view of mental illness took aim at providing "the most effective help to the greatest number of clients in the least possible time" (Nunley 1996, 170). Depression and other rising common mental disorders constituted an increasing public health concern, with the result that mental health care outside the mental hospital was perceived as a public health necessity.

It was only with de-institutionalization, the growth of GHPUs, the advent of antidepressants (1950s) and their wide use (from the 1980s) that psychiatrists became specialists in depression. India launched a National Mental Health Programme (NMHP) in 1982 with the aim of making mental health care universally available and accessible, but it was not actually implemented in most states. In 1996, the first District Mental Health Programme (DMHP) was launched that aimed to integrate mental health care into primary health care. There was then an effort to adopt this nationwide and make mental health care accessible to all by setting up psychiatric services in peripheral areas, training primary health care personnel and involving communities in promoting mental health, in effect formulating the priorities of the NMHP in a more concrete fashion. Yet this integration has not occurred in many districts of the country.

In Kerala, however, there have been active attempts to implement the DMHP in several districts since the late 1990s. Since then, primary and community health centres and *taluk* [sub-district] hospitals have been offered mental health services. Psychotropic medicines, such as the antidepressant fluoxetine, are part of the essential drugs list and the standard pharmaceutical equipment of every primary health centre in Kerala. Medical officers, nurses and healthcare workers are trained in basic psychiatric diagnostics and pharmacological treatment either by members of the district mental health teams or by other psychiatrists, often in cooperation with mental health NGOs. Additionally, schoolteachers and *anganwadi*[4] workers and other laypersons are trained in identifying children with mental health problems and in basic counselling skills. The DMHP in Thiruvananthapuram (Kerala's capital) started in 1999 and showcases what has been identified as "best practice" by the WHO. *Sampoorna manasikarogyam* [mental health for all] started in 2013 and is an ambitious targeted intervention project that aims to extend mental health coverage to all households in the district. Community-level workers are trained to detect cases and ensure appropriate follow-up in their respective communities and to improve mental health awareness in each household. Otherwise undetected cases in the community are identified through door-to-door visits by social workers or community health workers and then integrated into the primary care health system.[5] Mental health NGOs such as Maithri, for which laypeople and professionals volunteer to staff telephones to offer help to the "lonely, depressed, and suicidal", and outreach programmes for promoting emotional well-being and mental health are engaged in community mental health care. Psychiatrists in Kerala work with these organizations as well as with village *panchayats* [village or town councils] with the aim of achieving widespread emotional well-being and mental health.

The global standardization of diagnostic technologies such as the International Statistical Classification of Diseases and Related Health Problems (ICD) of the World Health Organization and simpler symptom scales enable mental health professionals, general physicians and even laypeople to quickly and easily diagnose depression. During a public programme on World Mental Health Day in 2012, psychiatrist Dr Indu V. Nair discussed depression and asked:[6]

> How can depression be diagnosed? If I am teacher, how will I be able to identify depression in my students? Or will an *asha*[7] worker detect that this person is suffering from depression? This can be done with help of two questions, which can easily be directed to anyone. First question is, "Are you experiencing sadness continuously for more than two weeks?" Next question is, "Are you experiencing disinterest?" These two key points, sadness and disinterest, will help you to conduct screening for depression. We all feel sadness and disinterestedness. But if it persists over two weeks, it is definitely a symptom of depression.

This diagnostic simplification parallels other similar efforts such as that of Vikram Patel who lists brief and simple symptom checklists for different mental disorders (Patel 2003). Under the rubric "To diagnose a common mental disorder (depression or anxiety)", Patel identifies three core symptoms that, should they persist for at least two weeks, result in a diagnosis of depression or anxiety: feeling sad, loss of interest in daily activities, and excessive nervousness or worrying (Patel 2003: 22).

Along with the institutional shift from the asylum to community psychiatry and from depression as a rare and severe psychiatric disorder to a mild or moderate common complaint came an increasing availability of training programmes for psychiatrists, psychologists and psychiatric social workers. The Kerala state branch of the Indian Psychiatric Society (IPS) had around 250 psychiatrists registered in 2012, and Kerala has a comparatively large proportion of psychiatrists working in government and private colleges, mental hospitals, general hospitals, nursing homes and private clinics. However, postgraduate training in psychiatry came late to Kerala. Most psychiatrists working in the state were trained elsewhere since opportunities to train in this area are limited. The state currently has only a few seats for the degree of Medical Doctor (MD) in psychiatry and the Diploma of Psychological Medicine (DPM) (Kishore, Shaji and Praveenlal 2010). Psychiatry is not a high prestige pursuit among the available medical disciplines in Kerala or in the rest of India. The strongest medical students choose specialisations in radiology, surgery or cardiology, which are the branches of medicine that are the most prestigious and lucrative. It became clear in my conversations with consultant psychiatrists and psychiatric residents that most of them would have preferred to practise in another field but either lacked the marks to do so or ended up in psychiatry by chance.

The medical students who end up in psychiatry study a somatic approach as well as drug prescription in their MBBS (Bachelor of Medicine and Bachelor of Surgery) classes. This matches what patients expect from allopathic doctors. Senior psychiatrists I spoke with vividly remembered the 1970s and early 1980s when psychiatry involved more psychoanalysis than biological psychiatry. Most spoke of this time somewhat dismissively, voicing approval of what they regarded as the scientific progress towards biopsychiatry as a more somatic psychiatry. The inferior status of psychiatry within medicine in India has several roots. Part of the heritage of colonial psychiatry is that practitioners struggled to be recognized as real scientists rather than "custodians of the mad" (Quack n.d.). Further, more than any other branch of medicine, other doctors look down on psychiatry as imprecise and lacking solidly discernable and treatable diseases. Until the recent neurobiological turn, psychiatry was perceived as characterized by vague and subjective classifications giving rise to doubtful conclusions. Lacking a somatic foundation, psychiatrists were often accused of being imprecise and missing a basis in scientific, evidence-based facts. This disparaging view mirrors wider asymmetries between sciences of the body and those of the mind as well as between the medical and psychosocial sciences. This pushes psychiatrists to orient towards somatic medicine (Fabrega 2009). Locating mental illness as imbalance of discernible neurotransmitters and thus within a specific organ of the body (the brain) and localizing treatment mainly in the prescription of medication promotes the somatic and scientific standing of the discipline. This status in turn relies on presenting mental disorders as somatic diseases treatable like any other physical disease, and encouraging the epidemic view of depression with the aim of treating as many cases as possible as rapidly as possible (Nunley 1996, 188).

The low prestige of psychiatry among the medical disciplines is not specific to India but is exacerbated there because mental illness and behavioural problems are widely seen as more religious or cosmological than medical. Ritual healers are sought to provide treatment before, parallel to or after allopathic psychiatric treatment. Therefore, psychiatrists in India and Kerala – to a far greater extent than their colleagues in Western countries – are strongly motivated to demarcate their treatment from the folk sector, which they often describe as superstitious. At the same time, the psychiatrists I interacted with are either largely ignorant of or dismissive towards Ayurvedic psychiatry. Quack developed a model that effectively captures the structural asymmetries and hierarchies in mental health care in India with regard to prestige, funding and credibility:

"somatic medicine trumps psychiatry trumps psychology trumps AYUSH trumps high Hinduism trumps folk healers"[8] (Quack n.d.). In Kerala, psychiatric social workers would be located between psychology and the AYUSH disciplines in Quack's model. As allopathic psychiatry struggles to achieve full recognition as scientific and somatic medicine, psychiatrists are actively policing the borders of the discipline to ensure exclusion of and differentiation from other "inferior" approaches. Indeed, to "sell psychiatry" (Nunley 1996, 170) to the public, one of the most effective tactics is to market it as scientific and somatic. However, psychiatrists are often stigmatized due to a reputation for dealing with "crazy patients". This stigma may also exist to an extent in some Euro-American settings, but is powerful and pervasive in India. Nunley (1996, 182) is correct when he makes a connection between this stigma and psychiatrists as "doctors of the mad" to scholarship on Indian notions of the self (Daniel 1984; Marriott 1976; Marriott and Inden 1977) as being permeable and more open to the physiological and moral qualities of others with whom they are in contact. The greater focus on milder conditions, mental health, outpatient practice and community psychiatry, the stress on evidence-based practice and the engagement of global mental health discourses all serve to elevate the status of psychiatry and bring it into the mainstream. This also includes efforts to sell cosmetic psychiatry not only for the treatment of mental distress but also to enhance human capacity (Kramer 1993) making subjects "better than well", as a new form of pharmaceutical governance (and self governance) to shape citizens to better fit neoliberal exigencies.

There is a special emphasis in training not only psychiatrists but also non-psychiatrists such as general practitioners, gynaecologists, neurologists and other MBBS-qualified doctors in basic psychiatric nosology, etiology and pharmacology. The IPS recently succeeded in increasing the teaching hours in psychiatry for MBBS undergraduate students from 20 to 40 hours and the clinical posting from two to four weeks (Kallivayalil 2012), justified by the increase particularly of depression and the presumed treatment gap in depression and other mental disorders in India. As the majority of patients suffering from depression in India are most likely to see a general physician (either in the first instance or as their primary source of allopathic diagnosis and treatment), scaling up knowledge of depression in general physicians is regarded as "cost effective and practical" (Kallivayalil 2012). Both psychiatry and depression are therefore entering mainstream medical training and practise as psychiatric expert knowledge is increasingly disseminated to non-psychiatric doctors.

Many psychiatric units in general hospitals in Kerala employ clinical psychologists and psychiatric social workers to provide clinical services. Further steps towards mental health professionalism included the development of psychology and psychiatric social work as degree and postgraduate courses of specialization at colleges in Kerala. Clinical psychology in Kerala was initiated in the 1950s by Malayali doctor V.K. Alexander, who was educated at Princeton University in the United States and trained the first PhDs in clinical psychology in Kerala (Halliburton 2009). Dr Alexander founded the Department of Psychology at the

Union Christian College of Aluva in 1965. It is the oldest psychology department in Kerala. Although many people I spoke with used the terms "psychologist" and "psychiatrist" interchangeably when referring to *manasika* doctors [doctors of the mind], psychologists in particular are increasing in importance in Kerala, especially in the fields of education and intelligence testing. Psychiatric social workers also play a role in both clinical practice and planning and initiating within community psychiatric care in Kerala. Working either as part of clinical institutions where they offer cognitive behavioural therapy and other clinical psychotherapeutic practice, in community psychiatry outreach programmes, or with psychiatric NGOs, they are engaged in expanding the infrastructure for psychiatric and psychotherapeutic services, fostering mental health awareness in the community, offering support and help for people in distress outside clinical settings, and are engaged in rehabilitation and family reunification programmes for patients with mental disorders. They participate in promotional activities including organizing stress management programmes, mental health care in schools and services to support effective parenting, life skills instruction, marital and family enrichment, and community-based rehabilitation. The initial focus of mental health NGOs in India was intellectual disability in children, then severe mental disorders, substance abuse, and rehabilitation and vocational therapy. More recently, their scope has broadened to encompass depression, stress and other common mental disorders that are increasingly perceived as major causes of disability. Interlinked with the aims of the Global Mental Health movement, this led to the mushrooming of mental health NGOs providing community-based counselling and suicide prevention, clinical care, rehabilitation and community outreach programmes. This was certainly the case in the psychiatric units of the two multi-specialty hospitals Syrian Christian Hospital and the Guruji Institute of Medical Sciences where I met a larger number of patients diagnosed with depression. In both institutions, I had the opportunity to sit in on outpatient consultations, accompany staff on their rounds, and talk to patients and their family members both in the wards and in the OPD before or after their medical consultations.

The Syrian Christian Hospital is a multi-specialty hospital in Alapuzha district with an attached medical college and over one thousand beds, situated on the outskirts of a large town in Kerala. Founded in the 1960s, the hospital has been part of policy efforts to develop and uplift health care in rural areas of Kerala. The psychiatry unit formed to address the needs of the mentally ill and emotionally disturbed was founded in the early 1970s and is one of the earliest general hospital psychiatric units in India. Three consultant psychiatrists see about 100 outpatients a day, and there are usually longer queues in front of the offices of the two senior male doctors who saw most patients for 3–4 minutes each than in front of the office of the younger female doctor who spent more time with each patient. The senior psychiatrists also saw patients in their homes in the evenings. Thus, the hospital is what a student called a "medium hospital": crowded, but not so much as government-run hospitals in which a psychiatrist might see up to 300 patients a day. Dr Matthew Kurien, one of the senior psychiatrists, told me: "You can sit with me, no problem. But you are wasting your time. I have only very short time for each patient. Go and sit with Dr Mona [the junior doctor] there you will learn more. She takes more time for her patients."[9] Indeed, the energetic Dr Mona spent an average of fifteen minutes with each patient. During the consultations, she not only spoke to the patients and their family members – together and separately – but also took phone calls, offered counselling over the phone, organized administrative tasks and explained things to me. On most days, she did not stop for lunch. Watching her, the social worker Saju who used to go home at around 1 p.m. each day remarked, "We should take care of our own health first. Then only can we treat the patients."[10]

Almost all patients arrived accompanied by a family member. Each consultation ended with a prescription. The psychiatrists were also responsible for the inpatient psychiatric ward that served around fifty patients in the general ward and a dozen in the private ward who stayed on average between two and four weeks. Apart from the psychiatrists, nurses, a psychologist, a social worker and an occupational therapist also cared for the inpatients. Patients could move around freely in their respective wards. Two secure rooms were reserved for violent and unmanageable patients. As is usual in wards in government-run and private general hospitals in Kerala, there was no privacy in the general ward, and this allowed the families and friends of patients to interact and develop a ward solidarity (although caste, gender and religious demarcations still had power). Dr Leena, a psychiatrist at the hospital, had an office in the general ward and called patients and families for counselling. With so many patients on the ward, I expected her office to be permanently crowded but most of the time it was empty. She told me that she tried to see each inpatient once during their stay, usually shortly before discharge when her main focus was psychoeducation, which meant educating patients and caregivers about the importance of compliance with treatment and only coming off medication with medical approval and support. She had another office in the outpatient department where the majority of patients she saw were children brought by their parents because of learning difficulties at school or "behavioural problems". The youngest patient I saw in the junior psychiatrist's office was a five-year-old girl who was diagnosed with dyslexia.

The private ward was located in another part of the building. There, patients had private rooms in which they resided with one or more family members. The cost per room was about ten times that of the cost of a bed in the general ward and although the hospital offered health insurance, it did not cover psychiatric treatment. Separate patient rooms in the pay ward created far fewer opportunities for exchange between bystanders, and they did not experience the intense interactions of the general wards. Psychiatric social worker Saju had his office in this part of the hospital. Although his official remit was "to take care of the psycho-social aspects", he seemed like more of an adjunct to the doctors. He explained,

> I have to spend time with the patients and have to give the report to the doctors. They [doctors] will only listen to me, not to the patient. If doctors

> spent more time with the patients, they won't have time for the outpatients.[11]

Like the psychologist in the general ward, it was his task to fill in patient charts on admission. Sitting in his office, he would call in patients or bystanders for counselling if it was needed. Apart from psychoeducation, he provided suggestions for behaviour modification inspired, as he said, by cognitive behavioural therapy. The bulk of the talk addressed the caregiver rather than the patient. Although he wanted to address family-based and other psychosocial problems and to do some psychotherapy, in practice, "most of the time, you can't do anything more with the patient than psychoeducation, psychotherapy only in some cases. Otherwise simple counselling or psychoeducation is more than enough". Although Saju was supposed to see each patient (and caregiver) every day, his office also remained empty most of the time. Next to the pay ward was the de-addiction ward. There, around twenty patients, all of whom were men, had beds in one large room. Their accompanying family members were mostly women (wives, mainly) who slept on cots rolled out next to the patients' beds. The diagnosis for all of these patients was alcohol dependency syndrome and the aim of their treatment was withdrawal from alcohol and management of the side effects of the withdrawal process. Two social workers were attached to the de-addiction ward. The unit's occupational therapist was officially responsible for all psychiatric patients but in practice offered occupational therapy only to some chosen patients ("those who are interested") in the general wards in the mornings, and in the private ward in the afternoons. Her sessions consisted of praying, singing songs, playing games, watching TV and improving patients' intellectual capacities, although she complained that she did not have the facilities available at other institutions that had special vocational rehabilitation programmes. In addition to the unit's staff, there was a group of MBBS students from the attached college serving their obligatory twelve-month rotational internship, of which they had to spend two months in psychiatry. Interns studying for a Masters degree in social work specializing in psychiatry had to complete a mandatory one-month internship in a psychiatric institution, and they also had an office in the general ward where they offered counselling for individual patients. For both groups of interns, the task was in the main to fill in patient charts while sitting in on consultations in the offices of the doctors, the psychologist or the social worker.

Patients came from the rural area around the hospital, from all religious communities, and were largely lower middle class (in the general wards) and middle class (in the private ward). Apart from the de-addiction ward, which was funded by a government programme, all patients had to pay for their accommodation and medicine. According to psychiatrists and social workers, increased mental health awareness resulted in an increasing number of patients coming directly to the psychiatric department, although most still came following referral from a general physician, neurologist,or gynaecologist.

Depression was one of the most frequent diagnoses of outpatients at the Syrian Christian Hospital. The majority of inpatients were diagnosed with psychotic disorders such as bipolar affective disorder or schizophrenia. Psychiatrists told me that widespread awareness of depression today results in sufferers seeking treatment in the initial stages of the disease, often making admission unnecessary. As Dr Mona explained:

> We don't admit depressive cases, unless they are very much depressed. Usually they will come in the initial stages of depression itself. So it is not necessary to admit them. We will give them medicines and send them back. The admissions are mainly psychotics, acute psychotics and alcoholics too. Depressive patients get admitted very rarely. They can be managed with medicine alone. So there is no need for admissions in the hospitals unless they are that much depressed and show psychotic symptoms.

Apart from depression (with and without psychotic features) the most frequent diagnosis in outpatients was bipolar affective disorder. Other frequent diagnoses included alcohol dependency syndrome, acute psychotic episode, adjustment disorder and (rarely) schizophrenia. The fact that the majority of inpatients were diagnosed with bipolar disorder was astonishing but corresponded to the numbers in other psychiatric hospitals that I visited where this was by far the most common diagnosis, followed by schizophrenia. Reflecting on the reasons for the high frequency of diagnosed bipolar disorder compared to unipolar depression or mania, Dr Mona voiced the assumption that unipolar depression was rare as most patients with depression were prone to switching into mania – arguably due to the high doses of antidepressants and polypharmacy they were prescribed and the observation that mania patients usually also experienced depression, making the diagnosis of unipolar mania extremely rare. Officially, the Syrian Christian Hospital employed what they called a "bio-psycho-social" approach; in practice, the bulk of the treatment was pharmacotherapy. "Before a patient is stabilized, there is no point in counselling," Saju told me.[12] "Only in a stable state, the patient can get counselling. Otherwise it's a waste of time." In an acute state, patients received pharmacological treatment and their family member(s) were given "psychoeducation" and advice to strictly monitor medication use. In the general ward I saw many patients drugged and calmed by large doses of sedatives, antipsychotics and antidepressants.[13]

The prestigious Guruji Institute of Medical Sciences is one of the leading private multi-specialty hospitals in Kerala. It serves thousands of patients each day and offers mental health services for inpatients and outpatients, hosts regular conferences and workshops, and offers postgraduate psychiatric training in the attached medical school. In contrast to the Syrian Christian Hospital, most patients are upper and upper middle class and come from all over Kerala (although there are some patients who fall below the poverty line who are supported by an internal fund). The psychiatrists at the Guruji Institute describe their approach as "comprehensive", with mental health services ranging from psychosocial treatments like counselling and psychotherapy to biological treatment modalities including pharmacotherapy and what is called modified electroconvulsive therapy (ECT under anaesthetic). In practice, however, the bulk of the treatment is pharmacotherapy. The five doctors and the psychiatric social worker in the department for psychiatry and behavioural medicine saw around fifty outpatients each day and were responsible for around thirty inpatients. Most of the patients came either referred by another department in the hospital or by other physicians, with an increasing number arriving on their own initiative. The psychiatrists were able to spend much more time with their patients than at the Syrian Christian Hospital or at the government-run institutions. The Guruji Institute was also a training institution with an MD course in psychiatry, so the hospital's doctors were involved in teaching a handful of postgraduate students of psychiatry. On their daily rounds on the mixed ward (women and men) and private rooms, doctors were accompanied by nurses, postgraduate psychiatry students and the psychiatric social worker. I sat in most often on Dr Lakshmi Nair's consultations. She spent between ten minutes and an hour with each patient and their accompanying family members listening, educating, explaining diagnoses, and providing counselling and cognitive behavioural therapy. She made a point of integrating religion and patients' understanding of mental health as peace of mind or inner balance into their psychiatric treatment. According to Dr Nair[14]:

> The western way of psychotherapy is more towards self-actualization or expansion of your potential. This is the way you can handle a patient with western education or western patients. Whereas in a patient who is not that exposed to western culture, you will have to put in terms of achieving peace or harmony inside, which is more in keeping with what they are thinking, closer to perfection in the sense of being closer to God. This would be in accordance with the religious texts. Reading parts of their religious texts should comfort them. Speaking to them along these lines makes it easier for them to accept what I am telling. When I give counselling I often say, this is what God expects you to do, this is written in the Gita, Bible or Qur'an. Put it across that way, it is more accepted. The target is the same as in Western therapy but put in a different frame. Perfecting the person or at least making the person more adaptable and more at peace with himself, that's the whole idea.

Compared to the Syrian Christian Hospital, the social worker at the Guruji Institute had little influence or power. Officially, she was assigned the care of the psychosocial aspects of those psychiatric patients admitted to the hospital, but her room was empty most of the time and referrals from the psychiatrists were almost non-existent. She also had no say during doctors' inpatient rounds. The status difference between the psychiatrists and the social worker in this situation was not only related to differences in training, but also to the young age and the gender of the social worker. In the main, patients were referred for counselling or psychotherapy to one of the four psychologists from the neighbouring department of clinical psychology, a department separate from the psychiatry department. Unlike at the Syrian Christian Hospital, psychologists at the Guruji Institute assessed, diagnosed and treated patients independently of psychiatrists. Psychologists told me that patients from all wards were referred to the department "if needed". Apart from that, they received outpatients who came to them directly for marital, professional, school-related and other kinds of problems. But were patients at the clinical psychology department being seen for depression? Many of the patients who came seeking help for somatic or relationship problems actually suffered from depression, psychologist Dr Savitri Menon told me.[15] The clinical psychologists treated children, adolescents and adults. In children and adolescents, their main remit was intelligence testing and the treatment of learning and behavioural problems, but they also addressed other mental health problems and adjustment issues. Adults received behavioural therapy and family therapy for depression, marital and family problems, and other kinds of distress in which they mainly learned to adjust and tackle stress factors in their lives. Only rarely did patients self-refer explicitly seeking help for depression. Most of them were either referred by other hospital departments (often for medically unexplained somatic symptoms), or they self-referred due to interpersonal problems within their family. Here, as is the case in other institutions, cognitive behavioural therapy – the epitome of evidence-based psychotherapy – was theoretically the treatment of choice. In practice, it was often transformed into behavioural therapy and even more often into family counselling. A good number of the psychiatry department's in- and outpatients were diagnosed with depression; many of them came from far away. Travelling for a psychiatric treatment and admittance into a general hospital were both strategies employed by families to avoid the stigma of mental illness.

Glocalization of depression in Kerala involves changes at the institutional, material and cognitive levels. For this reason, in this chapter I explored institutional shifts as a requirement for the stabilization and expansion of depression as a mental health category. A major transformation was the shift from colonial asylum psychiatry to community psychiatry, including the establishment of psychiatric units in general or multi-specialty hospitals. These, in turn, formed a major part of my ethnographic research in mainstream psychiatry. In contrast to the large asylums (or "mental health centres" as they are called today) that provide treatment mainly for psychotic patients with only very few in- and outpatients treated for severe depression, in the psychiatric units in general hospitals – especially in the outpatient departments – psychiatrists diagnosed many patients with depression. The relocation of psychiatry from the abandoned spaces of the asylum into the spaces of somatic medicine and the community was a prerequisite for bringing depression into the mainstream and the construction of depression as an epidemic. Psychiatry's entrance into mainstream paralleled that of depression. But how does this manifest specifically in Kerala?

From expert to popular knowledge: the myriad masks of depression, neurochemical imbalance and the denigration of ritual healing

Depression is a complex moving target constructed in part by institutional shifts in clinical practice, training, pharmacology, and the production and dissemination of expert knowledge. In Chapter 2, I examined the representation of depression in Indian media and the way psychiatrists have expanded their remit by encompassing aspects of everyday life and ever-expanding groups identified as predisposed or vulnerable to depression. Here, I extend this to investigate the expansion of psychiatry's increasing influence in everyday life, and explore how psy discourse on depression is vernacularized in Kerala. This process is most visible in the ways both psychiatrists and depression are portrayed in local media as a vehicle for the dissemination of allopathic psychological and psychiatric knowledge about depression. I pursue a project of exploring the discursive activity of psychiatrists in the public sphere initiated by Chua (2013) by focusing on psychologists and psychiatrists who engage the public as lecturers, authors, and guests on television and radio programmes in which psy professionals blur the boundaries between clinical and popular registers. Chua focuses on public performances of psychologists (and psychiatrists), but I place reports on depression published in Malayalam newspapers and health magazines in Kerala written by psychiatrists and psychologists at the centre of my analysis. How, I ask, is depression construed and vernacularized in these reports and how is psychiatry presented in this process?

Kerala has the largest per-capita circulation of newspapers and magazines in India. Despite the state's relatively small size, the two largest-selling Malayalam dailies *Malayalam Manorama* and *Mathrubhumi* have a larger readership than any of the other newspapers in India (Jeffrey 1997). High literacy rates, but also high *health* literacy rates in Kerala fuel a large media market (print, television, radio) for health-related subjects and for mental health issues in particular (cf. Halliburton 2005; Chua 2013). The main Malayalam monthly health magazines *Arogya Masika* and *Arogyam* regularly feature articles by psychiatrists and psychologists. Although dominated by allopathy, there are also non-allopathic medical practitioners who express their views including those from the AYUSH disciplines. Along with these, Malayalam newspapers, popular women's magazines such as *Vanitha*, TV programmes and the English-speaking national media regularly feature pieces and exposés on mental health. The cultural production and stabilization of depression as a problem of everyday life is closely intertwined with the production of mental health professionalism, authority and social prestige. The aim of psychiatric authorship of articles on depression and mental illness in the popular press (apart from contributing to mental health literacy) is to bring both depression and psychiatry increasingly into the mainstream in a process Pinto has called "enacting authority" (Pinto 2012).

This attention to depression builds on and promotes science, rationalism and somatic approaches. Psychiatry is presented in these pieces not as the discipline most closely related to asylums, lunatics or the bedraggled, abandoned and wretched. Rather, it is represented as a scientific, modern and desirable approach to common ailments such as depression described as physiological pathologies that can be easily corrected with medication. Psychiatrists, more than experts in any other field of medical specialization, are heavily involved in selling psychiatry as science to the public and differentiating themselves from religious and cosmological healers. Further, the media visibility of psychiatrists has proved an effective strategy for widening their client base. The dissemination of psychiatric idioms through print media has improved not only the status of psychiatrists in Kerala but also the expression of distress from possession to depression and tension (Halliburton 2005). In this way, media engagement with depression and mental health strongly influences and shapes public discourse on depression.

The emergence of depression as a favoured media subject not only stabilizes and expands the identification of new groups of sufferers but also produces new subjectivities and forms of citizenships that are related to neoliberal forms of governmentality. These give rise to what Ecks calls "pharmaceutical citizenship" (Ecks 2005), that is, the process of demarginalization and achievement of full citizenship through the use of antidepressants. They also produce psychological citizens as both consumers of professional health care and entrepreneurial managers of their own moods and mental health. This self-monitoring and management localizes the responsibility for mental health with individuals and their families. Health magazines and the news media are an important though largely unexamined site for the production of these new kinds of consumer and self-monitoring subjectivities and citizenships (Briggs and Hallin 2007; Rose 1996). These forms of care and monitoring take on a specific form in Kerala due to the particular involvement of families in care. New pharmaceutical forms of care are often an extension of familial care rather than – or in addition to – forms of self-care. This process is further exacerbated by a new conceptualization of public health defined in terms of proper education, and a regular flow of information required for subjects to consider and exercise choice.

By educating their readers about depression through reports and self-tests in health magazines and newspapers, mental health professionals as authors engage in a process of selling depression. In India, direct-to-customer advertising of antidepressants and other prescription drugs is not allowed, but media campaigns to "raise awareness" about depression are used as a way of directly addressing the customer (Ecks 2013). The "mongering" of depression[16] – that is, the marketing of a presumably under-diagnosed medical condition that was previously largely unknown – has been identified as a key tactic for promoting pharmaceutical products indirectly, but very effectively, to customers. Mongering depression often involves alliances between pharmaceutical companies, doctors and occasionally biosocial groups all of which have a vested interest in the condition. Knowledge about depression put forward in the media is therefore always "interested knowledge" (Lakoff 2005) in that it is deliberately intended to serve the interests of the pharmaceutical industry and other stakeholders.

Psychiatry expands its reach into everyday life by pathologizing an ever-increasing array of states and moods otherwise (or previously) regarded as a common part of the *conditio humana*. This pharmaceuticalization becomes especially obvious in light of the notion of masked depression. Under titles such as "Depression in Disguise" and "Depression in New Attire", psychiatrists and psychologists writing in magazines in order to reach ever wider audiences beyond clinical settings have made use of fictional examples of sufferers of masked depression to identify the symptoms of this covert threat. These include anger, aggression, quarrelsome behaviour, memory loss, somatic symptoms such as *vedana* [pain] (in the head, chest or lower back), *perippu* [numbness] in the hands or legs, sexual dysfunction or changes in sexual desire (Roy 2012; Nair, Kumari and Sandeep 2014). They also identify a "sudden expression of acute spirituality" (Roy 2012) or (in adolescents) tantrums, lack of concentration, learning difficulties, consumption of intoxicants, gaming, overuse of social media, obstinacy and impatience as signs or symptoms of masked depression. But the list does not end there: masked depression is also described as manifesting as obesity or slimness, laziness, changes in appetite or sleep, and digestive disorders.

In the articles mentioned above, psychiatrists advertise masked depression as a relatively recent phenomenon arising only in the last fifteen years. In "Depression in New Attire", the disorder is described as being "all around us, sometimes barely within arm's reach". The many symptoms of masked depression identified in these articles are linked in "Depression in Disguise" to stereotypical Malayali behavioural traits:

> Malayalis manifest some peculiar symptoms of depression. [...] Instead of listening to others we prefer to defend ourselves by arguing. Instead of agreeing we prefer to keep silent even when the evidence is against us. This particular behaviour sets Malayalis apart from other people. This may be the reason why Malayalis are different in the ways of showing symptoms of depression.
>
> (Nair, Kumari and Sandeep 2014)

Medical anthropologists and cross-cultural psychiatrists have described the tendency of South Asian patients to express depression in somatic idioms of distress. Psychiatrists in Kerala likewise told me that their depression patients often displayed somatic symptoms and behaviours that they understood as forms of masked depression. What are the implications of this novel and specific symptomatology of depression? It is no stretch to assume that somatic symptoms identified as signs of masked depression (such as pains, numbness, anger, irritation, consumption of intoxicants or sudden interest in spirituality) have been present in the population for some time. What seems to be new is the subsuming of these states and behaviours under the domain of depression that renders them targets for treatment by psychiatrists armed with antidepressants. In other words, what is new is that these commonplace symptoms and behaviours are being psychiatrisized, and that psychiatry is expanding its influence beyond the clinic into the realm of everyday distress.

But not all medical experts in the media participate in these medicalizing discourses of masked or mild depression. Psychiatrist Dr Ramdas and gynaecologist Dr Rameshkumar, in "Female depression through the seasons", ask instead:

> Is *vishadam* not a natural human emotion? Who hasn't experienced desperation and sorrow in this stressful journey of life? Haven't poets and artists made this state of mind as subject for their artistic creations? Aren't some experiences of depression bitter-sweet and provide an escape from the monotony of life? Then why is this condition projected as an unhealthy phenomenon or diseased state?
>
> (Ramdas and Rameshkumar 2014)

They then identify the difference between *vishadam* and *vishada rogam*. The latter is described as "different from the distress and depression we experience in our daily lives [vishadam]. The disease called *vishada rogam* is of a long term nature." They then attempt to educate their readers on the scientific understanding of depression, noting that if depression is a disease of the mind, and the mind is part of the body, that therefore "diseases of the mind are also diseases of the body." They argue that treatment for mental health should be based in science, as is treatment for physical health. In their construction, it is precisely the localization of depression in the brain (or the somatization of depression) that makes possible its scientific treatment.

At the same time, medical authors also depict mental health problems as moral-physiological weakness. Depression is described in vernacularized or popular psychiatric discourses as a weakness of the mind or lack of mental strength [*manodurbalam*]. Psychiatrist Dr Mohandas described mental health in a presentation of the IPS Kerala State Branch in just this way:[17] "Having a sense of values and showing love and decency are indicators of a healthy mind. The minds of people who don't have these qualities will have no peace of mind resulting in many mental problems." Following that thinking to its logical conclusion, attending to social norms results in mental health while deviation in behaviour or thinking from social norms results in mental illness. Most psychiatrists, however, have discarded this notion in no small part because it shifts responsibility for depression and its treatment to inherent patient traits and away from the framing of depression through a scientific, somatic understanding that allows for pharmacological treatment. In "Treatment Without Drugs", psychologist Anil Kumar (2010) elaborated a popular notion of the predisposition to depression in terms of passion and the experience of intense emotion that at once accords with vernacular Ayurveda and what has been referred to as "Indian psychology" that is largely built on the Bhagavad Gita. In this notion, strong emotions and attachments to persons, goods or ideas are understood as the root problem that gives rise to depression should those passions be unfulfilled. According to Kumar,

> If a person loves another individual or an object of interest more than himself he is more suitable a candidate for depression. Let it be an individual, an ideology, an aim in life, strong passions on any of these can lead to depression in the event of a failure, or unsatisfactory accomplishments. It can even annihilate the whole life of that person. This conclusion is backed by many a research.

However, such views are largely drowned out by the many mental health experts who promote their "scientific" construct of depression as both a growing and significant social threat and as a condition treatable exclusively by their profession.

And yet, psychiatrists speaking in the media identify a lack of understanding in Kerala's population about the treatments best suited to mental health problems. In "Before Seeking Treatment", psychiatrist Dr C.J. John (2009) argues:

> people are confused about what treatment to go for when it comes to diseases of the mind because they are not knowledgeable. The common belief is that all mental problems can be solved by giving an increased dose of pep talk, advice and consolation [...] It is very difficult for many people to accept the fact that medicines and treatment are necessary for curing mental diseases. [...] Treatment methods based on research and the feedback from case studies are giving relief and cure to the majority of patients. With treatment many patients could regain better standards of living. Recent medicines with little or no side effects have played an important role in this.

The underlying message conveys a hierarchical model of psychiatric authority in which the psychiatrist knows best. This is in opposition to what Briggs and Hallinn (2007) describe as a neoliberal consumer model in which patients are accorded agency to freely choose their treatment on the health care market, but accords with a fetishization of research. In fact, the mere mention of the word "research" in Malayalam and English popular press seems sufficient to shore up psychiatry's truth claims and its authority over mental health.

Not only psychiatry, but also clinical psychology (and especially its hallmark, cognitive behavioural therapy) are presented as scientific and rational through and through. As Kumar noted, "The most effective and well-known approach towards depression management is cognitive behavioral therapy (CBT). [...] CBT is a rational treatment in which [...] deeply embedded irrational thinking structures are rationally analyzed and convincingly corrected" (Kumar 2010). The fetishization of rationality in this depiction of CBT (and in the scientific understanding of depression more generally) is in line with the focus on rationality promoted by the *Kerala Yuktivadi Sangham* [Kerala rationalist association] and the communist parties of Kerala. Both the psychologization and psychiatrization of mental health care and the Yuktivadi Sangham share a common interest in denigrating "irrational" ritual healing as non-scientific and superstitious.

Hand in hand with the fetishization of rationality and scientific approaches to mental health is the denigration of what are represented as "non-scientific" treatments based in superstition, and "false assumptions" with regard to mental illness. "People read news stories and articles in magazines with great interest. But when it comes to seeking help for treatment this interest vanishes. Secretly they go to the fakes and quacks", complained the psychiatrist Dr C.J. John (2009). He warned readers against the allure of promises of fast cures peddled by quacks and those offering treatment without "any scientific study or clinical experience under an experienced therapist." Likewise, Drs Ramdas and Ramesh-kumar (2014) warned against "superstitious" treatments that were not only "unscientific" but also much more expensive than proper medical treatment.

> Even today there are so many people who go for *homam* [fire sacrifices], *badha ozhippikkal* [exorcism] and other primitive methods of treatment because they are afraid of modern treatment methods. When their pockets are empty after trying *mantravadam* [magic, sorcery] [...] only they go to a qualified doctor.

This theme was echoed in "Live Without Losing Balance", in which psychiatrist Dr Mohandas (2009) noted that when people are unable to find healthy outlets for mental stress, they blame their *nakshatram* [birth star], jinn, or evil spirits and turn to *elassu* and *mantravadam*. "Beliefs are good and they must have them", he continued, "But these beliefs are being used for exploiting people." Indeed, in the media, medical mental health experts often depict religious healing as cruel and violent. In "Before Seeking Treatment" Dr C.J. John warned his readers not to fall prey to practitioners of exorcism:

> The ancient generations believed that people who were unable to control their thoughts and emotions were possessed. Exorcism was practiced from very ancient times. Jesus Christ was a therapist who cured possessed people in a humane way. Before and after Jesus, and even to this day exorcism means cruelly assaulting patients.
>
> (John 2009)

Policing quacks and "superstitious" forms of religious healing is an important means by which psychiatrists emphasize their authority and solidify psychiatry as science in popular perception. On the other hand, both as authors and as clinical practitioners, psychiatrists display tolerance for certain high-caste religious and spiritual practices. This respect however is not so much motivated by a shared ontology but rather by a psychologization (Tarabout 1999) of the efficacy of ritual healing. To be recognized, it seems, religious practice must pass through psychology. "There are psychological solutions to counter depressive and negative thoughts," writes Dr C.J. John (2009). "Yoga and meditation are good for this. Prayers and religious practices are good to rekindle hope." He describes these high caste practices as psychological methods for tackling depression, or "culturally sanctioned stress busters". Some psychiatrists emphasized the physiological effect of religious practice as having a direct impact on neurochemicals in the brain. Psychologized and psychiatrisized, some religious and spiritual practices are tolerated or even recommended so long as they do not interfere with pharmaceutical treatment or the supremacy or the scientific discourse of mental health. "You must not take the attitude that where medicines have to be taken prayers or rituals will suffice," Dr John warned his readers.

ECT is also promoted as a useful and scientifically grounded treatment for severe depression and psychosis, contrary to popular perceptions that it causes brain damage leaving the patient "like a vegetable". Critiques of ECT have been voiced in the last decade, especially in the aftermath of the restructuring of psychiatry following the Erwadi tragedy in 2001. Although there has never been a significant antipsychiatry movement in Kerala, criticism of ECT is visible in representations of psychiatry in Malayalam films such as the blockbuster *Thalavattam* (1986) based on *One Flew Over the Cuckoo's Nest* and starring the famous actor Mohanlal as a patient who becomes mentally ill after the death of his girlfriend and in which unmodified ECT is portrayed as a brutal invasion.[18] Also other popular Malayalam films such as *Ulladakom* (1991) in which Mohanlal plays a psychiatrist, *First Bell* (1992) and others depict a negative image of "shock treatment" and patients are depicted in a zombie-like state after ECT.

Psychiatrists today try to counter anxieties about "shock treatment", as it is popularly called, and instead stress the efficacy and scientific basis of ECT. In "Anxiety And Neurosis", psychiatrist Dr Shureshkumar (2009) emphasized that patients treated with ECT feel no pain or discomfort during the procedure thanks to the use of mild anaesthesia and muscle relaxants. Further, ECT is used in combination with medication to prevent reoccurrence, and though side effects "such as loss of memory and articulation may be shown," they last "only for a short period." In an article appearing alongside "Anxiety And Neurosis", psychiatrist Dr Jayaprakash counters "misconceptions" that modern ECT is a dangerous treatment, explaining:

> Most mental diseases are caused by the improper functioning in the organic electric impulses and organic chemical activities in the brain. The shock is given to divert the mind from the disorderly functioning. It creates a seizure in the brain causing a convulsion and controls the functioning of the brain and brings it back to normalcy. This is the underlying principle of shock treatment.
> (Jayaprakash 2009)

ECT is presented as a treatment that cures mental disorder and especially depression by returning brain function to normalcy. According to Dr Jayaprakash, it "can be compared to other treatment methods like surgeries when patients suffer from diseases of the body." And, he argues, there are no serious side effects. Even the side effects acknowledged to occur are sometimes cast in a positive light. Although I have not encountered written reports, mental health professionals told me in conversation that short-term memory loss due to ECT is often considered a beneficial aspect of the treatment. A psychiatric nurse told me that the memory loss is seen as positive especially if traumatic events are causative factors for depression.[19]

Appropriating the focus on mental health rather than mental illness that is globally disseminated by the Movement of Global Mental Health, psychiatrists in Kerala describe the aim of treatment as restoring a healthy mind. Although this might seem obvious and universal, local notions of mental health in Kerala are closely related to culture-specific concepts of the mind and the self. In many popular mental health articles, the aim of treatment is formulated in terms of "peace of mind", "peaceful balance" or "calmness" on the one hand and manobalam and control of the mind on the other. These local notions are then linked to the pharmacological therapy of balancing neurochemicals. The fact that local concepts frame the mind as physiological facilitates the perception of mental illness as somatic or material. The embodied mind out of balance can regain strength and peace through a kind of physio-moral strengthening process. Antidepressants facilitate this physio-moral balance of mind in the same way as CBT or certain religious practices.

Several authors have stressed the gendered nature of popular articles on depression and advertisements for antidepressants in the USA, identifying an overrepresentation of women in texts and images (Metzl 2003). They show that beneath purported biological neutrality, these articles and advertisements convey messages about the need to "discipline" and "enhance" female bodies (Blum 2004). In the Indian context, Ecks (2005) demonstrates the over-representation of (fair middle class) women in antidepressant advertisements. Malayalam articles focusing on women and depression often assemble local notions of the female body or local gendered biologies and female gender norms to account for the higher prevalence of depression in women. In particular, hormones related to menstruation, pregnancy and menopause as well as thyroid problems are cited as making women vulnerable to depression, implying that depression lies somehow in the *prakrti* [nature] of women. Moreover, local cultural notions of womanhood further associate women with mental suffering. Dr John (2014) begins "Women Who Drink Tears" with the Malayalam proverb: "If you are a woman you must drink tears" and then analyses the "traps set by the society" for women. Many women, he argues, suffer physical and mental violence related to their husband's alcoholism, or domestic violence and sexual abuse. They are unable to cope because they are not supposed to talk about such troubles. Along with biological factors such as hormonal changes throughout the lives of women, it is these social factors that predispose women to depression. He continues: "These circumstances prevailing in the society present the ideal situation for the seed of depression to germinate and flourish very fast. [...] They have to pass through depressive times like menstrual periods, gestation, childbirth and menopause." Dr John then combines a discourse of women's empowerment with a medical or pharmaceutical humanism, asking his readers to seek treatment early. Seeking medical treatment, in his construction, becomes an emancipatory and empowering act that along with overcoming depression is equivalent to overcoming the subjugation and marginalization of women. "Women's roles should be rewritten to make her strong. This is the only way to save women from the traditionally defined role and traps set by the society", he writes. Despite articulating social causes of depression in women, his proposed solution is merely pharmaceutical.

In "The Mind Of The Malayali Woman" in the same issue, psychiatrist Dr Geetha criticizes local perceptions of the mind of women:

> Many poets have written poems and songs for movies describing the mind of Malayali woman. All the available words have been used to describe the beauty and softness of their minds. One poet even described Malayali woman's mind as a clear sky in which flowery clouds swim. This mind has now turned into a restless sea. A sea that is always restless with stress. The fact is supported by the increase in the number of women coming for treatment of mental diseases.
>
> (Geetha 2014)

Weaving a local biologism together with women's victimhood, she states, "although, as a species women are mentally stronger than men, women, regardless of age, are way back in the matter of mental health." Where women are described as predisposed to depression by local notions of gender norms and female physiology, increasing rates of depression are represented as a recent phenomenon, a product of unhealthy socio-cultural-economic and diet transformations in Kerala. However, this does not prevent authors from framing women's predisposition to depression in the biological terms of genetics and hormones. Psychiatrists and psychologists writing on depression in women are often involved in two contradictory processes: they reify biological differences in identifying female predisposition to depression while simultaneously presenting antidepressants as key tools for pushing back against gender norms.

As discussed in Chapter 2, depression diagnoses are increasingly frequent in children and youth in Kerala. The rise of depression in the young expands the spectrum of depression to encompass a part of the population in which it was only rarely seen before, a process of "selling depression" as a problem shaping Kerala's future. This expansion of depression corresponds to an increase of the symptomatology of depression. There is a great deal of "masked depression" diagnosed in children and adolescents. Symptoms perceived to be most problematic are those related to difficulties and disinterest in studying because studying is understood as the main activity for youth in Kerala. Along with typical somatic symptoms of depression, key symptoms of "masked depression" in children are aggressive behaviour and disobedience. A TV news report stated

> Telling lies and stealing are the main symptoms seen in these children. They also argue and talk back. Show disrespect to teachers and parents. Criticize and belittle others. They find it difficult to follow the norms and conventions of the society.[20]

After first describing the social causes of the rise of depression in children, Dr Krishnakumar shifts to a somatic narrative explaining that the neurological imbalance that gives rise to depression is expressed when children who are genetically vulnerable to this neurochemical problem experience "excessive tensions" and then become depressive (Krishnakumar 2010). Voicing a social critique, Dr Krishnakumar describes the epidemic rise of depression in youth as others would describe the rise of diabetes: as a physical condition resulting from changed life circumstances for children.

As with children and adolescents, the changing social circumstances of the elderly make them vulnerable to depression, writes Dr P.V. Indu (2014). Here also, however, follows a medicalizing appeal in an idiom of urgency: depression should not be taken as an existential problem of old age and the reorientation from joint to nuclear family living patterns, but as a disease to be treated by a professional as soon as possible. Depression is "sold" to the elderly and their families as a treatable problem and people are encouraged not to take symptoms lightly by saying "Oh, mother is old, these are the problems of ageing." Physical symptoms are cited as particularly important in elderly people and the recommended treatment deals not with social factors, only the somatic disease. Antidepressants, along with antipsychotics and benzodiazepines, are the treatments of choice.

Dr John ends on a comforting note, telling readers that if they think they are experiencing any of the symptoms he listed, "do not worry. Do remember that there are scientific solutions for all these. Seek help." Self-tests for depression in the form of quizzes or checklists ("If you answered 'yes' to any of the above questions…") are common in magazine special issues and articles about the condition (John 2010). Ecks (2005) describes self-tests as one of the most important disease marketing strategies for pharmaceutical companies. They rapidly and effectively instil a particular understanding of depression and the "cure" in the mind of the reader, aligning reader subjectivities to the symptomatology of depression as defined by diagnostic manuals such as the ICD or the DSM.

"A gramme is better than a damn":[21] marketing depression, marketing a "cure"

> We have seen that in certain key respects the most widely prescribed of the new generation of psychiatric drugs treat conditions whose borders are fuzzy, whose coherence and very existence as illness or disorders are matters of dispute, and which are not so much intended to 'cure' […] as to modify the ways in which vicissitudes in the life of the recipient are experienced, lived and understood.
>
> (Rose 2003, 58)

> Pharmaceutical corporations and the psychiatric profession are working hand in hand to popularize the notion of depression as a medically treatable disease.
>
> (Kirmayer 2002, 316)

Pills to endure a difficult mother-in-law

My research assistant Sujatha and I invited Reetamol, a Muslim woman in her thirties from a lower middle class family in a nearby town, to sit with us in our little room at the Syrian Christian Hospital while she was waiting to see Dr Mona for a routine check-up.[22] Her chart showed that she had been diagnosed with recurrent depressive disorder (RDD) a year ago when she had first visited the psychiatric unit of the hospital. The chart showed her husband had brought her in, and listed "anger problems with mother-in-law" and "episodic behaviour disturbances" as her main complaints. Her chart also enumerated (almost entirely in English) her symptoms, including increased sleepiness, decreased food intake, loss of interest, crying spells, feeling under pressure, an inability to cope with daily life, and feeling unable to socialize with others or enjoy pleasurable situations. It also reported that she felt weak and guilty, was not completing daily prayers, experienced heaviness in the chest, was constipated and was unconcerned for her crying children. The chart also noted that she spent a lot of time lying down and worrying about whether her children (in kindergarten) were studying well and whether she would be able to complete her housework. The chart included a note to the effect that Reetamol's mother-in-law criticized her for being *vatta* [crazy]. Dr Mona explained to me that she had prescribed Veniz (an SSRI and generic of desvenlaxafine), Zapis (a benzodiazepine and generic of clonazepam) against hyperarousal, and Risdone (an antipsychotic and generic of risperidone) for irritable outbursts and "some behavioural modifications".[23]

Reetamol came to the hospital on her own on this occasion. Her story started with her arranged marriage:

> I couldn't get along with my mother in law. She is of a nagging type. Whatever I do, she finds some fault in it. It is next to impossible to please her. Even if I did something very well she found some fault in it. All this weighed heavily [*bharam*] on me and finally forced me into *depression*.

After her marriage eight years ago, Reetamol's mother-in-law ignored her. She and her husband were the only children living in the house, the others having moved out to live elsewhere with their families. I asked if she quarrelled with her mother-in-law. "No", she said, "I am very patient. I don't respond in the same tone. I keep silent. I tried to keep everything inside me. That turned out to be dangerous for me." We asked why she initially came to the hospital, and she told us,

> I had no interest in anything. I didn't care about my children. I just kept myself in my room and cried. I had no appetite. I was very disappointed and distressed. I hid all my problems from all people. Everything I kept inside me. At last, when I stopped doing anything and sat crying only people realized there is some problem with me.

Did her natal family know about her condition? "No," she replied, "I didn't inform anyone in my family. I didn't want to sadden them." Later when we asked her if she used to pray, she said, "We used to pray *namaz* [daily prayers] five times a day. Then I lost my concentration. When I try to pray my mind is disturbed by the ill feelings and I can't pray." We asked about her husband. Was he supportive?

> My husband is a nice person. He would tell me to forgive her because she is his mother. He would always comfort me. She wouldn't listen to any one. That was her nature. That will not change. She thinks that she is a virtuous person. I treated her very well. But she wouldn't respond that way. Now I am angry with her. I thought, why should I be cordial to her when this is the way she treats me? I don't care what she is doing. Now we don't talk to each other. I go for PSC[24] coaching. Classes are held on alternate days. So I can escape from the torture on these days at least. The rest of the days only I have to suffer.

At the beginning of her marriage, Reetamol had been teaching for some time but could not continue because of the stress.

> At night after all the work I did the preparation for the class. She is *manic* about cleanliness. She's not satisfied with whatever others do. She's not satisfied with the food others make. She insists on cooking everything herself. She doesn't want others to touch what she has cooked or her things. Her behaviour borders on the extremity that it is very difficult to adjust with her. She is of a different culture. Now she will always ask me to do some kind of work. Not anything important. Cleaning, cleaning, cleaning. Nothing else. Only cleaning. How can we live only by cleaning?

Some time later she talked about the stigma of mental illness:

> When neighbours see me going to a hospital they ask me, why I am going to the hospital. I tell them that I have a headache and that's the reason for going to hospital. It's kind of shameful to tell them the real reason. So no one in the neighbourhood knows the real reason behind my hospital visits.

Sujatha asked, "You take the medicine because you think that you cannot control the illness without it?" Reetamol answered,

> I was not able to take care of the children and I was simply sitting and crying. I was not able to do anything. This is the reason for me to come here and get treatment. I know it cannot be cured. Just to get some relief by taking some medicines. Mentally I drifted away 100%.

I wanted to find out if she knew about depression.

> Yes, we had to study psychology for B.Ed. [Bachelor of Education]. There was vishadam in the syllabus. I used to tell my husband after the marriage that I will get vishada rogam if I go on like this. And finally it became a reality.

We asked her about her symptoms and she described feeling "as if there was a knot on the chest [*nenchil kettu*], like weight on the chest [*nenchinn bharam*]. Disappointment, indifference, I lost the interest [*talpariyam illa*] to live, but not longing to die. I lost the aim in life." In the story she shared that day in our little office, Reetamol demonstrated mental health literacy and that she was well informed about depression and its psychological causes, but also revealed typical somatic complaints that were frequently repeated in the other narratives of depression that I heard in Kerala.

Depression as a disease label is constructed in Kerala through glocal institutional, pharmaceutical and cognitive assemblages. However, it is also a "moving target" (Hacking 2007) co-constituted and stabilized by different actors at multiple scales. In this section, I focus on a key element of the stabilization of depression: antidepressants. This material focus connects the interests of the pharmaceutical industry to psychiatry through examination of the launch, globalization and local appropriation of antidepressants as disease-specific agents. The history of depression in modern psychiatry is closely tied to the creation and rise of antidepressants. In India as elsewhere (Kitanaka 2012; Healy 2004; Moncrieff 2008), pharmaceutical companies are involved in the mongering of depression including creating "awareness" or "mental health literacy" through media reports and "awareness programmes" in schools, colleges and communities. The development of new drugs went hand in hand with the shift from the asylum to outpatient care. The launch of the first antipsychotic, chlorpromazine, and the first antidepressant, imipramine, in the 1950s gave rise to the early efforts of Indian community psychiatry. In the late 1980s and early 1990s, the development and increased availability of SSRIs helped to push the integration of mental health into primary health care (Ecks 2011).

The expansion of antidepressants on the material level parallels the expansion of psychiatry on institutional level. The marketing of fluoxetine, sertraline and later desvenlaxafine has been critical to mainstreaming not only depression but also psychiatry. At the same time, the promotion, supply and demand of these drugs conspired to expand diagnostic boundaries creating an ever-growing set of indications for antidepressants (Zita 1998; Metzl 2003; Healy 2004). This is related to what Ecks (2005) has called "pharmaceutical citizenship": the promise of de-marginalization through the consumption of antidepressants that includes, I suggest, not only a promoted *right* to access the "monoculture of happiness" through the use of antidepressants but also an implicit *obligation* to participate in pharmaceutical consumption in order to avoid or recover from any socio-economic disability due to depression. In this section, I focus explicitly on the role and influence of pharmaceuticals in establishing depression as a disease label and as an epidemic in Kerala. In so doing, I examine the relationships between diagnosis, diagnostic boundaries and the marketing interests of pharmaceutical companies.

Psychopharmaceuticals are more than material objects with physiological effects. As "socially embedded phenomena" (Cohen et al. 2001) they are simultaneously representations and agents that carry and shape meanings, transform social relations and reconfigure notions of health, suffering and personhood (Montagne 1996; van der Geest, Whyte and Hardon 1996; Petryna, Lakoff and Kleinman 2006). In the anthropology of pharmaceuticals, a growing literature focuses on the role, production and use of drugs (van der Geest, Whyte and Hardon 1996), their "life circles" (Cohen et al. 2001), "biographies" (van der Geest, Whyte and Hardon 1996), "social lives" (Appadurai 1986) and their role in transforming social relations, reconfiguring notions of health, disease, self and care in shaping subjectivities and shifting forms of governance (Lakoff 2005; Biehl 2006). In the case of psychotropic drugs in particular, key literature critically evaluates the scientific claims made on behalf of drugs (Breggin 2001; Cohen and Jacobs 2007), the pathologization and pharmaceuticalization of everyday distress (Horwitz and Wakefield 2007), the redefinitions of ideas of social belonging (Ecks 2005) and care (Pinto 2014), and the creation of diseases that did not previously exist (Lakoff 2005; Hacking 2007). For India, the role of antidepressants as actors to "swallow policy" (Jain and Jadhav 2009) has been criticized for silencing community voices and dissidence.

Focusing on pharmaceuticals instead of medical systems enables scholars to critically explore "pharmaceutical pluralism" (Ecks 2013) instead of the more vague "medical pluralism". Just as other objects that traverse manifold networks through global assemblages, antidepressants and other psychotropic drugs have a "distinctive capacity for decontextualisation and recontextualisation, abstractability and movement, across diverse social and cultural situations and spheres of life" (Ong and Collier 2005, 11). And just like any other object, antidepressants and other psychopharmaceuticals as actors can be ascribed agency in forming notions of self and health, reinterpreting suffering and reformulating forms of care and self-care.

The influence of the pharmaceutical industry in the development of depression since the 1950s has been convincingly established (Kramer 1993; Healy 1997; 2004; Moncrieff 2008). By the end of the 1950s, imipramine was the first drug promoted as an antidepressant targeting depression and acting in a disease-specific manner rather than producing an altered (exalted or sedated) state of consciousness. From then on, antidepressants were presented as working by reversing an underlying physical pathology. The pharmaceutical treatment thus appeared as a "therapeutic, medical enterprise" (Moncrieff 2008, 2353). Like later marketing strategies of SSRIs (and SNRIs) from the 1980s, the companies marketing tricyclic antidepressants and Monoaminooxidase (MAO) inhibitors promoted a construction of depression as a common medical condition. Moncrieff (2008) analyses the creation of the concept of an antidepressant along with the development of what she calls the "disease-specific model" – the idea that antidepressants target an underlying biological cause and rectify an underlying chemical imbalance. Drawing on Foucault's argument that presumably scientific facts are shaped by political and economic factors and the mutual legitimization of powerful groups and knowledge, Moncrieff unpacks the "myth of a chemical cure" as deeply rooted in the psychiatric profession's desire to incorporate with general somatic medicine in order to improve its medical credibility through diagnostic categories and cures, and achieving the move from the asylum into the community. The pharmaceutical industry further strengthened the disease-specific narrative of antidepressants in order to distinguish psychopharmaceutical from illegal non-specific psychotropic drugs. The specific action of drugs was one of the main sources of evidence for the medical understanding of mental disorders. The disease-specific model of drugs supported the view that the psychiatric classifications were valid (Moncrieff 2008).

The idea of the antidepressant that came to the fore in the late 1950s both strengthened and was impacted by the notion that depression was an important and independent psychiatric category. After some debate, mainly in North America, over the question of whether depression should be regarded as a generic (single) category or differentiated into reactive (neurotic) and endogenous (responsive to antidepressants) categories, the assumption that any sort of depression might be responsive to one specific drug helped to cement depression as one generic disease entity. This idea was solidified with the publication of DSM-III in 1980 and an updated version of the ICD that formed the basis on which the pharmaceutical industry created an extensive market for new antidepressants in the 1990s. The launch of SSRIs and the mainstreaming of depression were also closely connected with psychiatry's abandonment of psychoanalysis and revival of the nineteenth-century tradition of psychiatry as neuroscience, a process that started with the invention of chlorpromazine and imipramine in the 1950s (Shorter 1997). These antidepressants and their generics have contributed to strengthening the concept of depression as a singular biological disorder and the idea that personal problems could be attributed to chemical imbalance. The psychiatric category "depression" found its way into Kerala's psychiatric discourse as *vishada rogam* from the late 1990s and later made its way into popular psychiatric discourse.

The older antidepressants of the tricyclic and MAO inhibitor types were rarely sold either globally or in India since depression was a rare diagnosis. The arrival of new antidepressants shifted the market from benzodiazepines to SSRIs as the most frequently sold psychopharmaceuticals – a move from the "tranquilizer era" to the "antidepressant era" (Healy 2004). Eli Lilly's blockbuster, Prozac, and other SSRIs were marketed as the new, safe, feel-good drugs without the danger of dependency. In the 1990s the anxiety market transformed into the depression markets: depression was diagnosed far more frequently than anxiety and patients who had so far been treated with tranquilizers were now treated with antidepressants (Healy 2006). Though this shift is evident in Kerala, it was not as significant as in North America. With the rapid success of

SSRIs in terms of market share, depression began to change from a rare condition often involving hospitalization to a common and more easily treatable malady.

The understanding of the people who suffered from depression changed significantly over the second half of the twentieth century. In the 1950s, the typical subjects featured in advertisements were older women and sometimes men, but in the 1990s the advertisements for SSRIs depicted much younger individuals (Shorter 1997). Rapidly, depression went mainstream. Ecks analyses how the images in brochures that he collected in 2003 promoting SSRIs in Bengal, India, portrayed not marginal, isolated individuals but attractive, smiling, fair, middle or upper class South Asian people in Western clothes and often in the context of the cheerful company of partners or children. These images targeted consumers at the centre of society. Further, their message was that antidepressants not only alleviated depression and its symptoms, but also social marginalization based on class, caste or gender (Ecks 2005). In 2014, I was struck by a poster advertisement I saw for Nexito, Sun Pharma's brand name for escitalopram, at the annual meeting of the Indian Psychiatric Society (ANCIPS). It showed an attractive young woman in her early twenties, fair-skinned and wearing a sexy Western t-shirt smiling under the headline "the future is now". This advertisement associated "the new generation of SSRIs" (per the heading) with a new generation of young women who are successful, desirable and Westernized.

Critical literature within medical anthropology and beyond has demonstrated the deep influence of pharmaceutical companies on clinical trials, the production of scientific literature including the DSM and ICD (Healy 2006; Sismondo 2009; Light 2010) and the transmission of psychiatric knowledge leading to an "unwanted marriage between market and science" (Sismondo 2009). The generation of evidence on which globalized psychiatric standards and rational care is based is controlled by economic interests (Healy 1997; Elliott 2001; Kirmayer 2002). Further, there is as yet no evidence for the thesis of depression as a deficiency of the serotonin or norepinephrine neurotransmitters (Moncrieff 2008; Healy 2015). Moreover, scholars in this area are concerned about the expansion of disorders such as depression into everyday distress and an ever widening of indications for antidepressants since the 1980s. Sadness is increasingly pathologized, becoming a medical rather than an existential condition. With the integration of an ever-wider suite of emotions and moods constructed as symptoms of depression, the psychiatric profession along with the pharmaceutical industry have reclassified normal human sadness and experience as abnormal. With DSM-III, when professionals started to diagnose depression based on symptoms, the context in which symptoms arose was increasingly disregarded, and so emotional distress as a reaction to upsetting events more easily led to a diagnosis of depressive disorder. Through the "loss of sadness" people lose their capacity for tolerating suffering and grief (Horwitz and Wakefield 2007). This critique intensified with the later editions of the DSM. Psychiatrist Allen Frances, former director of the DSM-IV committee, publishes extensively on "out-of-control psychiatric diagnoses" and the role "big pharma" plays in this process. Aiming at "saving normal", he writes against growing medicalization and pharmaceuticalization of everyday life and ordinary sorrow, sadness and despair (Frances 2013). There are also concerns about the expansion of the scope of antidepressants beyond depression to include prescription for social phobia, premature ejaculation, insomnia, obsessions and compulsions, and post-traumatic stress disorder. As Applbaum (2006) points out, the effects of SSRIs on the body are so ambiguous that there is great scope for marketing-driven reinterpretations and diagnostic expansions; a phenomenon Nikolas Rose (2006) calls "disorders without borders". In India the markets for different sorts of psychopharmaceuticals crisscross with one another as each drug's indications expand: antidepressants are used to treat bipolar disorder, obsessive compulsive disorder, anxiety and for all kinds of unexplained bodily sensations, and antipsychotics and benzodiazepines are prescribed for depression.

Another line of critique argues that the biological reductionism and pharmaceuticalization of suffering may lead to biological surveillance and depoliticization (Rose 2003; Mills 2014) in that they help to silence political dissent and politicize private outrage with regard to political, social and economic inequalities. A neurochemical reinterpretation of anger, sadness and despair under depressive social and economic circumstances deprives people of the historical and political implications and moral dimensions of their experiences and thus roots their experiences in body chemistry rather than in socio-economic inequalities and structural violence. Antidepressants then become what Jain and Jadhav call "pills that swallow policy":

> As the pill journeys from the Ministry of Health to the clinic, its symbolic meaning transforms from an emphasis on accessibility and participation to the administration of a discrete "treatment". Instead of embodying participation and access, the pill achieves the opposite: silencing community voices, re-enforcing existing barriers to care, and relying on pharmacological solutions for psychosocial problems.
>
> (Jain and Jadhav 2009, 60)

Access to psychopharmaceuticals often remains the only way mental health services are delivered. Antidepressants then serve – together with the neurochemical imbalance narrative of depression – as substitutes for structural solutions which are much more difficult to implement. In this way, the Movement of Global Mental Health also transforms complex social problems into issues of delivery and availability of psychopharmaceuticals (Kirmayer and Pedersen 2014). The global pharmaceuticalization of "existential imbalances" (Jenkins 2011) is also related to consumerism and the neoliberal exigencies of a "monoculture of happiness" (Kirmayer 2002, 316).

Kerala has not only reportedly the highest depression rates; it is also the largest market for psychopharmaceuticals in India (Chua 2014). A high-rank medical officer psychiatrist told me that more than 50 per cent of all prescriptions in general practice are for antidepressants that have replaced paracetamol as the top selling drugs.[25] These are not the branded products of multi-national pharmaceutical companies, but rather generics produced by the huge Indian generic industry. All prescriptions by psychiatrists and general physicians that I saw and all of the products I bought from *pharma wallahs* [pharmacists] when I asked for medicines for depression were generics produced by Indian companies. Most of the antidepressants prescribed and sold in Kerala are SSRIs, and escitalopram and fluoxetine are the bestsellers. When these drugs were first licensed in the 1980s and 1990s, India's Patents Act only protected the patenting of the processes of drug manufacturing but not the drug products themselves. Until 2005, when India signed the Agreement on Trade-Related Aspects of Intellectual Property Rights (TRIPS) that guaranteed the worldwide protection of the branded products of multinational pharmaceutical companies (Agrawal and Saibaba 2001; Ecks and Basu 2011; Halliburton 2009), this patent regime allowed Indian pharmaceutical companies to reverse engineer drugs and sell them as generics. These inexpensive versions of popular drugs permitted the Indian pharmaceutical industry to rapidly develop into the world's top producer of generics (Ecks and Basu 2011; Halliburton 2009). For this reason, generic antidepressants are widely available and easily accessible in Kerala. In 2014, 10 tablets of Prozac (fluoxetine) sold for $25 USD, while 10 tables of generic fluoxetine (Prodep or Fludac), generic escitalopram (Nexito) or generic sertraline (Daxid, Sertee) cost less than $1 USD. SNRIs such as generic venlaxafine were slightly more expensive and therefore less frequently prescribed. Generic benzodiazepines were even less expensive, costing only $0.25 to $0.5 USD for 10 tablets. The protection of different production processes under the old patent system gave rise to a market in which a proliferation of companies of various sizes produced nearly identical pharmaceutical products. This has led to fierce competition that has driven down prices, again contributing to the availability and affordability of antidepressants and other psychopharmaceuticals in India. Sales are robust, but profits are small compared with those of big pharma in wealthier countries. However, health expenditure in India is expected to rise significantly in the future with drugs related to "lifestyle" diseases such as depression are predicted to increase sales and profit (Ecks and Basu 2009).

The cross-cultural reliability of DSM and ICD diagnoses is debated largely within scholarly circles. In clinical psychiatric practice in Kerala, however, diagnostics are not a central concern. The clear-cut divisions between different nosological categories often becomes blurred by psychiatrists' pragmatic focus on getting the patient better as quickly as possible. In the clinical encounters I observed, psychiatrists were much more interested in treating symptoms such as irritability, suspicion, adjustment problems or crying than in formulating a diagnosis, and prescribed accordingly. In clinical practice, the aim was less to fit the illness with the pill but rather to fit different pills with different symptoms. It is symptoms rather than diagnostic entities that are targeted by the medication, though ICD terms are often hastily written in the patient charts. Insight into the disease and behaviour corresponding to or deviating from gender, class, caste and age norms were examined in terms of brain neurochemistry and drug effects. Complex emotions and thoughts based in complex social relations and experiences were then read not as causes of depression but rather as signs and symptoms of the disease malleable through careful pharmaceutical management.

Psychiatrists prescribed SSRIs for panic, sadness, crying spells or anxiety and SNRIs for lack of energy and concentration, tiredness, indecisiveness, adjustment problems and a host of somatic complaints. Rarely psychiatrists prescribed tricyclic antidepressants (TCA). The most frequently prescribed SSRIs were branded generics of escitalopram, fluoxetine and sertraline, and desvenlafaxine was the SNRI of choice. For escitalopram alone, around 170 branded products produced by 75 different companies are available.[26] Additionally, psychiatrists and general physicians prescribed the tricyclic antidepressant amitriptyline for more severe forms of depression or in cases where SSRIs or SNRIs had proved ineffective. Psychiatrists generally preferred to prescribe single drugs, but general practitioners frequently prescribed combinations of antidepressants and anxiolytics or antidepressants and antipsychotics. Because the effects of SSRIs and SNRIs take a week or two to manifest, psychiatrists usually also prescribed anxiolytics and antipsychotics "for immediate relief" as psychiatrist Dr Mona explained.[27] They prescribed benzodiazepines to improve sleep and reduce anxiety and irritability, and a mild antipsychotic in low dosage for anger, irritability, sleep improvement, prevention of psychosis and, interestingly, "for behavioural modification".[28] Both anxiolytics and antipsychotics are used to make "the mind calm" which is the stated aim of medical and religious intervention in mental distress in Kerala, related to local notions of mental health, mind and personhood. These drugs take effect rapidly, so doctors reasoned that prescribing them would make patients less likely to seek out other doctors or treatments because they had the impression that the treatment was already working.

Bipolar Affective Disorder (BPAD) was by far the most frequent diagnosis of inpatients, but most psychiatrists in Kerala did not follow the standard recommendation of the WHO to prescribe lithium or sodium valproate both in the manic and depressive states, but routinely prescribed SSRIs or SNRIs plus benzodiazepines in the depressive state for a quicker impression of positive result and more effective management. The risk for BPAD patents is that taking antidepressants can easily provoke a swing into mania. This, Dr Mona told me, requires careful patient mood monitoring by family, giving rise to what could be called pharmaceutical forms of care. It is not so much a pharmaceutical form of self-care as suggested by the terms "pharmaceutical selves" (Jenkins 2011) or "neurochemical selves" (Rose 2003) but more a pharmaceutical form of care by family members (Pinto 2014). The British psychiatrist Joanna Moncrieff (2014) speaks of "bipolar imperialism" and observes that bipolar disorder, once considered rare and seriously disabling, has been transformed into a much vaguer notion of the experience of mood swings that can apply to almost anyone including children and youth. The rise in the number and frequency of BPAD diagnoses is pushed by pharmaceutical companies, Moncrieff argues, to increase the market for antipsychotics. To classify patients in a depressed state as suffering from BPAD expands the market not only for mood stabilizers but also for antipsychotics, the latter leading to "chemical restraint" and people feeling like "zombies" (Moncrieff 2014).

It seems that the three groups of medications – antidepressants, mood stabilizers and antipsychotics – originally corresponded to depression, mania and schizophrenia, but psychiatrists increasingly prescribe these drugs for an expanding variety of conditions. From the perspective of prescription and use of psychopharmaceuticals, mental illness thus becomes less, not more differentiated from the trend in DSM and ICD to progressively fine-tune psychiatric diagnoses.

Psychopharmaceuticals are usually prescribed in large doses and inpatients typically receive injections in addition to tablets as patients and caregivers perceive them to be stronger and faster acting (Nichter 1983). The perception that treatment has a rapid effect seems to be extremely important to patients and caregivers in the early stages of treatment. A typical treatment for a depression diagnosis as illustrated in Reetamol's narrative at the beginning of this chapter entailed an SSRI (mostly escitalopram, followed by fluoxetine), and/or an SNRI (mostly desvenlaxafine), a benzodiazepine such as alprazolam or clonazepam, and an antipsychotic such as olanzepine. In this way, once a person was classified as a mental patient, psychiatrists reinterpreted complex moods, emotions and behaviours as manifestations of chemical states to be carefully managed through a host of pharmaceutical interventions and a patient's return to corresponding to social – and especially gender – norms were perceived as a sign of success. Ethnographers have shown Indian psychiatry's heavy reliance on drugs, whether during in- or outpatient treatment, at public or private hospitals, in clinics or community mental health care (Nunley 1996; Addlkakha 2008; Jain and Jadhav 2009; Pinto 2014). Ideologically, psychiatrists privilege what they call a "bio-psycho-social" model of depression which integrates biological, psychological and social factors in both the causation and the treatment of depression and which was introduced into psychiatry as a challenge to the biomedical model of psychiatry in the 1970s by the American psychiatrist George Engel (1977). In clinical practice, this model is often subverted and treatment largely consists of pharmacological management of emotions, moods and behaviours. One of the most important reasons for psychiatrists' heavy reliance on drugs is their "epidemic view" (Nunley 1996) of depression and other mental illness (Chapter 1). This leads them to bracket the social and focus instead on neurochemistry, basing treatment largely in polypharmacy. Constructing depression as an epidemic equates it with infectious diseases. The logical response, therefore, is to treat as many patients as possible in the least time possible. The epidemic view has transformed depression from a subjective experience into a public health crisis worthy of, and requiring, intervention.

This view is closely related to several factors specific to India: psychiatrists' huge daily patient load, the inferior status of psychiatry vis-à-vis other medical disciplines (and the associated struggle for credibility) and the need to "sell psychiatry" as a credible medical discipline and mental disorders as in fact physical diseases. Allopathic medicine's most visible successes in India occurred in the context of the treatment of infectious disease epidemics, and so to patients and their families, the best possible medical treatment consists of allopathic treatment, the use of multiple pharmaceuticals and a rapid change in the patient (Nunley 1996). Psychiatrists that I spoke with felt drugs were culturally appropriate for their patients. They were assumed to fit better into patients' daily routines, which were often incompatible with attending weekly appointments with a psychiatrist or psychologist. Drugs were relatively cheap, easily accessible and positively valued as the epitome of modern medical care. They were seen as compatible with understandings of Indian notions of mind and the self as embodied, fluent and inessential that were quite different from Western notions of the self, transported through different forms of psychotherapy. Moreover, the use of pharmaceuticals fit local notions of efficacy, which attributed much greater effectiveness to drugs than to other kinds of exogenous therapeutic agents and remedies. Finally, prescribing and especially administering drugs was seen as a form of care and idiom of concern.

Medical anthropologists have pointed out the worldwide association of images of well-being and health with access to pharmaceuticals. Psychiatrists in Kerala told me that their prototypical depression patient is middle class, educated, Westernized and urban. This is stereotypical, but the strength of this stereotype demonstrates that depression is a disorder popularly related to Westernization, consumerism and middle class lifestyles. Depression, then, is not a disease of marginalization but of belonging. Antidepressants are not a sign of marginalization; rather they are the "little helpers" of middle class consumers. The message is clear: depression is not a disease of the marginalized. With the help of antidepressants, it is a manageable affliction for both the members and the new gods and goddesses (celebrities) of India's consumer middle class.

Transnational and national agencies and antidepressant marketing promote pharmaceutical social belonging, dangling the promise of pharmaceutical citizenship and demarginalization. However my ethnographic evidence shows that the prescriptions, purchase, possession and consumption of psychopharmaceuticals cause patients to experience severe stigmatization. In practice, it is not social belonging and care but stigma that is embodied in the practice of consuming antidepressants. Drugs are the most concrete sign of a patient's mental illness, hidden as far as possible from husbands, in-laws and other family members. But it is both the pills and the act of visiting a psychiatrist that cement the status of a person as a *manasika* [mental] patient. Psychiatrist Dr R.V. Paul told me of a case where he did not prescribe antidepressants to a woman he had diagnosed with depression because it would have negatively impacted her already difficult relationship with her in-laws.[29] Thus, in spite of shiny promises of demarginalization, in Kerala the use of antidepressants contributes to the marginalization of depression patients, often forcing them to employ complex strategies to circumvent the stigma of mental illness. Just as patients "mask" depression under somatic complaints (Chapter 2), doctors "hide" depression diagnoses by prescribing antidepressants but telling the patient the drugs are intended to help with their physical complaints. Though somatization is often framed as a lack of mental health literacy, somatization theory serves the promotion and growth of depression to include an ever-wider range of symptoms. General physicians, it seemed, were quick to prescribe antidepressants for any somatic kinds of distress not obviously or immediately attributed to ailments. This contributes to high sales of antidepressants, and some physicians prescribed SSRIs almost routinely and prophylactically, especially for women. Dr Girishkumar told me that diagnosing a patient with a mental illness instead of a somatic complaint was risky because, fearful of the associated stigma, patients might question the doctor's expertise and seek a new diagnosis (and treatment) elsewhere.[30]

Pharmaceutical companies actively create conditions and their cures, and use sophisticated marketing techniques to sell both. This process involves alliances formed between drug companies anxious to sell a product, doctors eager to diagnose under-diagnosed problems, new "kinds of people" (Hacking 2007) and biosocial groups organized by and for those who (or are thought to) suffer from the condition. In India, awareness campaigns directly or indirectly funded by pharmaceutical companies include media reports and self-tests of depression that contribute to the growth and stabilization of depression, while simultaneously widening the market for antidepressants. These campaigns reference misery, economic cost and the threat of apparently undiagnosed conditions. They interpret the data that is available to maximize perceptions of the condition's prevalence, and shape public fears and anxieties into a clinical problem, for which they conveniently also present the solution. Articles deriving from these efforts often hint at the huge economic burden of untreated depression and the high number of cases as yet undiagnosed. With regard to Kerala, the pharmaceutical industry stokes then harnesses the discourse of crisis by medicalizing social suffering as individual biological disorder: one treatable with a drug that will help to restore control, happiness and productivity. Medical anthropologists have described the marketing strategies of pharmaceutical companies including the bribery of psychiatrists and physicians by pharmaceutical representatives in the form of gifts, travel, sponsorship and other incentives (Lakoff 2005; Healy 2006; Nunley 1996; Ecks 2013). Often the representatives are the main source of information regarding latest drug developments and research. This is why long-lasting, warm relationships of mutual interest are carefully cultivated between companies, representatives and psychiatrists.

With antidepressants so widely available, routinely prescribed, affordable and accessible in India, does it make sense to speak of the "treatment gap" that the Global Mental Health movement suggests exists in India? Is there really a gap between the need for and supply of psychiatric services for depression? I find the notion of "floating prescriptions" (Ecks and Basu 2009) useful for understanding this seemingly paradoxical situation. The prescription leaflet, which in India always remains with the patients or their family, is agentive not only in transmitting expert knowledge about the latest drugs to non-psychiatric and even unlicensed practitioners, but also in transmitting diagnoses. The bulk of prescriptions for antidepressants are written not by the approximately 3,000 psychiatrists in the country, but by doctors in other specializations. This is where the importance of marketing directly to psychiatrists as gatekeepers or opinion leaders is so important to pharmaceutical companies. They contribute to trends in branded products, which are then transmitted through various channels to others involved in prescribing medications (pharmaceutical representatives have recently started to general physicians directly).

Ecks and Basu describe prescriptions as floating downwards from psychiatrists to non-psychiatric medical professionals and rural medical practitioners in Bengal, and I observed this process in Kerala with Ayurvedic doctors and even with religious healing practitioners. For example, the Muslim thangal Yasir Thangal used to either prescribe or sell psychopharmaceuticals he stored in his desk.[31] His clients often preferred drugs sold and ritually empowered by him because they believed they would be more powerful than those purchased in a pharmacy, and there was no difference in price. In this way, expert knowledge regarding diagnosis and treatment trickles down, and is disseminated to various non-professionals where it is often recontextualized within other practices and frames of knowledge. Allopathic general practitioners, Ayurvedic doctors and religious healers use a psychiatrist's prescription for "reverse-diagnosis", concluding the diagnosis from the name of a branded product. In this way, prescriptions are agents of disseminating drugs and diagnoses and antidepressant prescriptions are actors that stabilize depression as a disease category.

In this sense, it is not only the psychiatric prescription patterns that are "floating", themselves heavily influenced by the marketing practices of pharmaceutical representatives. "Floating" also are the diagnoses. Prescriptions move between patients, retail shops, non-psychiatric allopathic doctors, Ayurvedic doctors and ritual healers.

This section has dealt with the expansion of depression as a common mental health category and the way it is closely interlinked with the launch, globalization and local appropriation of antidepressants as presumably disease-specific agents. In India as elsewhere, the promotion of antidepressants and depression "disease mongering" (Moynihan, Heath and Henry 2002) are two sides of the same coin. The availability of antidepressants, benzodiazepines and antipsychotics in Kerala and their affordability give rise to wide access to pharmacological treatment for depression. It is not only an increasing array of symptoms being included under depression and becoming the target of antidepressants but also the psychiatrization of suicide as depression that makes attempted suicide manageable with antidepressants.

Depression and the medicalization of suicide

Since the 1990s, Kerala's reported suicide rates have ranked among India's highest – as much as double or triple the national average (Halliburton 1998; Münster 2012). There are two prototypical "kinds of people" (Hacking 2007) in Kerala that figure in media reports and government statistics as well as in ethnographies as prone to suicide: farmers in Wayanad and Kerala youth who fail in their aspirations for the "good life" (Chua 2014). For the first group, an administrative category "farmer suicides" has been created (Münster 2012), but the construction of "student suicides" or "college suicides" as a category is a much more recent phenomenon. Mental health discourse frames Kerala's suicide problem as a problem of depression: suicide and suicide attempts appear as symptoms of depression, and contribute to growing depression as a mental health problem, increase its aura of urgency and boost sales of pharmacological interventions. Psychiatrists and psychologists quoted the high suicide numbers in Kerala as evidence of the lethality of depression and the urgency of prevention, detection and medical treatment. However, media reports, anti-suicide campaigns and awareness programmes often conflate suicide and depression figures to support an argument for the need to expand psychiatric services. Despite depression being identified as a causative factor in only approximately 10 per cent of all suicides and the difficulties of retrospectively tracing the mental health condition of a suicide victim, psychiatrists I spoke with attributed the majority of suicide cases to depression. Further, they were convinced that psychopharmacological interventions were the most appropriate and expedient way of addressing Kerala's suicide problem.

"Is suicidal tendency a sign of mental disability?" asked Dr Paul in a Malayalam-speaking training programme held for caregivers in private rehabilitation centres.[32] "Yes of course it is". He continued:

> Our mental health care delivery system is inadequate, that is why our suicide rate is increasing. The mental health care delivery system in Kerala is going in a wrong direction. Whenever we could direct it towards the right path, our suicide rates will automatically slow down.

Dr Paul deployed an understanding of Kerala's suicide problem that accords with the agenda of the Global Mental Health movement: the solution is to "scale up" psychiatric services in suicide-prone population groups and geographic areas. Such services are largely equated to increased psychopharmacological management. In fact, instances of dark humour betray the deep concern about suicide and unswerving faith in the medicalization of the problem in Kerala: a psychiatrist ironically advocated dumping "anti-depressants into the drinking water" (Chua 2009, 11); and psychologist Anand Kutty sarcastically suggested using antidepressants in the form of mass vaccination.[33] Social factors relating to the socioeconomic transformations experienced in recent decades are significant and causative in Kerala's suicide and depression problems, and although this is well known in medical and popular circles, the most expedient solution is still identified as increasing the provision and use of antidepressants. In this way, the shortfalls of the Kerala model of development, farmer suicides and failed youth aspirations, depression and the Global Mental Health agenda of expanding mental health services and pharmaceutical delivery are woven together into a powerful discursive frame.

Scholarly writing and popular understandings[34] consider the issue of farmer suicides through a critique of India's neoliberal reforms that began in the 1990s.

As Münster (2012) has observed, farmer suicides are either described as victims of the structural violence of globalization and neoliberal reforms or as politically motivated acts of protest. The first interpretation constructs farmers as victims while the second grants them agency and the power to use their deaths as acts of political dissidence. Both constructions treat the medicalization of farmer suicides as a form of either bracketing structural inequalities or of silencing political protest and dissidence. The psychiatric discourse of farmer suicides considers the phenomenon through a framework of the individual self and overlooks the multiple complexities of the lived realities of distress and poverty (Mills 2014). To categorize these suicides and attempts as symptoms of depression frames acute social problems such as poverty and violence as individual psychiatric problems, and by constructing these individuals as in need of psychological counselling and psychiatric medication, critics argue, the mental health discourse on suicide de-politicizes suicide acts. From this perspective, the psychiatrization and psychologization of farmer suicides interweaves neoliberal political governance, the economic interests of the pharmaceutical industry and the global agricultural industry, and the status-related interests of psychiatric and psychological professionals. The psychiatric discourse on farmer suicide in Kerala enables professionals to pharmaceutically target individual brains while at the same time acknowledging social inequalities and structural violence. In this way, a complex agrarian crisis has been reconfigured as a public mental health crisis and both problem and cure are located within the same neoliberal logic (Mills 2014). Mills and others criticize the medicalization of these suicides, but others argue against the structural explanation inherent in these critiques. Although Münster's ethnography of farmer suicides in Wayanad district (Kerala) does not argue for a psychiatrization or psychologization of rural suicides, he argues against "economic reductionism". He contends that an exclusive focus on neoliberal politics constructing the farmer who commits suicide either as a victim or as a political agent with resisting neoliberal policies overlooks the "social and psychological nuances" of rural suicides (Mills 2014). These nuances lie not only in the causal complexities of each case of farmer suicide that resist generalization, but also in the implications of the sociological and administrative construction of the category farmer suicides (Münster 2012).

Mental health discourse medicalizes not only farmer suicides but also youth who commit suicide in response to unfulfilled aspirations. Local mental health professionals often attribute the rising rates of suicide and depression to over-ambition and dissipated desires propelled by aspirations for social and material gain. In her ethnography on discourses of suicide in Thiruvanathapuram, Chua focuses on what she calls the "productivity of death". She explores suicide as a lens into aspirations as the "experiential and affective dimensions of development and global change" and into the "bitter fruits" of development (Chua 2014). Next to Wayanad and Idukki, Thiruvananthapuram reports the highest rates of suicide in the state. Chua analyses one of the dominating explanations for these developments in the popular imaginary, namely the attribution of the suicide crisis to a problem of aspiration in which suicide is "not only a rupture in the fabric of life but is in fact also woven into its very warp and weft". Socially and morally, suicide "inflects political, social, and familial life in the region" (Chua 2014, 4) provoking reflection on definitions of "the good life at the crossroads of development, liberalization and global change" (Chua 2014, 15) and the institutionalized production of non-suicidal subjects.

Medicalization of distress and neurochemical imbalance explained: the body, the brain and the (non)sense of suffering

I now turn to investigate more closely the cognitive level of the local appropriation of depression in Kerala and the ways doctors explain a depression diagnosis to their patients. Both allopathic and Ayurvedic psychiatrists do not usually explain diagnoses to patients for reasons of time pressure, the assumption that diagnoses are made for medical experts not patients, and the assumed primacy of reassurance over explanation. Doctors reassure or console patients and their families, saying "Don't worry, take these medicines and you will be alright." However, I was surprised to observe – more frequently than I expected – that though many did not, several psychiatrists did explain diagnoses. In this section I explore the ways in which those doctors who did convey a depression diagnosis to patients and their caretakers did so, and with what intention and impact. Although psychiatrists in Kerala think with global notions of depression as a neurochemical imbalance in the brain, in explanatory encounters with patients and caregivers they adapt these to local notions of self, body and mind and to local forms of stigmatization and marginalization.

Parvathi: pathologizing grief

I was sitting in the office of Dr Mona at the Syrian Christian Hospital on a day like many others when Parvathi opened the door, came in and sat down.[35] She came to the hospital seeking help for her eldest daughter Chandra and wanted her to be seen by a psychiatrist for what she regarded as behavioural problems. Staff had started a chart for Chandra but the young woman was sitting outside and refused to enter the consultation room. By rejecting the space of medicalization she was pushing back against becoming a "patient". Parvathi was a middle class Hindu woman in her late forties, from a rural area about two hours by car from the hospital. She was working as a government employee and had a diploma in civil engineering. Asked about what brought her to the hospital, Parvathi answered that she had lost her husband in an accident two months ago. Dr Mona asked about her family situation and Parvathi responded that she lived separate from her in-laws and had three children. Chandra, her eldest daughter, completed her MBBS in China but lacked the confidence to look for employment, and resided with her mother for the time being. Her second daughter was in the first year of study for her MBBS in a town far from her mother's house. The youngest child, a son, had completed his plus two and was preparing to repeat the entrance exam for medicine after failing on his first attempt. He also lived in another town. Chandra was of a marriageable age, and Parvathi worried that when her daughter married, she would be left alone.

Dr Mona then asked Parvathi what kind of problems she was experiencing. "Family issues", she replied, and began to explain starting with what is often called "cultural difference". In this case it was the financial difference between her natal family and her in-laws.

> I am the daughter of a school teacher. We are four children, relatively financially sound; never faced financial problems. My husband is one of nine children, he was the youngest and only he had a job. I came into his family with tremendous responsibilities, had to do the role of a mother.

Family issues are a ubiquitous complaint in Kerala, as it seems that in every family there are some problems. The particular form of Parvathi's problem was also not unique: her mother-in-law criticized her constantly and complained about her in front of her son "with a sullen face". Parvathi's husband joined in with his mother, who always "came first" for him. Understanding the nature and complexities of similar family problems in Kerala, Dr Mona asked whether there had been physical violence. "There were no physical assaults, but he always taunted me. Verbal abuse is more painful than physical abuses," Parvathi replied. However, for two years she, her husband and their children had lived separate from her in-laws "happily together". Dr Mona prompted her to say more about the concerns she had for her children after this change, but Parvathi instead shifted to another issue, an extramarital relationship she had with another man. Although not uncommon, in Kerala, extramarital relationships are taboo as they offend social norms and are therefore rarely discussed. Parvathi mentioned this issue without prompting because she identified it as a key cause of her daughter's misbehaviour.

There is an element of the confessional to the offices of psychiatrists and other doctors. These professionals are seen as highly trustworthy, and their offices as places where it is possible to talk about taboo subjects and highly stigmatized problems without endangering the social standing of their family. Parvathi's extramarital relationship, it became clear, was both the consequence and further cause of her husband's abusive behaviour. "It slowly developed into something that grew overboard. There were personal visits also", Parvathi explained. Dr Mona asked, "Was it a brotherly attitude, or was he someone who cared for you?" "It grew into that," Parvathi admitted. Switching into a moralist discourse and alluding to a possible internal conflict while at the same time offering a way to save her honour, Dr Mona asked, "Did you realize that it was against social norms? At one side, you did not like it and yet were being forced into it. Was it an ambivalent state?" Parvathi conceded, "It outgrew that stage, it outgrew the limits, I know that." She told the doctor that her husband caused problems when he learned about the relationship. They moved to another town but her husband never stopped blaming and accusing her. That "he continuously tainted me in front of the children" was Parvathi's main explanation for her children's worrisome behaviour. "My three children were emotionally pained. They were influenced by the long years of accusations against me." Dr Mona probed further: "Was it that children would disobey you or go against what you said?" Parvathi responded that Chandra was tense about everything, angered quickly and was even violent.

> That's why I wanted to bring her here. The second daughter, who kept hearing what her father told me, developed an *ishtam* [liking] for a man, he is Muslim. She regards the boy as someone with whom she can share her grief, someone who can console and support her. Similarly, my son also gets angry fast. He has several girls calling him for chit-chatting.

In the face of this culturally inappropriate behaviour, Dr Mona asked, "How do you control your three children? It must be difficult to manage three children of this age group. Don't you have anyone else, someone authoritative, your brother or your husband's brother to help with the children?" Control is a virtue, and perceived to be one of the main tasks of parents and other elder – usually male – family members. However, it turned out that neither the brothers of Parvathi's now-deceased husband or her own brother were interested in this responsibility. This statement points to a possible feeling of inadequacy, while at the same time suggesting that Parvathi – as a woman, a widow and an individual currently lacking mental strength – was perceived by the doctor to hardly be able to control them all alone.

The doctor returned to Parvathi's worries: "What are your concerns now? You have all these issues, how are they affecting you?" to which she replied, "I am concerned about my eldest daughter, she has developed an *ishtam* [liking] for a boy, who has also completed his MBBS." Though Dr Mona's task as a psychiatrist was to elicit the impact of a situation or problem on the mind and the body of the patient, Parvathi's main concern was the difficulties of her eldest daughter. Initially she only mentioned her daughter's inability to control her anger and occasional violent outbursts, but now a second "behavioural problem" came into view: Chandra had a romantic relationship with a fellow student. At the moment Dr Mona asked how these problems affected her, she transformed Parvathi's family problems into indicators of her mental state and shifted the problem from the social to the individual, which she later located in the mind and in brain chemistry. As in so many other cases, patients arrive at medical offices with problems and doctors transform them – or rather their impact – into individual mental health problems and symptoms of ICD-based diseases. I saw this shift in many initial consultations, a moment when after coming in to talk about difficult situations, problems were medicalized and the patient left with a psychiatric diagnosis and a prescription for psychopharmaceuticals. Yet Parvathi, resistant to this path, went on to talk about her daughter's problematic relationship, enumerating different factors, including: the geographical distance to her house which would mean sending her daughter far away; the social distance between the two families ("Their nature and lifestyle are quite different from ours"); the bodily (somatic) incompatibility ("She is well-built, the boy is very lean"); the language difference ("I cannot come to terms with him or his ways of speaking"); the political distance ("His father is a politician and none in my family has an orientation towards politics"); and the insubordinate behaviour of Chandra with regard to that boy and their lack of maturity. "She has become so adamant. 'If not for this, I don't want marriage,' she says." "My concern is", Parvathi concluded, "who will talk sense to my daughter?" Dr Mona reassured her and suggested sending Chandra to see the psychologist, whose main task was then seen as "talking sense to the daughter", to persuade her of the inappropriateness of this relationship.

After this, medicalization arose again. Seeming to perceive a need to fix the problem in her capacity as a psychiatrist, Dr Mona prompted Parvathi to speak of symptoms of a depressive episode. "All in all, this must be a challenging time for you. With all these problems, do you have difficulties with sleeping?" It turned out that Parvathi was experiencing poor sleep quality, loss of appetite, reduced interest in her work and was presently on leave from her job because it pained her to go as her husband used to visit her there regularly. Yes, she reported, she did household chores, though admitting she had cut down on the number of dishes she cooked. Reducing the number of dishes is a common idiom of distress through which Malayali women communicate their suffering to other family members (cf. Nichter 1981). The depression checklist interrogation continued. To the question, "During the day, are you inclined to lie down?" Parvathi answered affirmatively. "Do your eyes well up thinking about your husband and children like this?" Parvathi moved her head affirmatively. "Does *veshamam* [sadness] grip you? Have you been someone with reasonable *manobalam*? Could you handle your mother-in-law's criticism with sufficient courage?" "Yes," Parvathi replied to all these questions. "Do you feel you have lost your will power [*manobalam*]?" Parvathi started crying. This last is popularly understood as a symptom and cause for mental illness (while will power is generally an idiom expressing mental health and strength). Dr Mona dug deeper, "Is it a state of losing all hope of the future? Do you feel a lack of purpose in living?" Parvathi admitted that she had suicidal thoughts. "I go through all this. I told my children even yesterday, 'I think about you all, otherwise I'd go with your father.'" Parvathi did not seem to understand why the doctor asked her these questions about her emotional and cognitive state. Again, she returned to the reason for her visit. "What do you suggest for my daughter?" Dr Mona replied,

> Your daughter is caught in a conflict and she needs guidance to come out of that. Meeting Leena Madam [the clinical psychologist] can be construed as helping with her decision-making. After examination, if Madam feels that she needs medical support, she'll send her here. But because your daughter has completed her MBBS, it will be very hard to convince her.

Dr Mona recommended seeing the psychologist and noted that sending Chandra to see the psychiatrist might make her think she had a psychiatric illness.

Dr Mona's attention to avoiding suggesting to Chandra that she had a psychiatric illness may have arisen as a matter of practicality in her case and as a way to ensure she pursued treatment. However, this strategy was consistent with efforts I observed on the part of other doctors to use different registers to avoid ascribing patients the highly stigmatizing label of *manasika rogam*. "What we usually say is not 'mental illness'; we try to avoid this term," Dr Paul explained.[36] "I tell them this is an exaggerated form of stress. This stress leads to insomnia, anorexia, feeling sad." Dr George, another psychiatrist who worked in a general hospital without a psychiatric unit but saw many patients with common mental disorders, explained,

> I will tell the person, "You have *sankadam* [sadness] or you have tension. It is part of your mind". We won't say that he or she is a mental patient. The word *manasika* [mental] is a sacrilege here. They [patients and their relatives] don't like to hear that word. It is quite difficult to say too.[37]

"So how do you explain depression to your patients?" I asked.

> I will say things like "It is *veshamam* [trouble] experienced by the mind. Your mind does not have any illness. There are some problems in your mind. It will be over with the help of these medicines if you continue it and do not stop till I say so."

Dr George used the word *manas* when talking to patients diagnosed with depression and their family members, but not, he stressed, *manasika* or *manasika rogam*.

> We won't say, "You have a mental problem". We will say, "you have a little problem in your mind. You have to take medicines to ease it", "your mind should be relaxed". That is the thing they like to hear. You should feel relaxed in the mind. In this way, patients don't feel they have an illness. They are just feeling weak or tense because of some small problems in their life that occupy their mind.

Psychologist Dr Shaju Manalil, a Catholic priest who runs a counselling centre in Ernakulam, told me that diagnoses are for professionals to communicate with each other and for identifying an appropriate treatment technique, not for patients and their families.[38] Research in the 1960s identified that revealing psychiatric diagnoses to patients and family members runs the risk of stigmatization and therefore interfering with the recovery process (Goffman 1963).[39]

Having offered reassurance about Parvathi's daughter, and a palatable treatment path, Dr Mona then proceeded with the checklist of psychological and somatic complaints for a depressive episode. I quote this in detail to show the translation of the symptoms of depressive episode outlined by the ICD and

DSM into culturally meaningful terms. Parvathi had not come to discuss her own problems but Dr Mona identified a potential medical issue. The doctor began with an opening enquiry that I heard her use many times: "In the midst of all these problems, does a good thing make you happy? Some funny incident happens while travelling by bus, does that make you smile?" Parvathi answered, "yes, it does." "Are you able to watch a good movie or go to the temple and pray?" She sometimes watched movies but did not go to the temple since her husband was very devout and used to go there twice a day, and the place pained her. It turned out that she had lost faith in God – an identified symptom of depression, especially in the context of Ayurveda (Chapter 5). The doctor continued, asking about Parvathi's family history. Her father had a mental illness that made him quick to anger. After some probing, Dr Mona found out that he had suffered from bipolar disorder for which he had undergone treatment. After some talk about physical complaints, blood sugar and regular menstruation, Dr Mona began preparing her for a diagnosis.

> When one's loved one is lost, there is a phase called grief reaction; it is to cope up with the loss. Different people need different periods. In your case, there is a situation that doubles the challenges. Considering your nature, two months was more than enough if there were only that incident to cope with, and had others been supportive. You should have gone to work long ago but you find it difficult because you have an additional burden to confront.

The doctor then asked Parvathi about the relationship she had with her children. One of the things that she asked was if she used to punish the children when she got angry, to which she answered that she would indeed "beat them in order to make them study", which is normal for most parents in Kerala. Parvathi also talked about her children having become gloomy after their father's death, that they were not as energetic as before. Parvathi additionally mentioned difficulty making decisions, and a previous thyroid problem. Then, the doctor made a first step towards conveying a diagnosis not yet in disease terms, but with regards to her *avastha* [inner state]. "You are currently experiencing a state of *vishadam*. It could be due to hormonal imbalance." Some further questioning revealed that Parvathi did not have support caring for her children, experienced sleeplessness and also racing pulse. "Is it increased heartbeat or heaviness?" Parvathi answered, "I experience weakness of the body. At that time, I am invaded by some thoughts and I'd sit crying."

Dr Mona settled on a diagnosis:

> Presently you are going through *vishada avastha* [a state of depression]. The first stage of depression is grief. Generally, people can resolve the state of grief. Some people go into complicated grief, while others enter an episode of depression. During this time, some changes occur in the brain in the form of chemical imbalances. As part of this, many positive qualities

> are lost, such as ability to make decisions or take initiative, self-confidence, energy, enthusiasm, courage and happiness [...]. In spite of having positives in life, one tends to see the negative side and become preoccupied with that. Self-confidence is lost and it becomes a case of "I cannot go ahead." It is because of your current state that you are not able to address the other problems. Otherwise with your inherent smartness, you could somehow manage your three children. Now you are in a helpless state. To correct that chemical imbalance, I am prescribing some medicines. This doesn't mean you are a patient and will be one for the rest of your life. Unless you get over this crisis, your children will choose their own tracks. If they do so, it'll lead to greater problems. To avert that, I'll call Madam [the psychologist] and tell her. I am prescribing a medicine called Zyren 50 [alprazolam] which will correct the chemical imbalance and restore your earlier mood, energy and self-confidence. Zapis [clonazepam] will help you relax during the day and improve sleep quality at night. You can take half of this medicine in the morning and one at night. Whenever you feel uncontrollably restless, experience increased heart beat or have a feeling that something will happen to you, you can take half of this tablet, and take rest for some time.

Dr Mona explained the diagnosis to Parvathi in terms of psychosocial factors and their biological manifestation in the brain as neurochemical imbalance, but she prescribed the benzodiazepines alprazolam and clonazepam that are usually used to treat anxiety disorder. She described the first drug as if it were an antidepressant and the second as if it was designed to aid relaxation and improve sleep. As she explained to me later, the choice of an anxiolytic instead of an antidepressant was pragmatic. Benzodiazepines act immediately while antidepressants take at least two or three weeks to show any effect. She wanted Parvathi to calm down first, develop trust in her as a doctor and hoped that after a while she could start treatment with antidepressants. Still, she managed her new patient's expectations: these medicines were no magic bullet that would provide an immediate cure. "I have prescribed medicines for fifteen days. In this time, you will feel only a change of ten to fifteen per cent. Considering that you have other on-going problems, the rate of improvement might be even lesser." Dr Mona ended the consultation with some final advice:

> You can take the tablets by 9 or 9:15 p.m. and then can continue with your work, so that you can go to bed by the time you naturally go to sleep. The maximum time is 10 p.m. If you are awake after 10 p.m., avoid doing tasks that will tire your brain. If you do not get sleep, you can read difficult portions of ethics such as *Ramayana* and *Bhagavadatha* in order to make you fall asleep. Drink five more glasses of water and avoid sleeping during the day. Daytime sleep can disturb sleep at night.

She then asked Parvathi to wait outside and telephoned the psychologist, Dr Leena. She communicated her impressions of the new patient in Malayalam, and I quote here again at length. Dr Mona's side of this conversation shows what she as a psychiatrist regarded as the essence of this family problem, how diagnoses and problems are communicated between a psychiatrist and a psychologist, and how strategies were developed to conceal medicalization of the situation from the daughter:

> The eldest one passed MBBS. The next one is MBBS first year. The third one is repeating medical entrance test preparation. Here the problem is that each one has an affair. The youngest is a boy. He is getting a lot of phone calls from a number of girls. OK, never mind, because he is a boy. The eldest one has an affair with a boy who has finished his MBBS. When her father was alive he exercised some control over their relationship. Mother is not so assertive as to have any control over the affair. She gets very irritable. Sometimes she gets violent also. A chart has already been taken for the daughter. But she is not willing to see a doctor. It is hard to get her to see a psychologist or the psychiatrist. [...] Do something at least to modify the behavioural problems if not the pervasive depression. But the problem is she won't come in. She is saying that she has no problem. My patient [Parvathi] says that if her daughter could be brought in on the pretext of calling her to discuss the matter of the mother, there is a chance of talking to her. Is it possible to give them time today because they are coming from Cheriparambu [about two hours by car from the hospital]?

Dr Mona was worried that Parvathi and Chandra might leave before seeing the psychologist. So she called Chandra in and – following her strategy of presenting the psychological consultation as if targeting her mother while in fact focusing on the daughter – she named and explained her mother's diagnosis as one MBBS-trained doctor to another. She related her mother's depression to genetic factors, mentioned the death of her father as the most important triggering factor and alluded to other factors without being specific. At the same time, she admonished Chandra about the importance of her mother's recovery with regard to her own future and that of her siblings:

> Your mother has severe depression. The medicines prescribed are for depressive disorder. When there is a depressive episode there are some changes in the brain, in the neurotransmitters. There are some psychosocial factors also, loss of father. That is the most important psychosocial pressure. There are also some other psychosocial stresses going on. So even if we give antidepressants the chances of a full recovery are difficult. What can be done is to give medicine to correct the neurobiology. To correct the social psychology or the environmental factors you have to take some initiative. Your mother has a significant family history and a genetic predisposition. There were people who had depressive and bipolar disorders in your mother's family. If she doesn't recover from the disease it will repeat every year. It will affect the future of each of you. By now you have no

> other caregiver. You have to take decisions and take care of yourselves. That's your situation.

In order to "discuss the psychosocial problems", Dr Mona suggested breaking for lunch and that the women come back after to see the clinical psychologist. She had spent about an hour with Parvathi and Chandra and written a six-page report.[40] For the diagnosis, she wrote "depressive episode severe, plus psychotic". Now she was exhausted and took her lunch in her office.[41]

Although Dr Mona identified socio-economic and psychological causes in this case, she located the main pathology in the brain and therefore in physical factors. This is in line with the approach of all psychiatrists in Kerala with whom I spoke or whose practice I observed. Neurochemical changes in the brain are the most fundamental etiology used to account for depression and to be addressed with treatment. "Though depression has many socio-economic reasons, there will be a chemical change in the neurotransmitters in the brain of the patients who suffer from depression. That means a biological reason is always there," explained psychiatrist Dr Indu V. Nair to the audience of mental health professionals and laypeople at the celebration of Mental Health Day 2012 "Depression – a global crisis" in Thiruvananthapuram.[42] Although many patients come seeking help for unresolved problems that call for psychosocial solutions, their issues are mainly constructed as neurochemical imbalances and dealt with chiefly through pharmacological treatment. As sociologist Nikolas Rose has identified,

> all explanations of mental pathology must 'pass through' the brain and its neurochemistry – neurons, synapses, membranes, receptors, ion channels, neurotransmitters, enzymes, etc. Diagnosis is now thought to be most accurate when it can link symptoms to anomalies in one or more of these elements.
>
> (Rose 2003, 57)

"Do you explain about neurochemical changes?" I asked Hindu psychiatrist Dr Lakshmi Nair of the Guruji Institute of Medical Sciences.[43] "Yes, some of the people want to know why this is happening," she replied.

> Then I tell them, there are certain chemicals in your brain which make you feel happy or motivated. So these chemicals have some kind of effect for developing depression along with other factors such as genetics or experiences in your childhood. This is why you have a tendency to develop the illness when you are exposed to some stress or sometimes by itself. That is how I explain it to them. Many of them, if you sit and explain, then it pays off because then people are more compliant with medications. Otherwise what happens is that they don't take the medication or they take it for one week and they say, nothing happens, then they stop it.

Through neurochemical imbalance of the brain, as serotonin and norepinephrine insufficiency, depression is formulated in terms of a disease entity. At a training session for lay caregivers at private (often religious) rehabilitation centres for people with mental illness, the aim was to teach these individuals basic knowledge of psychiatric, nosology and pharmacology. In this programme, psychiatrist Dr Paul explained a local version of the global biopsychiatric notion of depression and underpinned the professional authority of psychiatrists:[44]

> There's not much difference between mental and physical illnesses. You all know about heart disease, it involves damage in the heart. You know about liver disease, or that a kidney can have problems. You all know about the cause of diabetes; it is because of the reduction of the insulin level in the body. Similarly, human beings have an organ called *brain*. If there are some problems in the *brain*, especially any *imbalance in its chemicals*, it gets manifested as behavioural variations. Since the term *manasika rogam* [mental illness] has been in vogue a long time and since people think about the phenomenon called mind, this term (*manasika rogam*) has taken shape. In truth, it is a brain disease, similar to kidney or heart disease. As such, it has no differences from physical illness. The only difference is that its symptoms are shown through behavioural variations.

Dr Paul went on to counter local misconceptions and false beliefs about the cause of mental illness. He first addressed the vernacular explanations that I also heard discussed when people reflected upon the reasons for behavioural changes and emotional distress, namely fear [*peti*] and weak character:

> Why do mental diseases occur? Many people say, "I got scared [*petichu*], or my wife's behaviour is part of her character, or there are many financial problems", many reasons are attributed. All these are superficial things. In truth, mental illness happens due to imbalances of chemicals in the brain. Until about twenty years ago, even doctors were unaware of the presence of chemicals in the brain. It is only in the last ten, fifteen, or twenty years that we have come to understand about the chemicals in the brain. Similarly, what are the changes that happen in the brain when one gets angry or laughs? Now because medical science understands the neurochemistry of the brain and the impact of chemicals on behaviours, my colleagues and I can authentically say that it is brain disease [*brain rogam*] more than mental illness [*manasika rogam*].

He then shifted towards popular psychological explanations that locate the cause of mental illness in childhood experiences. "Does it happen because of incidences during childhood? No! People should clearly understand this." Then followed a question and answer session with the audience who asked about the neurochemical narrative Dr Paul explained: "Doctor, you said that mental illness occurs due to problems in the brain. So the notion that the cause of mental illness is due to tradition and environment is wrong, isn't it?" "Yes, that idea is wrong," he answered. "Tradition and the environment can influence the disease. But the fundamental cause of mental illness is always the structure and function of the brain." After a few more questions, another psychiatrist spoke about false conceptions as opposed to the scientific view of the nature of the mind. What were presented as misconceptions or superstitious assumptions about mental illness in training programmes like these including possession, occult violence, or depression arising from a lack of *manobalam* were very interesting for me because these were the conceptions and etiologies that I encountered time and time again in patient and family narratives in the course of my fieldwork. With regard to local conceptions of *manas*, people pointed to their heart or chest for both heart *and* mind when they used this term. Dr Paul wanted to replace the notion of *manas* with a scientific concept of the mind as arising from the function of the brain. Proposing "Now, what do you mean by 'mind'," he continued:

> Where is it located? What is it? Can we locate it or show it to another person? Is it an organ? All of us talk about mental health and mental illness. What is mind? The function of the brain could be basically called the mind. It comprises many parts of brain. Mind is one of the functions of brain. Mostly we point out to our chest when we say something about mind. But really it is the function of brain.

Just as in the present era of neurochemical conception of depression all explanations must pass through the brain (Rose 2003), so too do non-medical procedures designed to address the condition. Psychiatrists, both allopathic and Ayurvedic, were quite tolerant of religious healing practices for their psychological or neurochemical effects – so long as they did not interfere with medical treatment. However, this is how Dr Harilal, another psychiatrist at the training programme mentioned above, explained the utility of religious healing practices to the audience:[45]

> Through imaging studies it has been scientifically proven that psychotherapy, belief in God and so on can create favourable alterations in the brain. Any act that can calm the human mind like prayer or meditation plays a significant role in soothing the mind and the brain. All these have their impact on the brain in that they stabilize the brain just like antidepressants. But that doesn't mean that in severe cases of depression, you will have to skip antidepressants and resort to these methods.

Religious healing practices thus become not only "culturally sanctioned stress busters", as Dr C.J. John called them in "Before Seeking Treatment" (John 2009), but also effective in addressing faulty brain chemistry.

Critical scholars of psychiatry and neuroscientists (Rose 2003; Insel 2014) have argued that the construction of depression as arising due to neurochemical imbalance is not a verifiable scientific fact.[46] Cultural psychiatrist Kirmayer and philosopher and psychiatrist Gold make the critique that many psychiatrists, rather than focusing on the complexities of neurological networks, "follow a 'neo-humoral' approach of treating disorders as the result of too much or too little of some neurotransmitter" (Kirmayer and Gold, 2011). This neo-humoral model is a "metaphor" (Jenkins 2011) and a kind of "neuroreductionism" (Kirmayer and Gold, 2011). Kirmayer and Gold distinguish three forms of neuroreductionism: *Methodological reductionism* assumes that it is necessary and sufficient to "break down complex systems and phenomena into simpler components or analogous to study" and to approach pathological behaviour in terms of neurobiological processes; *ontological reductionism* claims that mind is nothing beyond the brain or the brain at work; and *epistemological reductionism* replaces first person narratives by measurement through brain imaging devices such as "ceroscopes" (Kirmayer and Gold, 2011) The reduction of neurological networks to "neohumoralism," the authors stress, is not only a form of simplifying complexities for popular consumption, it is also used in psychopharmacological texts and research but ignores the lack of a straightforward relationship between neurotransmitters and specific behaviours or disorders. This neuroreductionism, however, fits well with the technologies and economic interests of the pharmaceutical industry. Moreover, the neurochemical construction of depression fits with popular ideas about the importance of balance and harmony to well-being (Kirmayer and Gold 2011). Ecks (2013) shows how psychiatrists in West Bengal merge the notion of neurochemical imbalance with the paradigm of humoral imbalance. Probably more than for North America and Europe, the importance of balance and harmony to well-being is a critical component of local conceptualizations of mental health in Kerala. The aim of interventions – pharmacological, psychological and religious – is usually formulated in clinical encounters and in psychiatric writing in the media in terms of bringing peace and balance to the patient. This is based on the underlying assumption that neurochemical balance equals psychological balance, and that correcting imbalances in the brain results in mental peace and social well-being. With regard to harmony, psychiatrists often mobilize a dichotomy of Western and Indian psychiatry (cf. Pinto 2014). This is how psychiatrist Dr Nair explained this difference:

> The Western way of psychiatry or psychotherapy is more self-actualized, to expand your potential. That is the way you can handle a patient with Western education or a Western patient. Whereas in a patient not very exposed to Western culture, you will have to put it in religious or spiritual terms. Something like achieving peace inside or harmony which is more in keeping with what they are thinking, closer to God, closer to perfection in the sense of being closer to God.[47]

Depression as somatic imbalance not only reflects Ayurvedic ideas (Chapter 5) but also allows for different kinds of emotional and social issues to be reconfigured as somatic imbalance resulting from a lack (or excess) of certain chemicals.

Local ideas of mental health frequently refer to notions such as peace of mind, balance and mental strength regarded as synonymous, and often related to religion or spirituality. Further, anthropologist Tanya Luhrmann described local ideas of the mind in South Asia as transactional and social rather than private (Luhrmann 2012). Calmness, peace and balance thus characterize strong *manobalam* and mental health in South India. In accordance with Ayurvedic notions of the mind, vernacular ideas in Kerala regard the mind in more physiological terms. Moreover, the mind, as much as the self and the person, is understood to be permeable rather than bounded. In the anthropology of South Asia, significant attention has been accorded to this sociocentric conception of personhood – in particular, the way it differs from the Western, circumscribed construction (Marriott 1976; Marriott and Inden 1977; Dumont 1980). Recent studies transcend this dichotomy and show that both notions of bounded *and* permeable selves exist and are performed, staged and evident in different contexts and institutions in South Asia (Mines 1994; Lamb 2000; Sax 2009; Basu 2014; Quack 2014). Although most of my interlocutors were not aware of the philosophical ramifications of the notion of manas, I rarely found a notion of mind or emotions to be a reflection of a stable and essential inner self in the way that has been so important in Western early twentieth century psychiatry and psychotherapy. Local vernacular ideas of the mind – just like neurochemical notions, despite the differences between the two – construct it as a product of chemical processes or external agents, as something more contingent than the Western popular notion of mind. I argue that it is this physiological, permeable and non-essentialist notion of the mind that enables the neurochemical imbalance narrative of depression to fall on fertile ground in Kerala

Patients told me that if psychiatrists or other doctors explained depression to them, it was in terms of a chemical imbalance or a serotonin or norepinephrine deficiency. Most patients I met swallowed this narrative along with their antidepressants and handily combined neurochemical imbalance with other medical and religious explanations. But the idea of depression as arising solely from somatic imbalance has not gone without question in Kerala. Subhash (see Preface) who was being treated at the Government Ayurveda Mental Hospital at Kottakkal when we met was sceptical about the neurochemical imbalance narrative. "What came first they [the psychiatrists] don't know," he stated.

> First of all they have seen many patients with depression who had good serotonin levels. Secondly, even if the patient had a low serotonin level, they don't know whether the low serotonin level causes depression or the depression causes low serotonin level. So serotonin is not a help. It's high time that they realign, that they admit they have made a mistake.

Indeed, critical scholars of psychiatry have deconstructed this "unproven" scientific explanation (Healy, 2006), called it a "myth" (Moncrieff 2008) or identified it as a symbol (Jenkins 2011). What the model does accomplish is conveying a therapeutic urgency: it endorses a pharmaceutical solution, making treatment with

SSRIs appear both logical and indispensible. According to Ayurvedic psychiatrist Dr Joseph John,

> Doctors often say that there is a lithium deficiency in your body, so we are giving Lithium to you. That is wrong! Lithium is a medication to stabilize the mood, the mind. They pretend that Lithium is essential for all people. This is one trick of Kerala doctors. I am not against that. I am just explaining that they have some tricks in order to convince patients to take the medications. Otherwise the patient will not accept.[48]

This likely holds true for how some doctors present depression as a serotonin deficiency.

While Dr Joseph John and others object to the conception of mania as lithium deficiency or depression as serotonin deficiency, clinical psychologist Anand Kutty went further and criticized the excision of the mind from modern psychiatry in India:[49]

> Here in psychiatry mental illness is considered like any other physical illness. Basically there is no mind in mental illness in India. As far as psychiatry is concerned it had a soul, it lost it. It had a mind, it lost it. Then there is only behaviour. I don't believe in that whatsoever. So we don't have mind here. Mental illness is basically biochemical imbalance, hormonal problems in your brain, an organic problem. So the treatment would be what? To correct the imbalance or to rectify the brain damage, whatever. Basically it is just like any other physical illness. Just like diarrhoea we have depression. So the psychiatric job would be a little bit easier in India. Like you don't have to spend a lot of time with the patient. The patient is smiling a little more, the patient spends his time wandering outside, patient hears some voices, you can diagnose very easily BPAD, mania with psychotic symptoms, whatever. Just because certain biochemicals you are feeling like this. I will take out the biochemicals and you will be all right. It's simple.

Kutty, who received his M.Phil. in clinical psychology from the prestigious National Institute of Mental Health and Neurosciences at Bangalore, used a metaphor for the relationship between the mind and the brain that helped him in his own work and in the explanations he gave to his patients:

> The brain can be thought of as something like a car and the mind is something like the driver. Definitely, the driver cannot move an inch if the car is not functioning. But the car cannot move an inch forward if the driver doesn't want to drive it. So the mind, according to me, rises from the brain, no doubt. You have to have a neurobiological system. [...] But much of mental illness originates from "psychosocial accidents" [...]. Unfortunately, they are just treated biologically by psychiatrists. Instead of motivating the driver to drive, you are unnecessarily repairing the car, you

are trying to push the car. It will move, one kilometre. After that, it will stop, unless the driver takes any action.

The psychiatrist, in his critique, focuses only on the body (the car) while as a clinical psychologist, his job is to focus on the mind (the driver).

Anthropologists have also addressed the neurochemical model of depression and other mental illnesses from the perspective of lack of personal or cultural meaning. Luhrmann (2000) distinguishes between essential and inessential suffering: essential suffering is part of the *conditio humana* and belongs to the sufferer; inessential suffering arises from external forces and is treatable or curable. Central to her critique is the premise that mental illness is inherently different from other kinds of illness in that it is part of essential suffering. In mainstream psychiatry, Luhrmann identifies, essential suffering is turned into inessential suffering and targeted for eradication through the use of pharmaceuticals. Luhrmann is concerned about a decreasing ability to meaningfully encounter psychic suffering due to the ascendancy of the biomedical model (Luhrmann 2000). In a similar vein, Jenkins criticizes the representation of mental illness as biochemical imbalance because it "not only obviously oversimplifies the neuroscientific basis upon which it draws, but also falls flat as an existential and cultural matter of subjectivity" (Jenkins 2011). The neurochemical imbalance narrative, other than psychodynamic or religious framings of depression, provides no existential orientation. This is why Jenkins calls the neurochemical notion of depression a "dead metaphor" that, she argues, for laypeople affords little in terms of the "work of culture" (Obeyesekere 1990) for transforming suffering into meaningful personal subjectivity. Moreover, the neurochemical imbalance narrative as a brain deficit over which a person has little control deprives patients of agency. Jenkins and Luhrmann are pessimistic about implications of this model, but sociologist Nikolas Rose stresses the productivity of neurochemical imbalance narrative with regard to self-governance and agency (Rose 2003). Rather than relocating agency from patients to drugs, Rose argues that this model of depression and pharmacological mood modification produces new forms of agency and enables patients to actively monitor and manage their moods with the help of pharmaceuticals (Rose 2003).

I share this critique of the neurochemical model of depression as bereft of existential meaning and as de-essentializing suffering; however, in my view this critique also overlooks the potential productivity of this model. It is exactly the neurochemical model of depression as a dead metaphor that is experience-distant and removed from the realm of lived reality that encourages local interpretations to flourish. The neurochemical imaginary then serves, as Kitanaka has observed, as an empty symbol "into which rich meaning can be inscribed making local interpretations ever more diversified, creative, and evocative" (Kitanaka 2012, 68). In the Japanese context, Kitanaka identified that the neurochemical language of depression merges with a discourse about the social nature of depression, and gives rise to an idiom of critique (Kitanaka 2012). The same is true in Kerala. Further, Chua (2009) argues that with regard to the psychiatric categories of *samsayarogam* [the illness of doubt] and adjustment disorders in Kerala that the discursive or metaphorical flexibility of psychiatric terminology both enables vernacular forms of meaning making and carries with it the heightened danger of pathologization and stigmatization. Beyond the opposition of psychiatric and locally meaningful expressions of suffering, depression as a neurochemical imbalance can provide an idiom for articulating locally relevant experiences of distress and social suffering for mental health professionals and laypeople alike (Chua 2009). Following Chua and Kitanaka, I argue that it is the ontological instability, "diagnostic liquidity" (Lakoff 2005) or malleability of the neurochemical imbalance narrative of depression and its capacity to merge with other models of affliction and to be appropriated in local discourses that constitutes the nature of what is "at stake" (Kleinman, Das, and Lock 1997) in depression in Kerala.

The relocation of psychiatry from the abandoned spaces of the asylum into the spaces of somatic medicine and the community was a prerequisite for bringing depression into the mainstream and the construction of depression as an epidemic. In this chapter I traced the appropriation and glocalization of depression in mainstream psychiatry on institutional, material and cognitive levels that was closely tied to the increasing creation and acceptance of institutions of treatment and education, drugs intended to cure or manage, clinicians, expert and public knowledge, and a concomitant enlargement of the number and types of people diagnosed with depression. I then examined the ways professional knowledge and expertise about depression are disseminated to the wider public and into popular knowledge by focusing on how psy professionals represent depression in the media and how they selectively translate expert knowledge into the vernacular in a sort of pop psychiatric and psychological discourse. Media representations in Kerala promote depression as a brain disorder or, more specifically, a disorder arising due to neurochemical imbalance in the brain. By constructing depression as a somatic disease psychiatrists aim not only to destigmatize depression but also to secure psychiatry's place in scientific and somatic medicine. In medicalizing behaviours that deviate (even slightly) from local norms and expectations, psychiatrists and psychologists increasingly bring new population groups such as children or adolescents under the purview of the psy disciplines.

Psychiatrists and psychologists in the media often engage vernacular notions of depression as a moral-physiological weakness thus blurring the boundaries between professional and popular framing of depression. In the ways and means that professional knowledge is disseminated to the Kerala population, it is clear that the expansion of the symptomatology of depression and identification of the vulnerable not only produces psychiatric authority but also stabilizes depression as a localized health category. I have further showed that the expansion of depression as a common mental health category and the way it is closely interlinked with the launch, globalization and local appropriation of antidepressants as presumably disease-specific agents. In India as elsewhere, the promotion of antidepressants and depression "disease mongering" (Moynihan,

Heath and Henry 2002) are two sides of the same coin. The medicalization or psychiatrization of suicide as depression is also important to understanding mental health discourse in Kerala. Finally this chapter shifted focus to the cognitive level and explored how psychiatrists frame depression and convey diagnoses to patients and their family members in consultations. This brought into focus the specific forms and processes of the local appropriation and effectiveness of the neurochemical imbalance narrative of depression in Kerala. Although the neo-humoral model of depression is a global narrative, the framing of depression as a neurochemical imbalance in the brain becomes locally embedded by interweaving with local notions of self, person, mind and body in Kerala. It is the ontological instability and fluidity of the neurochemical model of depression that contributes to the stabilization of depression on local level in Kerala, not least due to the malleability of other local discourses of suffering. In the next chapter I investigate the impacts of the glocalization of depression on the subjectivities of those diagnosed with depression, and explore how it feels to be depressed in Kerala.

Notes

1 Dr Ashraf and Dr Girish, Kozhikode, 15 February 2010.
2 An exception is the renowned National Institute of Mental Health and Neurosciences (NIMHANS) in Bangalore.
3 The Little Flower Mental Health Centre is an elegant building housing around 100 inpatients. It is located in the middle of a large green compound where patients walked freely during certain times of the day with caregivers and one or two staff standing by.
4 Anganwadi are institutions that are part of the Indian public health care system and provide basic health care.
5 Blogsite for community psychiatry@NIMHANS,14 March 2013, https://communitypsychiatrynimhans.wordpress.com, accessed 2 July 2015.
6 Dr Indu V. Nair, Thiruvananthapuram, 10 October 2012.
7 *Asha* is an acronym for acquainted social health activist. These are grassroots health care providers. Asha workers are trained to detect cases of common diseases and bring them to health care facilities. They are especially engaged in immunization programmes and health care for women and children.
8 AYUSH is an accronym for Ayurveda, Yoga & Naturopathy, Unani, Siddha, Homeopathy and, since 2012, Sowa Rigpa (Tibetan Medicine). These are the medical systems promoted by the Ministry of AYUSH which replaced the former Department of AYUSH of the Ministry of Health and Family Welfare that again has replaced the former Department of Indian Medical Systems & Homeopathy created in 1995.
9 Dr Matthew Kurien, Ernakulam, 3 October 2012.
10 Saju, Ernakulam, 14 January 2013.
11 Saju, Ernakulam, 5 October 2012.
12 Saju, Ernakulam, 9 October 2012.
13 Electro convulsive therapy (ECT) was not in use after being discontinued two years before due to popular and intense critique.
14 Dr Nair, Ernakulam, 30 January 2013.
15 Savitri Menon, Ernakulam, 1 February 2013.
16 "Disease mongering" or the selling of sickness is a key marketing tactic in the pharmaceutical industry. As Moynihan, Heath and Henry (2002) and others have recently

described, this process involves alliances formed between drug companies anxious to market a product for a particular condition, biosocial groups organized by and for those who suffer from a condition, and doctors eager to diagnose under-diagnosed problems. Mongering includes awareness programmes produced overtly or covertly by the public relations departments of drug companies. These aim to attract the attention of the public, and shape their fears and anxieties into a clinical form (Moynihan, Heath and Henry 2002; Rose 2003).

17 Dr Mohandas, Vythiri, 15 September 2012.

18 If ECT is practised, it is now in modified form using anaesthesia in private institutions, leaving the asylum-like governmental mental hospitals such as Oolampara in Thiruvananthapuram the only places where unmodified "shock treatment" is practised.

19 Priya, Ernakulam, 26 September 2010.

20 Health News, Vishada rogam, www.malayalamtele.com/health-news-vishada-rogam-33-video_f2824ee08.html, 1 April 2014, accessed 20 November 2015.

21 This phrase comes from Aldous Huxley's famous *Brave New World* (1932), in which the drug soma is used by all members of society to deal with unpleasant emotions. In this (fictional) society soma supports key principles of instant gratification, the creation of workers who enjoy their work, happiness as the ultimate goal, and science and technology as the foundations of a good life.

22 Reetamol, Ernakulam, 16 January 2013.

23 Dr Mona, Ernakulam, 16 January 2013.

24 Public Service Commission. All government job vacancies are filled through the PSC. Selection is on the basis of written tests conducted by the PSC

25 Dr Sridhar, Thiruvananthapuram, 20 July 2016.

26 Drug Escitalopram Prize List, www.medindia.net/drug-price/escitalopram.htm, accessed on 1 June 2016.

27 Dr Mona, Ernakulam, 5 September 2012.

28 Dr Mona, Ernakulam, 5 September 2012.

29 Dr R.V. Paul, Ernakulam, 19 September 2012.

30 Dr Girishkumar, Kottayam, 22 January 2013.

31 Yasir Thangal, Kozhikode, 25 February 2010.

32 R.V. Paul, Ernakulam, 28 September 2012.

33 Anand Kutty, Kozhikode, 12 February 2014.

34 See the work of the journalist P. Sainath and the films *Gabhricha Paus* (The Damned Rain, 2009) by Satish Manwar and *Peepli Live* (2010) by Anusha Rizvi.

35 Parvathi, Ernakulam, 8 October 2012.

36 R.V. Paul, Ernakulam, 6 September 2012.

37 Dr George, Aluva, 7 September 2012.

38 Shaju Manalil, Ernakulam, 22 January 2013.

39 There are parallels to the way psychiatrists and psychologists in Kerala avoid sharing diagnoses of mental illness with patients to the way Luhrmann (2012) describes the way schizophrenia is dealt with in North India: "Many of the doctors didn't mention a diagnosis. Many of the families didn't ask. There was a good deal of deception – wives grinding medication into the flour for the daily chapattis they made for their husbands, doctors explaining to patients that they were completely well but should take strengthening pills to protect themselves for the ravages of their youth. As a result, none of the patients thought of themselves as having a career-ending illness, and every one of them expected to get better. And at least compared to patients in the West, they generally did."

40 Dr Mona invested considerable time for her patients. Her and several others' clinical practice of psychiatry that I saw contradicts homogenizing narratives of Indian psychiatrists spending little time for their patients.

41 I did not attend the psychological consultation as Dr Leena regarded outpatient consultations as too private and sensitive. The difficulty for social scientists to get

permission to participate in psychotherapy sessions suggests not only that neurochemical changes in the brain may be easier to share. It could also be a reason why psychosocial issues may be less visible in ethnographic accounts of mental health care in India.

42 Dr Indu V. Nair, Thiruvananthapuram, 10 October 2012.
43 Dr Lakshmi Nair, Ernakulam, 29 January 2013.
44 Dr R.V. Paul, Ernakulam, 28 September 2012.
45 Dr Harilal, Ernakulam, 28 September 2012.
46 Indeed, scholars of Science and Technology Studies (Latour and Woolgar 1979; Mol 2002) have demonstrated that all scientific facts are indeed "made" (as the Latin root word *factum* suggests) through practice such as in the laboratory.
47 Dr Lakshmi Nair, Ernakulam, 30 January 2013.
48 Dr Joseph John, Ernakulam, 6 September 2012.
49 Anand Kutty, Kozhikode, 15 February 2010.

4 Appropriating depression in institutionalized Ayurvedic psychiatry

1 Introduction

This chapter follows depression into the context of an indigenous medical system. I explore the appropriation and translation of the concept of depression and its underlying theories, psychiatric framings and mind/body distinctions in (re)invented Ayurvedic psychiatry. How, I ask, are mainstream psychiatric categories and their etiologies translated into Ayurvedic theory? How is the hegemony of modern psychiatry negotiated, mimicked or contested? How do the institutional regimes of depression come under the purview of, or become mirrored in Ayurveda? How is *bhutavidya* [knowledge of the bhutas] as a branch of Ayurveda reconfigured as Ayurvedic psychiatry and how is the appropriation of depression related to this process? Is there anything on the material level to mimic or resist antidepressants and how is this related to global and local policies? Which medicines and procedures are researched, presented and marketed as being Ayurvedic "antidepressants"? How is depression treated in Ayurveda?

The translation and reframing of depression in Ayurveda can best be described in conjunction with the (re)invention of institutionalized Ayurvedic psychiatry as an emergent field of specialization. The (re)invention of Ayurvedic psychiatry as a separate theory, practice and academic discipline in Kerala demonstrates the ontological power of mainstream psychiatry, as does investigating the ways Ayurveda reproduces and partly resists its categories and associated logics. Faced with resistance from mainstream psychiatric *and* Ayurvedic practitioners and authorities, Ayurvedic psychiatrists are not only busy inventing, defining and professionalizing this field, they are also involved in a politics of recognition with regards to Kerala's public mental health. This chapter traces the establishment of Ayurvedic psychiatry as a separate discipline, and considers the processes involved in its legitimization as scientific and authentic. This includes investigating teaching and clinical praxis, the ways practitioners and teachers engage with the hegemonic discourse of mainstream psychiatry, the reproduction or contestation of the mind-body dichotomy, and the ways professional Ayurveda is demarcated from undisciplined forms and also from religious healing. I show that the asymmetrical translations of mainstream psychiatric nosologies in general, and depression in specific, give rise to important strategies for establishing and legitimizing this discipline not only as scientific and rational but also as credible actors in the network of depression and mental health care in Kerala.

The glocal network of depression involves processes of translation, as does any network comprised of diverse actors. Using a Latourian conceptualization, I argue that the "translation" of depression into Ayurvedic categories serves to enrol Ayurveda into the network of depression and psychiatric care while at the same time maintaining its basic incompatibility and difference. Following Latour and Callon (1981), translations in this sense are:

> all the negotiations, intrigues, calculations, acts of persuasion and violence, thanks to which an actor or force takes, or causes to be conferred on itself, authority to speak or act on behalf of another actor or force. "Our interests are the same", "do what I want", "you cannot succeed without going through me". Whenever an actor speaks, s/he is translating other actors into a single will, of which s/he becomes spirit and spokesman.
>
> (Latour and Callon 1981, 279)

It is through such processes of translation, they suggest, that diverse entities and agents – laboratory researchers, academics, practitioners and social authorities – are linked together (Latour and Callon 1981). This idea of translation is central to actor-network theory:

> Actors in locales separated in time and space are enrolled into a network to the extent that they come to understand their situation according to a certain language and logic, to construe their goals and their fate as in some way inextricable.
>
> (Rose 1999)

Through this kind of translation, Ayurvedic psychiatry is established as a credible actor in the glocal mental health network of depression. By translating Ayurvedic notions and practices of mental health care into allopathic psychiatric language, diagnostic categories and notions of evidence and validity, Ayurvedic psychiatrists confer authority to Ayurveda (its texts and clinical practice) "to speak on behalf of" allopathic psychiatry and thereby integrate into the network of mental health care dominated by allopathic actors.

I deal more specifically with the double processes of translation and purification later in this chapter, but here, suffice it to say that this engagement with mainstream psychiatry – also described as syncretization (Leslie 1992), hybridization (Frank 2004) and creolization (Naraindas 2014a) – is specifically intended to regain autonomy of this reconfigured and invented field of Ayurvedic psychiatry. The endeavour is to produce a fresh, alternative healing system that will be recognized and supported as a key – and distinct – actor in mental health in India. Ayurvedic psychiatry as a (re)invented tradition preserves difference through practices that appear to render dissimilar elements as compatible. These processes of translation in the Latourian sense make incommensurable frames of reference once again commensurable, but it is translation that keeps elements and actors separate and autonomous because of the work of brokers and mediators operating in this crowded space, in the gap shaped by relations of institutional, economic and epistemological power.[1]

The five key aspects of my research and analysis that arise from following depression into this indigenous medical system, which also serve as the organizing themes (and subsections) of this chapter, are: the production of Ayurvedic psychiatric expertise and the professionalization of this field; embodied minds; the politics and pragmatics of nosologies and their translations; Ayurvedic psychiatric treatment; and the politics of recognition. Therefore, in this chapter, I will first describe education and practice within the context of institutionalized Ayurvedic psychiatry at GAMH and the Ayurveda College, Kottakkal (subchapter 2). I will then proceed to deal with the Ayurvedic notion of depression as a physio-cognitive-moral problem (subchapter 3) before I come to the reconfiguration, translation and autonomy of Ayurvedic psychiatry in which I deal with the double processes of translation and purification both towards mainstream psychiatry and towards occult violence (subchapter 4). This chapter then elaborates on Ayurvedic treatment of depression with a special focus on three different kinds of treatment and concludes with a description of the Ayurvedic politics of recognition (subchapter 5).

2 Institutionalized Ayurvedic psychiatry: education and practice

Institutionalized Ayurvedic psychiatry is mainly practised at the Government Ayurveda Mental Hospital and the Ayurveda College in Kottakkal, Malappuram district in Kerala. The Government Ayurveda Mental Hospital (GAMH) was established in 1974 on the joint initiative of a member of the Arya Vaidya Sala and a member of the Legislative Assembly in Trivandrum. The first superintendent was an institutionally and *parampara* [family tradition]-trained medical officer hailing from a family of *vaidyas* [traditional Ayurveda practitioners] that had been treating mental illness for generations. Under his management, the hospital joined the state system and became subject to the direct authority of the Directorate of Indian Systems of Medicine in Tiruvananthapuram. First housed in a smaller Malabar-style mansion on the premises of Arya Vaidya Sala in Kottakkal, it shifted into a larger, modern facility in the late 1990s. Today, GAMH accommodates up to fifty patients, including children (since the 2010 establishment of a child psychiatry unit). The institution boasts free wards and pay wards for inpatients and a daily outpatient facility that attracts patients from different social and religious backgrounds from nearby villages and towns, other parts of Kerala and even other states. The inpatient treatment takes around forty days after which patients return for regular outpatient check-up and treatment.

I first came to GAMH in 2012 and, at that time, the institution comprised a superintendent and three other medical officers – one trained psychiatrist and two general physicians (one with a PhD in psychology). By my later visits, one of the medical officers had assumed the post of superintendent after the retirement of Dr Sundaran. It was perhaps no surprise that Dr Sarasvati became superintendent as she grew up in a family long involved in a healing institution specialising in mental health that combined Ayurvedic medical treatment and mantravadam. Other family members worked in allopathic psychiatry and ritual healing, and she once joked "We used to say that the mental health of Malappuram district was in our hands." On my subsequent visits in 2013 and 2014 Dr Sarasvati was represented by Dr Kumar, a former postgraduate student of Ayurvedic psychiatry at the Ayurveda College, Kottakkal. Two general practitioners without formal psychiatric training were serving as medical officers (staff physicians) and the position of a specialized medical officer was vacant. As staff physicians who do not occupy the post of specialized medical officer are transferred every three years, there is constant fluctuation in the hospital's medical team. Other staff members included Ayurvedic therapists, nurses and other attendants and security staff. So far, no psychologist or psychiatric social worker has been employed although, physicians told me, this is a future goal. A 2014 newspaper report in one of Kerala's largest Malayalam dailies took a critical view, terming the complement of mental health professionals at GAMH insufficient and calling on the government to appoint "psychiatric social workers and a psychologist" to improve the situation.[2] The article also criticized the requirement that GAMH patients be accompanied (by a bystander) as this is difficult for poor patients – who constitute the bulk of the patients at GAMH – to afford or arrange. Finally, the article cited the lack of a rehabilitation programme at GAMH as problematic, although, as Ayurvedic psychiatrists explained me, Ayurveda has a lot to offer in mental health rehabilitation.

On the occasion of the opening of the child psychiatry unit in 2010, doctors employed at GAMH presented a position paper, *Vision 2020,* to the Minster of Health and Family Welfare for Kerala. The paper noted that although the institution's official name is the "Government Research Institute for Mental Disorders" no research takes place there apart from the small-scale work of students.[3] The vision the authors articulated for the future involved dividing the hospital into a research wing and a treatment wing. The research wing would host national and international scientists and support research activities and publications. GAMH and Kottakkal were ideal sites for such research, Dr Kumar argued, as they already brought together patients, college students and the Oushadhi pharmacy.[4] The aim behind developing GAMH as a proper research site and institution, Dr Chandra stressed, was to become a key actor in mental health policy in Kerala and in India more broadly.[5] "India's and Kerala's mental health policy," she argued,

> now revolve around modern psychiatry. All mental health plans, programs, everything is for modern psychiatry. There are no recommendations or

> suggestions regarding how Ayurvedic psychiatrists can contribute to mental health programs. There is nothing in there for how Ayurveda should be operating in the mental health area. There is no mention of Ayurvedic psychiatry at all. If there are policy recommendations, everything else follows.

It was a Wednesday morning in mid-March 2011 when, as usual, I went to the P.S. Varier Ayurveda College, Kottakkal to attend the general *manasika OPD* [psychiatric outpatient clinic] conducted by students on the postgraduate course in Ayurvedic psychiatry. Before shifting to the outpatient block attached to the college hospital (built in 2014) where each department had their own outpatient room, the psychiatric outpatient clinic had been located separately from the outpatient block in the rooms of the department of *Kaya Chikitsa*[6] located in a small flat building at the rear of the College campus. The psychiatric outpatient clinic opened in 1997, three years before the postgraduate course *manovigyan avum manas rogam* or simply "Ayurvedic psychiatry" (three-year programme) was established which produced its first graduates in 2003. This course accepts six students a year, and completion qualifies students to teach in Ayurveda colleges and practise as Ayurvedic general doctors or psychiatrists.[7] By 2014, approximately sixty candidates had received their MD (Ay)[8] and were qualified in psychiatry. As in biomedicine, students of Ayurveda are granted a place on a postgraduate course according to their marks and rank and apply through a central tender procedure. In Ayurveda as in allopathy, psychiatry is not a prestigious specialization (Chapter 1). Allopathic psychiatrists are fighting to establish the status of their discipline as scientific medicine, but Ayurvedic psychiatrists in addition face the burden of negative connotations associated with Ayurvedic psychiatry (i.e., that it is based in superstition, backward or related to spirit possession). Unlike allopathic psychiatrists, however, fewer of those who study Ayurvedic psychiatry go on to work as psychiatrists, and not all Ayurveda practitioners who work with psychiatric patients have completed a postgraduate qualification in psychiatry. There are several reasons for this situation. One is the stigma associated with psychiatry. If an Ayurvedic doctor specializes in psychiatry and writes it on the practice board, patients are likely to feel stigmatized on entering the clinic. Moreover, Ayurvedic psychiatry is still not very well known beyond Kottakkal and people seek Ayurvedic treatment mainly for other somatic complaints, mostly aches, pains and allergies. In general, the number of Ayurveda patients is less than that of allopathic medicine. Young doctors of Ayurveda who start their own clinic by necessity must treat all kinds of diseases. Though specialization is required in the BAMS degree (Bachelor of Ayurveda, Medicine and Surgery), most do not practise as specialists – either in psychiatry or in other concentrations – and students told me that specialization mainly serves academic purposes. A third reason is the lack of posts for Ayurvedic psychiatrists. Apart from GAMH in Kottakkal, there are no other government mental hospitals and less than a handful small private clinics that specialize in psychiatry in Kerala. Although the recently founded Association of Ayurveda

Psychiatry and other organizations such as the allopathic Kerala State Mental Health Authority (KSMHA) demand the establishment of psychiatric units in Ayurveda general hospitals, these institutions do not have any beds officially designated for psychiatric patients. I say "officially" because in almost all Ayurveda general hospitals that I visited I found patients diagnosed with depression or anxiety. One college hospital in a larger town had a doctor who was well known for her expertise in mental illness and saw many patients with mental health problems although she had no special training in psychiatry and the hospital officially had no beds for mental patients. Similarly, many of the non-institutionally trained vaidyas also used to treat people with mental health problems.

The Ayurveda College psychiatric clinic is run by first, second and third year students, supervised in the first years by a senior doctor of the college. Patients arrived, usually accompanied by one or more family members, and spoke first with the head of the outpatient department (OPD). Then they were entrusted to one of the second or third year students who would take over their case either as part of their postgraduate research or because they had already had contact with the patient. The student doctor took the patient to a separate room establish the patient's history and follow up. As late as 2009 students and patients would all sit together in one large room, clustering together in what could hardly be glossed privacy. In 2010, however, I was surprised to see students taking their patients to a separate room. The board outside read "counselling unit", and though the furnishing was rudimentary there were large curtains that separated the room into three spaces, which provided a modicum of privacy. The door of the general consultation room was always left open, and the line of patients waiting to be seen began at the room's entrance so these consultations were usually observed by other patients and their family members. However, the longer, more extensive interviews students conducted with their patients were conducted in the relative privacy of the curtained-off areas. Students and teachers had been trying out various systems for managing the OPD.

One experiment was to devote the morning hours of each day to specific kinds of patients. The kinds of diseases, formulated and clustered together in modern and popular psychiatric terms, had also changed over the years. The Wednesday that I visited in March 2011 was one of two *ellam manasika* [all mental disorders] days, whereas Mondays were devoted to alcoholism, Tuesdays to *vishadam* [sadness, confusion], *utkanta* [anxiety] and *tenshan* [tension], and Fridays to child psychiatry (dedicated mainly to children who suffered from learning disabilities or autism). Yet, most patients were not aware of this arrangement and in any case were unlikely to know their diagnosis, so patients came with any problems on any day of the week, though the OPD was always particularly busy on Wednesdays.

This Wednesday morning, however, neither the students nor their mentors were in the psychiatric OPD room. Instead, they gathered in front of the department, equipped with placards and ready to join the campus-based strike that had been initiated by college's Postgraduate Students Association (PGSA). In this strike, students demanded a dedicated psychiatric department with posts for full, assistant and associate professors. Student strikes, mostly organized by one of the student parties associated with the Marxist or Congress parties, are a common phenomenon in Kerala colleges. At these times, the empty college becomes what Lukose calls an "evacuated public space" (Lukose 2009). Like other public spaces such as roads, shops, schools and public transit, the college is "an embattled terrain, a technology of citizenship in which struggles over its proper functioning constitute a struggle over the meaning of democratic citizenship" (Lukose 2009, 142). The psychiatric OPD was empty that morning as students and teachers marched through the college campus and the hospital, some with fists clenched and raised, shouting slogans like *Inquilab zindabad!* [long live the revolution!] and voicing their discontent and demand for solutions: "Where are the teachers, where are the classes? Arrange teachers and classes, arrange patients and departments!" Accusing the CEO and the principal of the college they shouted: "You are P.S. Varier's dream! Aren't you shameful? Simply sitting on easy-chair under the fan, open your eyes!" A student speaker added:

> In Kottakkal College, there is a PG psychiatry course! Even after thirteen years, there are no teachers and no classrooms! There is no department![9] Officials sit with closed eyes! Studying for entrance test after crossing the hurdle of entrance students joined the PG course. Negligent officials! Shame, shame management! You took 15,000 rupees fees from us! You have filled your box with it!

When they finally ended up in the entrance hall of the college's administration building, the representative of the PGSA presented their key concerns:

> The prevalence of mental diseases has increased very much due to the changed circumstances of our lives. As more people are affected by mental diseases the supply of health care delivery needs to be increased. The relevance of having a large number of qualified doctors has been steadily increasing.

In this way, the global mental health discourse of an increase in mental disorders, of a treatment gap, lack of spending in mental health care delivery plays out in political demands made by students of Ayurvedic psychiatry. They stress the importance of producing qualified allopathic but also Ayurvedic psychiatrists as mental health experts. Although the *manasika* [psychiatry] postgraduate course – the only one in Kerala – had been established thirteen years ago, there was still no manasika department in the college, no head of department and no professor specializing in psychiatry. The PGSA demanded one full, one associate and one assistant professor. However, the Central Council of Indian Medicine (CCIM) was against the establishment of a manasika department, students later told me.[10]

Every day, class was supposed to be held from 2 to 4 p.m. After completing their morning work either at the College or GAMH and having their lunch, students gathered in the library of the kaya chikitsa department, chatting, working on their theses, preparing presentations and waiting. "Will there be a class today?" I used to ask. Often, the students did not know. It depended on whether one of their senior colleagues, the second or third year students, had prepared a class, whether a professor from the college was inclined to give a class – which was rarely the case – or whether an allopathic psychiatrist, a psychologist or somebody from outside had been invited to teach for the afternoon. On many days we waited in vain. When there was a case presentation, students gathered in the classroom. With a professor of kaya chikitsa in charge, the senior student presented a case or spoke on a subject such as "Depression, the modern view", "Depression, the Ayurvedic view" or "The Ayurvedic management of schizophrenia", and afterwards students asked a few questions. Most of the cases the senior students presented were GAMH inpatients.

Although there have always been Ayurvedic practitioners who also treated mental health problems, the establishment of Ayurvedic psychiatry as a distinct field of specialization is a recent phenomenon, closely associated with GAMH and the Ayurveda College, Kottakkal. Students complained that there was no department for Ayurvedic psychiatry and that although the course had been running for more than a decade and state regulations for Ayurvedic colleges required a separate department for a postgraduate course, that it was still housed in the Department of Kaya Chikitsa. Dr Kapur, then in charge of the manasika course, told me that apart from providing students with professors and regular classes, the establishment of a manasika department would also impact patient admissions at the college hospital.[11] Legally, aggressive or suicidal patients cannot be admitted to a general hospital. A separate psychiatric ward with trained staff and security based on the model of allopathic general hospital psychiatric units would be required. This also depended on the establishment of a manasika department at the college because at that time, only patients with mild depression, anxiety or alcohol dependence could be admitted to the college hospital. A psychiatric unit would also provide postgraduate students with the facilities for their research, as otherwise most relied on GAMH inpatients, Dr Kapur explained. This made it difficult for students as they had to follow GAMH protocols. "They [doctors at GAMH] don't use single medicine, they are using treatment packages. But we have to do research on single drugs or single combinations," he said. As Pritha, a postgraduate student complained, in the college the students did not have access to enough cases.

> We don't get much exposure to psychiatric patients in the college. Teachers are not interested. If they wanted they could get much more patients, but they treat them at home. Our training is almost a purely academic endeavour only. We study books and texts but we have only little clinical experience. That will come only once we start practising.[12]

A department of psychiatry and regular classes were just two of a suite of demands made by practitioners of Ayurvedic psychiatry who formed the

Association of Ayurveda Psychiatrists (AAP). Because there are not enough posts in the field of mental health to employ the students who qualify in Ayurveda psychiatry, their expertise and the potential benefits for public mental health are lost. This is why another key demand was for every Ayurveda district hospital to create one psychiatrist post. The Kerala State Mental Health Authority (KSMHA), a mainstream psychiatric body, also supports this demand. The AAP was founded in 2012 as a forum and a lobby for those doctors who practised Ayurvedic psychiatry in both government and private settings, and either specialized in psychiatry or engaged in general practice. The founders of this association were mainly young, engaged practitioners, and most had not settled in permanent jobs. The main goal of this association and of those participating in the strike described above is the promotion of Ayurvedic psychiatry. One of the main hurdles they have to overcome is that Ayurveda is popular in Kerala, but mainly for the treatment of pain, psychosomatic diseases, skin problems and what are known as "lifestyle disorders". For most people – allopathic mental health professionals, religious practitioners and laypeople – the use of Ayurveda for the treatment of mental health problems is still largely unknown outside Kottakkal.

Although with regard to professionalization, Ayurvedic psychiatry has grown significantly there are still major obstacles on the path to wide public recognition. I now investigate the complex processes of translation and purification that are involved in the professionalization of Ayurvedic psychiatry before moving to consider in detail the Ayurvedic treatment of depression and the politics of recognition. But before doing so it is necessary to describe the Ayurvedic notion of depression.

3 The physiology and morals of depression[13]

My fieldwork in Ayurvedic psychiatry began with several weeks of intensive instruction in Ayurvedic theory and practice. Each time I met a new doctor, I introduced myself and my interest in Ayurvedic understandings and treatment of depression. This introduction involved several layers of translation. For example, the incompatibility of Ayurvedic notions of mental illness came across in responses from doctors such as "There is no concept in Ayurveda that is the same as depression" or "you won't find a system of psychiatric classifications as you find in the ICD [International Classification of Diseases of the World Health Organization (WHO)]. What we have are umbrella terms". At the same time, doctors, college instructors and students in class, in clinical practice, and in researching and writing their MD theses were constantly involved in translation processes. The double process of incompatibility and translation so characteristic of institutionalized Ayurvedic training stood out clearly. I deal in greater detail with these processes of translation and purification below,[14] but in this section I focus on those Ayurvedic concepts that are translated into or correlated with mild, moderate and severe depression in training and clinical practice. In the pages that follow, I present an introduction into the Ayurvedic notion of depression or more precisely an introduction into the etiology, pathogenesis and symptoms of *vishadam, kaphonmada* and *adhijonmada*[15] as they are taught and practised in Kottakkal. Scholars of Ayurveda have dealt with Ayurvedic notions and treatment of mental illness and occasionally touched upon depression (Langford 2002; Giguère 2009; Halliburton 2009; Naraindas 2014a), but to date the Ayurvedic approach to depression has not been described in detail. I begin this subchapter with a brief introduction to notions of Ayurveda required to understand the theory that follows. Then, I elaborate on the notions of vishadam, kaphonmada and adhijonmada and their *nidana* [etiology] and *samprapti* [pathogenesis]. Finally I provide an analysis of depression as a physio-cognitive-moral problem and situate this within anthropological theories of self and person in India.

This subchapter explores a theory of depression as it is negotiated and practised in institutionalized Ayurvedic psychiatry. Ayurvedic practitioners understand and treat depression as a problem at once physiological, moral and cognitive. This approach is deeply intertwined with the Ayurvedic concept of mental health as *doshic* [humoral] balance and involving mental strength, self-control, equanimity and clarity. Although in this elaborated form it is part of an Ayurvedic scholarly discourse, this concept is in its basic assumptions shared by vernacular physiology and embodied experiences of mental health in Kerala. Most Malayalis are not familiar with Ayurvedic psychiatric theory but do have an understanding of mental illness as heat in the head or in the body, as lack of mental strength or as weakness. Since applications such as oil or medicated mudpacks have long been part of folk medicine for mental illness in Kerala, most Malayalis are at least somewhat familiar with many of the Ayurvedic psychiatric procedures. Moreover, many Malayalis share a notion of mental illness as a product of physio-moral imbalance. Malayalis speak of an "imbalanced lifestyle" or "imbalanced food". The notion of imbalance provides a popular idiom for talking about both physical and mental illness in Kerala. It is, as Rhodes notes is the case in Sri Lanka,

> an idiom in which moral and physical balance can be talked of in the same breath, so that excess in the sense of 'transgression of moral limits' and excess in the physical sense often go together and provide mutually reinforcing meanings for the events of daily life.
>
> (Rhodes 1980)

The three texts that are regarded most authoritative for the teaching and practice of Ayurveda, are the Caraka Samhita, Susruta Samhita and the Asthangahrdaya Samhita of Vaghbata. The earliest of these texts have been written before 200 BCE and 400 CE while the Asthangahrdaya Samhita has been dated around 600 CE. These texts are closely associated with the philosophical traditions of Samhkya, Yoga, Nyaya and Vaisesika (Weiss 2015; Halliburton 2009). The focus on the Asthangahrdaya Samhita in Kerala rather than the Caraka and the Susruta Samhita elsewhere in South Asia is a characteristic feature of Kerala

Ayurveda. In these "great three" Sankrit texts mentioned above and in the clinical practice of Ayurveda, illnesses of the body and of the mind are understood in relation to the *doshas* [humours or principles], *dhatus* [tissues], *agni* [digestive fire] and *prakrti* [constitution] of the patient. Additionally, for practitioners of Ayurvedic psychiatry the *gunas* [qualities] or mental doshas are of salient importance. The three doshas may present either in their normal or physiological state according to individual constitution or in their faulty or harmful state. They are called "dosha", which in Malayalam means "fault or harm", because they can cause problems or illnesses, Dr Rasheed explained.[16] The doshas are both principles and substances governing the physiological functioning of the body and the mind. Health requires their balance while illness is the result of their imbalance. The three doshas – *vata, pitta* and *kapha* – are often translated as the humours (wind, bile and phlegm) of Greek humoral medicine. However, this translation is problematic because it carries the connotation that the three doshas are physical substances, and this is only part of their meaning. Many scholars of Ayurveda describe doshas rather as "principles" (Langford 2002), "principles of relationship" (Halliburton 2009), or ways of thinking about the body. These principles are "linked through an elaborate system of correspondences not only to somatic processes, but also to processes in the environment" (Langford 2002, 29). The idea of dosha circumvents, as Langford (2002) stresses, the conceptual split between the body and the world. My Ayurvedic interlocutors translated vata as the moving principle, pitta as the transforming and kapha as the stabilizing principle. Many types of pain, emotional upheaval and distress are related to vata. Additionally, vata is dry, pitta is hot and kapha is cool. Yet doshas are not only an abstract but also a concrete part of the physiology of the body. I often heard practitioners speak of kapha when referring to mucus or of pitta when referring to vomit. Healing consists of pacifying the vitiated doshas and bringing them back to their physiological, normal or balanced state. Depression as an illness is, then, a deviation from an individual's normal physiological state.[17] Other important notions are dhatu and *agni*. Food is converted into seven dhatus[18] with the help of agni, [digestive fire]. If agni is too weak or disturbed, the metabolic process that transforms food into tissues does not work smoothly. This may lead to depletion of any of the seven dhatus with *ojakshaya* [depletion of the vital essence of the metabolic process] being the most problematic form. The emphasis in institutionalized Ayurvedic psychiatry, however, is not so much on the dhatus because, in the words of Dr Nayar, "the dhatus refer more to the somatic levels. You cannot relate the mind to the dhatus."[19]

More important for Ayurvedic theorizing and clinical practice of mental illness are the three gunas: sattva, rajas and tamas. Sattva indicates a healthy or pure mind, whereas rajas [activity and change] and tamas [darkness, heaviness, plumpness, ignorance] are viewed as nocuous qualities that can cause mental illness. In this sense, *hina sattva* [deficient sattva quality] constitutes the predisposition for all mental disorders, whereas *sattvabalam* [mental strength] prevents them. Ayurvedic psychiatrists also describe their patients with reference to sattva. Persons with *pravara sattva* [a high level of sattva] have robust mental health and are morally strong while persons with a low level of sattva lack these qualities and are therefore more vulnerable to mental illness and more difficult to treat. Enhancing these qualities and increasing the level of sattva is thus a key part of rehabilitation or preventive treatment once the acute problem has been addressed through purifying and pacifying therapeutic procedures. Although the gunas are often termed "mental doshas" and thus psychologized, they are in fact physio-moral qualities of the material and intangible material world according to Samkhya philosophy.

Depression of two kinds

Three terms are drawn upon in the context of glocalizing and translating depression in Ayurveda in Kerala: kaphonmada, vishadam and adhijonmada. Rather than being a categorical distinction, the difference between kaphonmada and vata vitiation is a continuum, similar to the continuum of mild, moderate and severe depression. Mild depression is correlated with vata vitiation and severe depression with a predominance of kapha dosha and a more significant impairment of the mental faculties. During their academic training, students of Ayurveda are taught the theoretical possibility of diagnosing severe depression and other mental disorder along with certain *graha* diagnoses,[20] but this has little clinical or diagnostic relevance. Students and practitioners do not think in terms of graha categories but in terms of vishadam, kaphonmada and adhijonmada and also in terms of mainstream psychiatric notions such as depression, schizophrenia and bipolar disorder.

In the Ayurveda College, students and teachers of the manasika course mainly differentiated between two kinds of depression: vishadam and kaphonmada. Vishadam was described as a symptom of vata vitiation while kaphonmada is used to refer to a syndrome or illness category. Vishadam, I was told, can be translated as the mild or neurotic form of depression or as reactive depression.[21] It manifests mainly as emotional disturbance or tension in reaction to external stressors including depressed mood, crying spells, anxiety, anger, agitation, sleeplessness and excessive worry. It is further characterized by sleeplessness, physical fatigue, difficulties thinking and speaking, and mild psychomotor retardation or agitation. Some practitioners also translated vishadam as confusion related to a lack in mental strength closely associated with Arjuna's *vishada yogam* [yoke of suffering] in the Bhagavad Gita.[22] The warrior Arjuna's predicament when he was confronted with his relatives and teachers as adversaries on the battlefield is often framed in terms of confusion about which path to take rather than in terms of sadness, hopelessness or despair. "In my opinion, depression is confusion," Dr Hari Namboodiri, a general Ayurveda physician "traditionally" trained in a *gurukula* [traditional school], answered when I asked him about depression.[23]

> This confusion could come in many ways; confusion because of fear of what will happen in the future or confusion because of too much desire. If

we don't follow *dharma* [righteous path, often related to one's predestined fate], we get into confusion.

In the course of our interview, he often used the term "confusion" to refer to depression. Similarly, Dr Manikandan (a doctor of Ayurveda and college teacher at Kottakkal) understood depression as confusion to be caused by a lack of sattva.[24] "In depression, a person is confused. His thoughts are covered with something, no proper thoughts are there, proper knowledge is not there, sattva is much less."[25] Both framings of vishada as sadness, despair or anxiety on the one hand and as confusion on the other indicate a somatic, cognitive *and* moral understanding of depression.

Vata vitiation and emotional disturbance are closely interrelated. Grief, anxiety and confusion can vitiate vata, while vata vitiation may manifest in excessive crying, anxiety and other signs of emotional disturbance. On the other hand, vishadam can "manifest in pure somatic symptoms such as aches and pains only", as Dr Krishnan explained.[26] By framing depression as an impairment or reduction of vata, Ayurvedic doctors elaborate an integrated understanding of "somatization" that contradicts mainstream psychiatrists' interpretation of somatization as a process of masking what are assumed to be psychological symptoms behind the expression of somatic symptoms. As vata vitiation, depression manifests at both the mental and somatic levels. Depression as vishadam is not perceived as a mental illness and does not require purifying inpatient treatment but can be managed with pacifying and mind-strengthening formulations and applications, counselling or psychotherapy, and (more rarely) yoga. In mainstream psychiatric and popular psychiatric discourse, vishadam and vishada rogam are the Malayalam translations of depression and depressive disorder, but for Ayurvedic psychiatrists vishadam is not a disease category per se but one of many symptoms of vata affliction. However, as many practitioners stressed, if vishadam persists it may develop into kaphonmadam.[27]

Vishadam is a symptom, but kaphonmada is a syndrome and a specific illness. *Unmada* [madness, mental illness] is characterized, I was taught at the college, by dysfunction of the mind, intellect, orientation of self in time, place and person memory, desire, habits, psychomotor activities and morals. Five forms of unmada are described in the classical texts relevant to the teaching and clinical practice of Ayurvedic psychiatry: in addition to *vatonmada* [a state characterized by unsteadiness of thought and emotions and psychotic features], *pittonmada* [a state characterized by excessive emotions or passions] and kaphonmada, the texts mention *sannipadonmada* [mental illness involving the vitiation of all three doshas], *vishonmada* [mental affliction due to toxins] and *adhijonmada* [mental illness following a loss]. The signs and manifestations of these doshic forms of unmada in the classic texts are described in physical, cognitive and emotional terms (Langford 2002: 236). Ayurvedic psychiatrists correlate kaphonmada with severe or endogenous depression that may or may not involve psychotic elements. Vishadam affects the dysfunction of *manas* [mind and emotions] only but kaphonmada additionally includes dysfunction of other mental faculties such as intellect, consciousness, memory, desire, manners, behaviour and conduct. Then, Dr Krishnan explained,[28] the person becomes "like a chariot without a charioteer", a phrase I heard often. In the development of kaphonmada, both kapha and vata are aggravated or vitiated and the accumulated kapha spreads to the mind-carrying channels that I describe below.[29] Gloominess, desire for solitude, disobedience and depressed mood are mainly related to vata, in combination with kapha dosha. If vata is vitiated, Dr Krishnan said, nothing is there to control the mind. This leads to depression and other mental diseases. For treatment, he continued, kapha has to be removed by *shodana* [purification] treatment and vata has to be pacified by *samana* [pacification] treatment. Vishadam does not require inpatient treatment and can be managed with Ayurvedic drugs and counselling alone. Kaphonmada, however, requires more intensive treatment, through purging and purifying procedures including internal and external oileation of the body, sweating, therapeutic vomiting and nasal treatment.

Dr Nayar specified the relationship between vata vitiation and kapha accumulation, integrating the modern concept of depression as the manifestation of neurochemical changes in neurotransmitters.[30] "If kapha blocks the *manovahashrotas* [mind-carrying channels]", he explained, "then vata cannot pass through. Vata is responsible for the regulation of the mind, and stimulates the connection between a sensory object, a sensory organ, the mind, and discriminating intellect." "Modern" (allopathic) doctors, he said, express the carrier function of vata in terms of neurotransmitters. Like vata, serotonin and noradrenalin carry information from one neuron to another. For allopathic as well as Ayurveda doctors, according to Dr Nayar, the carrying function of vata, or serotonin and noradrenalin, is disturbed in depression. In Ayurveda, this disturbance is conceptualized as a blockage caused by aggravated kapha. "By reducing the blockage of kapha", he concluded, "Ayurvedic practitioners stimulate the neurotransmitters as vata and the neurotransmitters are functionally the same." As becomes clear in Dr Nayar's explanation, the pathogenesis of depression is framed in a hybrid fashion drawing on both Ayurvedic and allopathic knowledge. Ayurvedic pathogenesis, then, becomes just another way to describe biochemical processes in the brain.[31]

Ayurvedic psychiatrists recognize kaphonmada when the symptoms correspond with kapha vitiation and follow a diurnal course typical for kapha afflictions such as aggravation in the morning or immediately after taking food.[32] The symptoms of kaphonmada largely correspond to the symptoms of severe depressive disorder (depressive episode or severe depression).[33] Some others – such as aggravation after taking food or in the night, or increased sexual desire – do not. However, most Ayurvedic psychiatrists agreed that mental illness always involves all three doshas at the same time, just to different extents. Dr Sarasvati explained,[34]

> Unmada with a single dosha is rare; also pure kaphonmada is rare. More often, there is kapha-vata-paittika or kapha-paittika unmada. If it is

> kapha-paittika, anger is there, the patients are quarrelling with others, and the kapha symptoms are also there.

On the other hand, vata is involved in other forms of mental illness besides depression, as Dr Shaila (who also held a PhD) at GAMH told me:[35]

> Vata will definitely be there in all types of mood disorders. Mood, we say, *vega* [emotions]. For the appropriate expression of mood, we need vata. Vata is the moving force that gives energy. Mood is actually energy or emotion. And that requires vata. That is why people say that vata is definitely impaired. So there will be vata impairment also in kaphonmada. Because sometimes this depression is a lack of expression of emotions. Even though they will have sadness, they won't express.

Dr Kumar, then the superintendent in charge of GAMH, disclosed the clinical pragmatics of single dosha diagnoses.[36] "We don't say it is purely kaphonmada because in all the cases of unmada it is said it is sannipad, three doshas are involved. For the convenience of the treatment modality only we differentiate between vatonmada, pittonmada, and kaphonmada."

Kapha dosha can manifest as many different problems according to where it has localized, but for kapha dosha to reach the mind and to develop a kapha-related mental illness, specific causative factors and predispositions are required. Ayurvedic psychiatrists take different levels of causation of depression or related Ayurvedic categories like kaphonmada into consideration. At GAMH, Dr Rasheed elaborated on the causal chain of kaphonmada:[37] excessive eating or over-nourishment and a sedentary lifestyle precipitate kapha dosha. External factors such as tension, bereavement, loss or unavailability of a desired thing, guilty consciousness related to social norms, different forms of poison, or an incorrect diet could trigger the disease. With regard to diet, food that is improperly cooked, spoiled or incompatible (such as fish and curd) and food that is regarded as *rajasika* [of rajas quality] or *tamasika* [of tamas quality], such as spicy food and meat, is understood to precipitate depression. Passions and intense emotions such as sadness, grief, anger, lust or the desire for material goods that result from too much attachment, false sensory perceptions or faulty judgment also cause kaphonmada. In contrast to Western theories, *all* intense emotions, passions and desires are considered to be causative factors of mental disorders. In order to develop kaphonmada, a certain psychic predisposition or vulnerability expressed in the terminology of the three gunas is required. In the words of Dr Rasheed:[38]

> Sattva is the healthy factor. If sattva guna is there, the mind will be strong, no mental disorder will occur. Rajas and tamas are the factors that are causing ill health for a mind. What may be reason, how many stress factors may have occurred, how many problems the patient has, if only the mind of the person becomes hina [weak] sattva – that means unhealthy – then

> only the mental disorder will occur. That is the principle in Ayurveda. Stress is for everyone. Everyone is having stress. High social person, high businessman has stress. Low socio-economic status people have stress. But all are not getting mental disorders. Life is always stress. Only very few are getting mental disorders. And that is because of ill-mindedness, mental unhealthiness. This mental unhealthiness is caused by rajas and tamas. If the tamas or the rajas part is predominant in a person that person is vulnerable to a mental disorder. If the same stress occurs to a person who has sattva guna, mental disorder may not occur. Sattva guna will create mental strength.

In this sense, deficient sattva quality constitutes the predisposition for all mental disorders, whereas mental strength or willpower prevents them. Some practitioners explained it the other way around: the aggravation of kapha or phlegm leads to a derangement of consciousness, intellect and memory, which again increases the proportion of rajas and tamas. In the case of kaphonmada, the proportion of tamas is increased. Only in a hina sattva predisposition can certain external factors give rise to a mental disease. The dosha that is predominant in the body of the patient at the time the triggering external factor is experienced determines the manifestation of the disease as wind, bile or phlegm forms of mental illness. Due to the mutual influence of the physical and the mental dosha, an excess of tamas facilitates the pathological aggravation of phlegm in the mind-carrying channels.

Dr Krishnan related the differentiation of vishadam and kaphonmada at the Ayurveda College to the academic engagement of international psychiatric diagnostic tools such as the ICD-10.[39]

> Academicians say it is vata, practitioners say it is kapha. In depression, mainly people see that depression is total depressed mood, withdrawal from society, sitting lonely somewhere. That is one angle of depression. Actually, depression has two domains. Agitated mood is there and depressed mood and self-withdrawal is there in depression. Two extremes are there. We can never say depression is only depressed mood or only this [agitation]. The other area is also there. Depressive patients sometimes lose their sleep, sleeplessness is there. Same time oversleep is there. So two domains are there, either no sleep or oversleep. ICD classification, in severe depression all extremes are there. So this type of discussion comes in the academy only. Practitioners feel it is a depressed mood, keeping in silent, going sitting somewhere. That is the only depression according to practitioners. They don't have ICDs, they don't have classifications. When we discuss, we discuss all the extremes, depression has got two domains, one is kapha-dominating, the other is vata-dominating. The kapha-dominating is the depressed mood and all. Vata-dominating is agitation, restlessness, no sleep at all, self-destruction, tearing the clothes and all; that type of agitation is there. That is vata dominant.

Dr Krisnan's statement that practitioners diagnose depression mostly as kaphonmada, while academicians differentiate between vata and kapha forms of depression is not supported by my research according to which many vaidya and Ayurvedic general physicians do indeed diagnose depression as a vata affliction (cf. Langford 2002; Smith 2006). Thus, his argument is best understood as a statement of the superiority of the scientific approach in academia, which is characterized by relating Ayurvedic theory to mainstream psychiatric, "modern" diagnostic tools. By differentiating vata and kapha forms of depression and relating them to ICD-nosology, this clinician and college professor claimed the participation and contemporaneity of Ayurvedic psychiatry in allopathic scientific discourse. In sum, mild depression with mainly somatic symptoms is discussed in relation to vata and not interpreted as *unmada* [mental disorder or madness], while severe depression, characterized by the involvement of mental faculties, is related to kaphonmada. This differentiation also has an impact on the choice of treatment.[40]

Another Ayurvedic category that is sometimes engaged as a translation for depressive disorder is *adhijonmada*, one of the six forms of unmada described in the classical texts. Teachers and students of the manasika course and practitioners at GAMH described adhijonmada as a rare reaction to the loss of a beloved person (or in exceptional cases, the loss of an object or ideology), and translated it as bereavement or sometimes as post-traumatic stress disorder. I never found this diagnosis in the patient charts at the college or GAMH. However, in the private clinic of the Ayurvedic psychiatrist Dr Joseph John, a BAMS-trained practitioner who specialized in psychiatry after his training with an allopathic psychiatrist,[41] adhijonmada was the most frequent psychiatric diagnosis. It was his diagnosis for patients with what he called "reactive" or "agitated depression". Other than kaphonmada – which Dr John described as endogenous, inherited severe depression that mainly affects tamasik personalities, the main symptoms of which were tiredness and social withdrawal – he maintained that patients with adhijonmada have no family history of mental problems. In a Malayalam pamphlet Dr John used to give to his patients, he included both acute and chronic stress as causative factors of adhijonmada:

> What are the common symptoms of adhijonmada? All the symptoms are akin to the symptoms of kaphajonmadam. Sudden crying spells, abrupt loss of consciousness, hysteric fits, sleeplessness, restlessness, intense internal turbulence, and so on are the common symptoms. The loss of some things people are too fond of or situations in which one has to bear some horrible things and the acute stress or chronic stress evolved from situations like this are the main causative factors of adhijonmada. [...] The sudden death of some close relatives or fond friends, unexpected financial disasters or loss of properties, severe diseases, family feuds, professional problems like unexpected transfers or punishments, etc. causes acute stress. On the other hand, the stress that a person has to bear for a long period of time is called chronic depression. The stress felt when you have to work hastily because

> of lesser time at your disposal, or when you have to work for longer time, overtime, the stress due to chronic incurable diseases and so on are examples of chronic stress. The stress due to your unquenchable desires and the frantic quest you undertake for the fulfilment of those desires can also cause chronic stress. All these phenomena can cause depression and can badly affect a person's physical and psychic health, and can precipitate a condition called adhijonmada.

This was Dr John's idiosyncratic way of interpreting adhijonmada. Like vishadam, it is mainly related to vata vitiation (with some kapha also involved), but unlike vishadam, adhijonmada is a syndrome of its own kind. Dr John's framing of adhijonmada as depression related to "stress and strain"[42] enables an easy dialogue with popular psychiatric notions of depression as related to the increased stress and tension Malayalis are experiencing as a result of major socio-cultural-economic transformations in recent decades. Further, it offers an Ayurvedic framing of depression as a widespread problem or even an "epidemic" as the flipside to the Kerala Model of Development. Stress and strain are problems so common in Kerala today that one Ayurvedic hospital has started offering outpatient treatment in a weekly "stress and strain clinic".[43]

Embodied minds

Although on institutional, educational and clinical levels a new field of specialization with a focus on mental diseases is being established, Ayurvedic theory and clinical practice do not separate mental from physical diseases. Mind and body are seen as closely interrelated.

Dr Ganapati (at another Ayurveda college) explained, "All diseases are both *sharira* [body] and *manasu* [mind]".[44] They are part of what anthropologist Mark Nichter calls a "resonating system":[45] what happens in the body resonates in the mind, and what happens in the mind resonates in the body. "Basically Ayurveda is a materialistic science and it has got a very materialistic outlook towards the nature, mind, everything", Dr Praveen, a general practitioner who focused on autism, explained:[46]

> As far as the pathological viewpoint is concerned we are approaching the mind from a very materialistic basis. We have a very solid concept that the lifestyle, especially the food habits, has got a very direct impact on the status of mind. It can influence negatively the status of the mind and obviously it can be influenced positively as well. Interestingly once you start going through the literature of the so-called psychiatric illness in Ayurvedic classics, one of the basic etiological features is *pathyahara* [unhealthy food habits]. They can influence negatively the status of the mind. And so obviously it can be influenced positively as well. So basically in that way Ayurveda is a materialistic science and it has got a very materialistic outlook towards the nature, mind, everything.

In Ayurveda, the mind cannot be treated directly. So Ayurvedic psychiatrists treat the mind by treating the body. Ayurvedic psychiatrists frequently used the metaphor of water in a vessel to describe the relationship between the mind and the body in Ayurveda. You cannot cool the water in a vessel directly, but by cooling the vessel the water also gets cooled. "By purifying the body," Dr Sundaran explained, "the mind gets clear."[47] Consequently, until recently there has not been a separation in Ayurveda between practitioners and disciplines treating the body and those treating the mind. The (re)invention of Ayurvedic psychiatry as a separate theory, practice and academic discipline in Kerala is influenced by the epistemological and institutional power of allopathic psychiatry. It establishes and institutionalizes a Cartesian dualism separating body and mind that did not previously exist in Ayurveda. The permeability and distinctiveness of Ayurveda with respect to allopathic psychiatry are part of the process of producing new institutions, experts and knowledge regimes in order to enter into the broader glocal network of mental health. As such, Ayurvedic psychiatrists are working to establish the compartmentalization of body and mind both institutionally *and* pedagogically.

The Ayurvedic notion of manas is often translated as but does not fully correspond to "mind". One of the basic characteristics of manas is that it is part of matter or the material world that is organized into different levels according to the degree of density. Samkhya philosophy, one of the schools that inform Ayurvedic concepts and practices, does not make a sharp ontological distinction between mental and physical domains. Rather than locating a split between body and mind, Samkhya philosophy distinguishes between consciousness without content or quality [*purusha*] on the one hand and matter [*prakrti*] which is imbued with the three gunas (sattva, rajas and tamas). The different mental faculties *buddhi* [discriminating intelligence], *ahamkara* [self-identification, ego] and *manas* [mind and emotion – the faculty that comprehends sensory objects] are part of matter [prakrti], not opposed to it. They are on a continuum from subtle (ahamkara and buddhi) to more palpable materiality (manas) (Langford 2002).

In a healthy person, there is a chain linking the sensory objects, senses, manas and buddhi. To perceive a sensory object, the senses attach to the object and send the information to manas that receives and aggregates the sensory information. If the linkage between manas and buddhi is disrupted or blocked, information cannot be processed or analysed, and it is impossible to construct a rational response. Depression, therefore, involves the disruption of this connection, which in turn is related to local moral worlds and local ideas of societal functioning. As such, it both results from and leads to *prajnaparadha* [an offense against wisdom]. Manas, therefore, is both a sensory organ and responsible for organizing and controlling the other senses. It is, as Zimmermann remarks, "the 'common sense' over and above all the organs of the empirical senses, the internal organ ensuring the link between the *atman* [inner self, soul] and the life of experience" (Zimmermann 1987, 195). At the same time manas is able to control and substitute thoughts and emotions. In this latter sense, it has, as Dr Devan of the Ayurveda College identified, "two roles: direction of the senses and self-control".[48] Distinct from discriminating intelligence, ego-consciousness and consciousness, manas is a mental faculty that is lower, more dense and more of an epiphenomenon than an agentive organ. Its emotional and cognitive content can be influenced through the same material means as other physical diseases. Emotions and thoughts thus can be changed and replaced through a process of physio-cognitive self-control.

In the Ayurvedic pedagogic and clinical practice that I observed, "manas" is used interchangeably with "mind". In spite of this apparent synonymy, it does not match the psychological aspects of the Euro-American concept "mind" because manas lacks the connotation of a deep, essential, true, inner, authentic expression of the individual self. Instead, it is understood as somehow more material, epiphenomenal and inessential than "mind". In fact, manas more closely resembles the contemporary mainstream psychiatric approach to the mind as an expression of the brain. Both allopathic psychiatry and Ayurvedic psychiatry have a material approach towards the mind but they differ in fundamental ways: allopathic psychiatry's materialism is the product of a long history of reductionisms. The ancient trialism of soul, mind and body was reduced to a mind-body dualism, which now is being further reduced to a materialism that extinguishes the mind by reducing it to a mere epiphenomenon, manifestation or "function" of the brain. The Ayurvedic concept of manas, on the other hand, incorporates mental faculties into the realm of matter and sees the body and the mind as two sides of a resonance system. Other than the biopsychiatric reduction of mind into matter, the Ayurvedic conception of mental health problems is not reductionist. Physiology in Ayurveda, based on doshas and gunas, transcends allopathic physiology by including morals, values and sometimes spirituality and differs from it by its strong emphasis on *pathiyam* [diet and daily activities] that are again related to South Asian notions of permeable selves. In classical Ayurvedic texts it is not the brain but the heart that is the seat of the mind and emotions. Manas includes both mental and emotional processes that affect the humoral balance in the heart, the vessels and other parts of the body (Zimmermann 1987). According to Zimmermann, in the classic texts the link between mind and body is established through the concepts of purity and non-violence. Purity of the mind and an absence of distress and anger are seen as essential for the health of the body (Zimmermann 1987, 178–179). In Ayurvedic theories of the mind and mental illness, physiology, morals, lifestyle, existential questions, and (for some interpreters) religion and faith are interwoven. Manas and mental dis-order for that matter can be manipulated and treated in the same way as are bodily and somatic diseases. That is, through purification and diet, but also through cognitive and moral controls (Obeyesekere 1977; Langford 2002) again targeting physiological processes.

It is true that Ayurvedic theory regards both mind (and mental disorder) physiologically, but there is more to it: Ayurvedic theory and practice provide a complex depiction of manas and the problems affecting it, whether physiological, moral or cognitive. I take up this point again in the next section in the context of considering depression as a physio-moral problem.

Manovahashrotas and the grammar of the Ayurvedic body

The interconnectedness of the somatic and the psychological further becomes obvious in the idea of *manovahashrotas*. These are specific channels carrying thoughts, ideas and emotions. Manovahashrotas can be affected by a blockage of accumulated kapha dosha that effects a vitiation of vata, pitta or both and leads to depression or other forms of mental illness. Dr Krishnan, one of the teachers at the kaya chikitsa [general medicine] department, drew a picture showing a tube obstructed by huge blocks to symbolize kapha obstructing the mind-carrying channels and preventing the transmission of vata.[49] "The channels are blocked. This will cause vata kapha. Because of the obstruction only vata is vitiated," he explained. In this sense, depression is described as the result of a blockage in specific channels. The blockage of the manovahasrotas can be removed first and foremost through purifying treatment of the body or, as I occasionally heard, by counselling, psychotherapy or *pranayama*[50] or even by consolation or a sensible smile. Basically, all these impact thought and emotional processes by pacifying the vata dosha or, as Dr Namboodiri expressed it, by opening the manovahashrotas.[51]

In the course of many discussions with Ayurvedic practitioners on the subject of manovahastrotas, it became clear that they thought of them as a helpful concept or part of a cognitive map. Many emphasized that manovahashrotas are "a concept only", useful to think with but with no concrete material reference in the physical body. Although manas is described as flowing through channels, Ayurvedic practitioners clearly differentiated between *shrotas* [channels] carrying visible body substances and manovahashrotas. "We have got a concept known as manovahashrotas," Dr Nayar explained.[52] "That means the channels for mind, transmitting the actions of the mind. When these are getting blocked that will result in unmada including depression." "Can you translate it as mind-carrying channels?" I asked. "Roughly," he replied. "Is there a chart for the channels?" "No, it is a concept only. You cannot dissect a human body and show it. It is not a structural thing but a purely functional concept." Likewise, Dr Ganapati pondered my question regarding the nature of the manovahashrotas, and pronounced:[53]

> I think it is a concept only. We cannot see or detect the manovahashrotas by surgery or anything. Other channels such as *raktavahashrotas* [blood carrying channels] you can see. Manas is present throughout the body, it travels. I think because of that the concept of manovahashrotas evolved. And also to interpret the samprapti of mental illness it is said that the vitiated doshas reach the manovahashrotas.

The Ayurvedic body cannot be neatly mapped onto the biomedical body, as I heard Ayurvedic practitioners repeat time and again. Most Ayurvedic academics and practitioners have appropriated this discourse of parallel yet incompatible bodies. This incompatibility or parallelism of Ayurvedic and allopathic epistemes and ontologies usually refers to the body in general, but some Ayurvedic notions such as doshas or manovahashrotas seem particularly resistant. Since most institutional Ayurvedic teaching does not deny allopathic truth claims, one way out of this dilemma is to categorize the Ayurvedic body or parts of the Ayurvedic body as functional and the allopathic body as structural. The manovahashrotas would then be serve a functional description as "concepts only" which means that they have no ontic reality. With the metaphor of language and its grammar, Dr Nayar gave me a useful model for understanding the relationship between empirical observation and concepts of the body:[54]

> Which one was first formed, language or its grammar? At first, language was formed, and then people started to make uniformity. Grammar is a by-product of language. Likewise in Ayurveda there are constant methods of trial and error observation. In this way, they have found out things, developed concepts, came back to their trials and errors, refined the concepts..

In this sense, the manovahashrotas are part of an Ayurvedic grammar of the body that helps to understand its function. As a grammar, manovahasrotas do not map the structural body but are rather a mental map of the Ayurvedic functional body, a figure to think with. A grammar is normative yet invisible and one of the implications of Dr Nayar's grammar metaphor is that Ayurvedic practitioners treat pathologies of the body and mind with the grammar as the underlying yet unknown basis. They treat these pathologies *as if* the Ayurvedic body existed, as if the Ayurvedic body was the basis of their clinical practice.

Another way out of the dilemma of moving from the Ayurvedic into the allopathic body is employing translation in the Latourian sense to make discordant elements compatible with one another. It was in this sense that Dr Nayar spoke about manovahashrotas, testifying at once the dual training of students in Ayurveda and in allopathic physiology and anatomy:[55]

> I will tell you one modern concept. In the brain, you have got an internal communication between the various areas. In the frontal area of the brain the highest centre for the cerebrum is located. That will analyse all your facts, information, everything. In the back of your brain there is the occipital lobe where your visual information is analysed. Actually communication is between this occipital lobe and the frontal lobe. Only through this communication the frontal lobe can get correct information. The visual information should be communicated to the frontal lobe. Such a vast network of communication happens in your brain. It also has the amazing capability to build up new communication networks in brain. Today you close the book and stop working as an anthropologist and say, I am going to become a mathematician tomorrow. A reconfiguration of you brain will occur. It is very elastic, plastic. New connections will be there; new areas will get in touch. Likewise there are numerous channels. How is this communication going on? Through nerve fibres and neurons. We can roughly equate these

> nerve fibres, neuronal networks, and other associated structures to the manovahashrotas. I am equating the manovahashrotas that my *acharias* [preceptor, teacher] taught me about to certain chemical transmitting channels. By the term manovahashrotas we mean those channels that help us to communicate between various areas of the brain, not only carrying information from the sense organs to the brain. They are less mind-carrying channels but rather information-carrying channels.

Mind-carrying channels are another case where the Ayurvedic body transcends the mind-body binary. The ontological difficulties of mapping this binary onto Ayurvedic bodies that become obvious when doctors tried to translate or correlate manovahashrotas to allopathic neurophysiology are resolved by either designating them as conceptual only or by translating them into the neurobiological body.

Gunas, sattvabalam and mental health

> The result of virtuous activities in sattva is declared purity, the result in rajas is misery, and the result in tamas is nescience.
>
> (Bhagavad Gita 14:16)

Ayurvedic psychiatrists frame predisposition and vulnerability to depression and other mental illness in terms of the three qualities [gunas] and mental strength [sattvabalam]. According to Samkhya philosophy, one of the philosophical schools that inform Ayurveda, the gunas are qualities that pervade the material world [prakrti] including the mind.[56] Ayurvedic psychiatrists describe the gunas as qualities, tendencies or, as did Dr Sundaran, "personality traits".[57] In Ayurvedic psychiatry, sattva indicates a healthy or pure mind or constitution, while rajas and tamas are viewed as harmful qualities that can cause mental illness if pathologically increased. Ayurvedic psychiatrists often describe the gunas rajas and tamas as mental doshas, capable of causing mental suffering, distress and illness. In this sense, deficient sattva quality (hina sattva) and an increase in rajas and tamas constitute predisposition to mental disorders, whereas mental strength prevents them. In the words of Dr Praveen, the gunas are the hardware while the actual life circumstances and stressors are the software.[58] "Sattva is the healthy factor", Dr Rasheed explained.[59] A weak mind and external stressors can trigger mental disorders. Dependent on the dosha that is predominant at the time of stress, this will lead to unmada, vishadam or other forms of mental pathology. In the absence of such a guna-based vulnerability, the same stressor might lead to more physical diseases, dependent again on the predominant dosha.

Clinical psychologist Anoop Kumar was one of my main interlocutors in clinical psychology in Kerala. In his research (Kumar 2006), he explored the relevance of the gunas as an "Indian approach for personality" for assessing patients with depression. "Indian psychology" is a marginal subfield in the training of clinical psychology at the National Institute of Mental Health and Neurosciences (NIMHANS), Bangalore. The characterization of sattvik, rajasik and tamasik personalities that Kutty employs in his work was informed by his teacher Kiran Rao's reading of the Bhagavad Gita, and is not only relevant to clinical practice but is also largely congruent with the description I got from Ayurvedic psychiatrists.

People with a high level of sattva have a tendency to be wholesome, self-controlled, equanimous, tolerant, kind, honest, devotional, modest, wise and intelligent. Those with high rajasik are predisposed towards activity and passion, hyperactivity, immodesty, arrogance, insincerity, malice, selfishness, sensuality and stubbornness. Individuals with tamasik are inclined towards inertia, ignorance, delusion and impurity and are depressive, disrespectful and lethargic (cf. Langford, 2002: Giguère, 2009). Deficient sattva quality constitutes the precondition for all mental disorders, whereas a high proportion of sattva or mental strength prevents them. The key characteristics of a pravara sattva personality are seen to have intelligence, good memory, fearlessness, strong problem solving capacities, the ability to bear pain and suffering without complaining, and display behaviour in accordance with social norms. Hina sattva personalities are described as stubborn with unchangeable and incorrect convictions, no capacity for critical self-reflection and a false pride that prevents them from sharing their worries with others. In those who have pravara sattva, "These people will learn things from their life, from their own efforts they will overcome the problems coming in the future, with their own thinking, with their own experience" (Kumar 2006). Those who have hina sattva, "will not learn from they have already gone through. They will not learn from others' opinion. They will not learn by thinking what the consequences will be" (Kumar 2006). Thus, weak sattva is not only a predisposition or a risk factor for mental diseases but also an impediment to recovery.

The sattvik notion of mental health is closely related to sattvabalam. Sattvabalam literally means strength of sattva, which in this context is often used as synonymous with "mind", many Ayurvedic psychiatrists told me. It is thus translated as mental strength or, more often, as willpower. "If you analyse the depressive patients", Dr Nayar explained while introducing the concept,[60]

> there will be some weak-mindedness in all these patients. A strong mind means you are equipoise. You are not depressed when you are sad nor are you over thrilled when you have joy. A strong mind means a strong character. But these patients have some type of weak-mindedness, some problems persisting in the back of their mind; subconscious mind is there. Subconscious mind means there will be certain feelings that may have created in you during your childhood, and they may repeat that.[61]

Dr Devdas, a college instructor of Ayurvedic psychiatry, related mental health and sattvabalam to local moral worlds[62]: "Whenever the individual loses the mental power, sattvabalam, then definitely the diseases come. All our gurus, goddesses, gods, they are all sattvika, they didn't have any disease at all. Our aim in life is to attain sattvika level." "Everyone," he went on engaging Hindu ideas of dharma, "has his or her own duties and responsibilities in the society. If you do these perfectly you will become sattvika. That is what the gurus and gods are saying." "How do you do this in your clinical practice," I asked him "We have to be a role model," he replied invoking cultural norms and ideals of the good or righteous life. "We have to become like Lord Rama or Lord Krishna. People will realize what their responsibilities are. Role models work very well if a parent doesn't want to work any more due to depression." "That works," he stated. "Beyond the limits of drugs these words are working". He concluded in telling fashion: "Psychotherapy is very fast developing in America."

The concept of sattvabalam closely resembles the vernacular Malayalam notion of *manobalam* [mental strength, willpower]. Both can be seen as a culturally shared notion of vulnerability to mental illness. Family members often draw upon the notion of mental weakness [*manodurbalam*] as one cause of mental illness. It is also the mental weakness narrative that doctors engage when framing the problem to patients and families in consultations, and to explain the mode of action of the treatment and the Ayurvedic medication as mind-strengthening. Many mainstream psychiatrists explicitly and vigorously refute the narrative of mental weakness as a cause for depression and seek to replace it with a neurochemical imbalance narrative. However, Ayurvedic psychiatrists engage a shared cultural notion of mental illness as mental weakness. Sattvabalam is also one of the fields that doctors have to complete in the case record for each patient at GAMH. After biographical details, a physical examination, an allopathic psychiatric examination, an Ayurvedic assessment and the allopathic and Ayurvedic psychiatric diagnoses, the case sheet has a section on "etiological factors". Here, the constitution of the doshas (vata, pitta, kapha), the constitution of the mind (sattva, rajas, tamas) and the sattvabalam are assessed and noted. In this last field, practitioners are supposed to tick off excellent, medium or low. Usually, however, this field is left blank.

How does a guna-related predisposition or vulnerability to mental illness evolve? To answer this question, Ayurvedic psychiatrists take not only the socialization of the child into account but also go back to a person's birth, the pregnancy that produced them, and sometimes even to previous lives. The theory of predisposition to mental illness is closely related to other Ayurvedic fields of paediatrics and gynaecology and to the Ayurvedic notion of child development. "There are several factors that play a role", Dr Shankaran, a teacher at another college in Kerala, explained.[63] One factor is the guna constitution of the parents at the time of conception. "If the guna of the father and mother is rajas and tamas predominant then the child will also be rajas and tamas predominant. Then the child is a vulnerable person." A second factor is the atmosphere experienced by the mother during pregnancy. "If the mother has severe mental stress or tension then that will also affect the progeny; then progeny will be rajas and tamas predominant." He elaborated:

> Whether the mother is living a happy or joyful life, the baby will also become that much with a stable mind. And if always this quarrel and this restlessness is happening, the mother will be restless and it will affect the development of the baby also.

A final factor in sattvabalam is socialization, including the family atmosphere and child rearing practices. Thus, for Ayurvedic psychiatrists, mental health care and prevention of mental diseases begins not only with the socialization of the child but already much earlier with the mental health of the parents.

Thus, the family can be a site of the prevention but also the precipitation of mental health problems. Enhancing the sattvik proportions can be done as part of Ayurvedic treatment. But, as many Ayurvedic psychiatrists emphasized, this is also part of the *culture* of Kerala. Ayurvedic mental health care that is basically the promotion of sattva guna, then, corresponds to an idealized "traditional" family life. This is what Dr Rasheed identified:[64]

> It happens in the families, unknowingly. In Ayurveda we know the scientific side but everyone at home practises it. That is why in a good family, in a good culture people will behave well. They will understand each other's problems and they will have a wonderful family life. We are big families, the society and Indian family system is like that. So after the marriage several functions are there. When the lady becomes pregnant, then the mother-in-law, father-in-law and lady's father come to the son's house with sweets and everything. By the eighth month they will be taking the lady to their parents' home. At that time they will be happy, be given sweets and presents, and they will be shifted to their home. After marriage they will be staying in husband's house. When they become pregnant by the eighth month they will be taken to their natal families. Such social customs are there. That is actually the basis of what the science of Ayurveda says, that is unknowingly practised as per the society, social rules, and cultures here in Kerala.

But the family can also be a site where mental health problems are precipitated by the promotion of rajas and tamas guna:

> The child will try to imitate. If the father and mother have a good relation, the child will also see, and unknowingly the sattva guna will increase. If the father will always quarrel with the child its rajas guna will increase. Also if the father keeps saying, don't do like that, don't speak like that, this is not good, abuse words are not good, and before the child they use to fight, using abuse words against each other or against the neighbours, the child seeing this will try to imitate, he will practise what he sees from father and mother. So slowly the rajas guna will arise.

Most Ayurvedic psychiatrists drew a connection between tamas and depression. As Dr Kutty, a BAMS-trained practitioner who specialized in psychiatry and ran his own private clinic, said quite often when I asked about the relationship between depression and the gunas, "basically, depression is because of tamas guna."[65] Dr John described tamas in a way that almost resembled depression:[66]

> A person in whom the tamasika guna is predominant will be melancholic, will have an unreasonable fear, will be depressed almost all the time, fatigued, will have an overwhelming tendency to lie down, will be ignorant and will have diminished memory power.

Similarly, the Ayurvedic psychiatrist Dr Mary related depression to selfishness, egocentrism and narrow-mindedness that corresponded to rajas and tamas qualities.[67]

> In depression patients we see more selfishness. They always think, "What will happen to me?" They are very narrow-minded people thinking about themselves only. They don't appreciate others. This is what Ayurveda, allopathy, and psychology tell, also the Bible, the Bhagavad Gita, all tell the same thing. The basis of all mental problems is moral, I think. These people are very hina sattva, they have no *bhakti* [devotion]. Bad things we have done in the past are the reason for depression, the reason for all diseases. The more bad things we have done, the more our *bala* [strength] is decreased. We also get the karma from our forefathers.

Can sattva be learned? Can a pravara sattva or sattvabalam be developed? Ayurvedic psychiatrists and other Ayurvedic physicians emphasized that it is not possible to lift a patient from a condition of hina sattva to a state of pravara sattva but that sattva might be developed or somewhat improved by counselling, a change in lifestyle, education, the company of righteous people or, according to Dr John, devotion and a strong belief in God. To my question of whether and how the gunas can be changed, Ayurvedic physicians stressed that it is difficult though possible. Many emphasized a change in diet and lifestyle first and foremost. Others suggested counselling and yoga exercises to address the gunas. Thus, while the doshas can be corrected in the hospital, a healing based on change in the gunas has to take place not in the hospital but at home with the family.

Doshas and gunas are mutually related. Doshic imbalance may lead to an increase in rajas and tamas and their pathological increase can vitiate the doshas. The aggravation of kapha leads to a derangement of consciousness, intellect and memory, which again increases the proportion of rajas and tamas. In the case of kaphonmada, the proportion of tamas is increased. Due to the mutual influence of the physical and the mental dosha, an excess of tamas facilitates the pathological aggravation of kapha in the mind-carrying channels. This mutual influence was brought home to me by Dr Deepak.[68] According to him, the doshas and the gunas are interrelated and are just two points of view, with the doshas being denser than the gunas.

> Vata, pitta, kapha deal with the body, rajas and tamas deal with the mind. If a person is depressed we can interpret that as a doshic problem like kaphonmada but a stronger focus is on the mental doshas. They are the manifestations of the same thing from different perspectives. We can consider body and mind as two different compartments, but from another point of view, from another dimension it's one and the same. When it comes to more evident and material, it is more body, when it's more subtle it is mind, atman, and all other, this is the concept. And when we consider these two, we can consider them on a vertical axis. The most palpable thing is kapha. Then still subtler is pitta, and even still subtler is vata, then comes tamas, then rajas and most subtle is sattva. I can treat a depressive patient by reducing the kapha, if I reduce the kapha the tamas also will be reduced.

In this way, the purifying treatment that reduces kapha likewise reduces tamas and the patient will become more active and their mental faculties will be strengthened.

It is important to note that gunas and sattvabalam are not purely psychological. The Ayurvedic framing of mental health in terms of gunas and sattvabalam blurs the boundaries of body, mind and morals. It offers a somato-psycho-moral concept of vulnerability to mental illness that is largely informed by high caste Hindu notions of biomoral purity and Buddhist notions of suffering. The tripartite division of the three gunas is also related to other aspects of Hindu daily life in Kerala such as diet and activities. As Osella and Osella (2008) note, Hindus in Kerala reinforce food hierarchies by distinguishing between "hot" and "cold" foods, or by using the Samkhya philosophy model of categorizing foods according to the three gunas. Social hierarchies map neatly on to this classification: people who eat sattvik food are sattva, those who eat rajasik or tamasik food are rajasik or tamasik. Sattvik characteristics such as vegetarianism is one of the central aspects of ritual superiority and inferiority that is still highly significant in Malayali Hindu social life.[69] Thus, with a notion of mental health in terms of gunas and sattvabalam, Ayurvedic psychiatrists engage a Brahminical, high-caste ideology of physio-moral purity. Gunas are then physiological, psychological and moral qualities or tendencies, often related to high caste Hindu values or purity and impurity that are acquired through the physio-psychological-moral status of the parents at the time of conception (or what is increasingly understood as inheritance or genetics) and the mental status of the mother during pregnancy, including socialization, lifestyle and diet. Since the guna constitution is also influenced and determined by that of one's parents, Ayurvedic mental health care takes an intergenerational approach. Treatment and prevention of mental disorder always impacts the mental health of the generations to come. Some Ayurvedic practitioners relate gunas to genetic make up. The mental strength [sattvabalam] of the parents is understood to be inherited by their children, passed through the genes.

Dr Sundaran spoke of the relationship between the decline in mental health and a decline in "culture" or "traditional" family life and practice.[70]

> Mental health awareness has been a part of our lifestyle. Previously it was. Nowadays, we have no regular prayer in our houses. Previously, twenty-five years ago, every Indian house, especially in Kerala, we used to light the lamp and recite some prayers in the evening. These prayers made up the mental health. Through this habit, regularly at 6:30 p.m. lighting the lamp, we used to keep discipline and it reflected the total life of that person. And early morning also, 4:30 or 5 a.m. we recited lines of prayers. If we go through the lines of that prayer, praying please God, help my husband for good life, and so on. This is linked with our mental health. Now also we are doing the lamp lightning but not regularly, no punctuality, no prayer.

Thus, a physio-moral notion of mental health is closely associated and tied up with a normative "traditional" family life involving habitual and regular practices.

Not all Ayurvedic physicians agree with the focus on gunas as a predisposition and etiology of mental illness in Ayurvedic psychiatry. The main criticism is that practitioners and students of institutionalized Ayurvedic psychiatry mimic the compartmentalization of mind and body, of mental and physical diseases, and that the translation of allopathic psychiatric concepts into Ayurvedic ones remains superficial. Dr Praveen addressed this issue:[71]

> The major problem these days with Ayurvedic practitioners is that they take the allopathic information as the basic and try to solve the problem with an Ayurvedic treatment. They do not take the case as such and try to derive it with Ayurvedic principles keeping the allopathic explanation apart. They take the allopathic explanation for granted and then they try to match them with whatever possible information is there in Ayurveda. I don't think it is the right way of approaching Ayurveda. For explaining these things in Ayurveda we have to keep the allopathic explanations away first and we have to see the case unbiased with your own basis and assess the situation. You see, once you ask most Ayurvedic practitioners about depression, immediately they turn their senses toward the explanation of mind which is given in Ayurveda, then they make the stage with sattva, rajas and tamas. They are ready to fight with sattva, rajas and tamas.

Dr Praveen's critique goes to the heart of contemporary institutionalized Ayurveda. It targets the translations that ostensibly render Ayurveda and allopathy commensurable. Ayurvedic psychiatrists, he implies, mimic allopathic distinctions between the body and the mind, somatic and psychological diseases, medicine and psychology. Somatic diseases are then described primarily in terms of the doshas, dhatus, agni and so on while for mental diseases the gunas are extracted from the Ayurvedic repertoire. Instead, Ayurvedic classical texts suggest a dichotomy of spiritual and physiological diseases, and Ayurvedic psychiatrists mimic a distinction between mental and physical diseases that is currently being transcended in current neuropsychiatry when mind or consciousness is reduced as a mere function of neurochemical processes in the brain.

Another important notion for the Ayurvedic etiology of depression and related mental disorders are the manovikaras[72] [mental or emotional[73] pathologies, inner turmoil]. The understanding of manovikaras is an important element in the syllabus of the Ayurvedic psychiatry course and appears in the etiology section of almost every MD thesis on depression or related Ayurvedic notions. For example Abraham notes, "When the *manasika bhavas* [mental states] become excessive or inappropriate this is termed as vikaras" (Abraham 2009). The potentially pathogenic emotions listed in the classics are considered in assessing and constructing the etiology and pathogenesis of depression. In contrast to Western theories, intense emotions, passions and desires that disturb the balance of the mind (whether negative or positive) are considered to be causative factors of depression and other mental disorders. Accordingly, recovery consists of purifying the mind by removing or replacing the passions and intense emotions rather than ferreting out their deeper meaning as a manifestation of one's inner self. Like manas, manovikaras are not expressions of a deeper self but epiphenomena, aberrations from a normative healthy physio-moral state (cf. Langford 2002). Manovikaras as part of the etiology of mental illness are closely related to South Asian notions of mental health as *shantam* [a balanced mental and emotional state, peace] and to Hindu philosophical notions of emotional over-involvement and attachment as pathogen. In the Upanishads, passion inhibits self-realization that is dependent on non-attachment to the phenomenal world. In the Bhagavad Gita, uncontrolled passion is the impediment to equipoise and wisdom while control of passion and the severing of the self's attachment to the world is associated with salvation (Bhattacharyya 1986). Accordingly, in Ayurvedic theory, mental health as mental peace is attained through control of the senses, the mind and the passions. It is the passions and overflowing emotions *and* their frustration that are regarded as causative for mental health problems.[74] Many Ayurvedic psychiatrists with whom I spoke about the cause for depression referred to frustration, disappointment, disillusionment and the dashing of dreams as main causes. The Ayurvedic solution is either the satisfaction of such desires or emancipation from passion in order to achieve a cure.

Depression as a problem of perception

So far I have described depression in Ayurvedic psychiatry as a physio-moral problem, accommodated in the course of the re-interpretation of Ayurveda and its notions of health and disease. Students and teachers of the manasika course in the Ayurveda College, Kottakkal have further an elaborated theory of depression accommodated into Ayurvedic theory as a cognitive problem. I rarely heard this elaborated theory of perceptual disruption discussed by Ayurvedic clinicians, but it was an important element in the classes and often elaborated in MD theses. Depression was conceptualized as a doshic problem related to the vitiation of vata, kapha or rarely pitta (as discussed at the beginning of this subchapter). Depression evolves when the mind-carrying channels are blocked and manas cannot flow freely and function well. This impaired function leads to a disruption of the chain of perception between *artha* [sense objects], *indriya* [senses], manas and buddhi. Proper perception and knowledge results only if all elements in the chain are connected smoothly and united. Since the transmission from one element to the other is governed by vata, a vitiation of vata leads to disruption. Zimmermann (2014), based on his readings of Ayurvedic texts, argues that all causes of disease are recognized in Ayurveda as either of insufficient, perverted, or excessive union [*yogam*]. As Dr Sundaran (1993) identified, this means,

> The mental diseases are born out of the excessive thinking, undesirable or unwanted thinking; and unreal thinking distorts the indriya which are working in unison with the mind. The union of the mind and indriya is jeopardized here. And this ill union ruins the buddhi. The excessive, insufficient or perverted union of the thinking process is of course an undesirable effect; it goes without saying.

A blockage in the manovahashrotas arising from vitiated doshas may lead to a disrupted connection of the elements of the chain of perception as much as this disconnection may lead to imbalanced doshas. This disrupted union includes mind and emotions as well as morals and habitual behaviour. According to Dr Nayar, disobedience of social norms may be a sign of mental illness:[75]

> These people lose discipline in their lives. They will not do what we tell them. They don't obey the rules of the society. If you tell a psychiatric patient you should not speak there they will not obey. They can hear our voices; they can see us. But something happens in their analysing mind. Their buddhi, their manas is getting deranged. Manas does not properly accept the sensory stimulus. They may hear but they do not listen. Our words are not being processed to their mental faculties.

As Dr Nayar makes clear, the cognitive in Ayurvedic mental health is closely associated with the moral.

It is through the purifying and pacifying procedures and medications that I describe below that the perverted union of the chain of perception produced by a blockage in the manovahashrotas becomes normalized.[76] "By making the body purified, the mind gets clear and good thoughts occur," Dr John explained.[77] This assumption – one shared by many Ayurvedic psychiatrists I spoke with – is based on the notion that mental illness hinders clear perception, correct morals, and good behaviour and reflects a positivistic epistemology (cf. Halliburton 2009). Like a tainted mirror that cannot reflect its image clearly, depression and other forms of mental illness are seen as obstacles that hinder a person from perceiving the world "as it is" and from behaving according to social norms. It is the disruption in the chain of perception described above that leads to wrong cognition, wrong conclusions and wrong behaviour. In other words, depression is described as a state of ignorance.[78]

Prajnaparadha is often described as one of the main causes for depression.[79] The Sanskrit term literally means offence or crime [*aparadha*] against wisdom or intelligence [*prajna*]. With this term, Ayurvedic practitioners usually refer to a deliberate or wilful behavioural error or transgression that leads to illness resulting from improper union of the sensory objects, the senses and the mind (cf. Langford 2002; Smith 2006). Dr Devdas specified, "Prajnaparadha are crimes against wisdom, violating inner consciousness, going against common sense, going against the good sense, imprudent conduct, mistakes against wisdom, lifestyle diseases, impulse control disorders, faulty judgments, faulty actions, and so on."[80] In turn, following the daily regimes [*dhinacharya*] as laid out in the classical texts is seen as preventive to any diseases.

In the anthropological literature, prajnaparadha is often glossed as "improper engagement of the senses with the sense organs" (Langford, 2002, 277). Smith describes this term as an "extreme transgression of one's better judgment wherein one's ordained life, style, religious vows, and proper behavior are transgressed, may be due to lust and so on" (Smith 2006, 493). In the context of Ayurvedic psychiatry, prajnaparadha is either related to moral transgression or sin or psychologized or internalized as guilty consciousness resulting from the first. This guilty consciousness is then brought in and aligned to feature as one of the symptoms of depression per the DSM and ICD. In this latter sense, it is the faulty behaviour as such *and* the guilt resulting from it that are referred to as prajnaparadha. In this way, prajnaparadha figures as a connective link between Ayurvedic and allopathic theories of depression. The difference is that prajnaparadha constitutes a *cause* while guilty consciousness is a *symptom*. The characteristics and symptoms [*lakshana*] of a disease, the disease itself and causative factors are seen as a web of signs referring to each other instead of to an underlying referent in Ayurveda. As Langford (2002) has shown, notions of the self or the unconscious are also interwoven into a web with other signs and become rhetorical devices to denote modernity and science rather than representing "a stable signified" (Langford, 2002, 258) or an underlying cause. Prajnaparadha then easily moves from behavioural fault to guilt to mental illness, or else from cause to characteristic to symptom and back. The transformation from faulty behaviour to internalized guilt marks a shift from behaviour to psychic configurations: from the violation of social norms to psychology and the inner feelings produced through this behaviour.[81] Whether conceptualized as faulty behaviour, sin or guilty consciousness, it is moral transgression or "non-dharmic action" (Smith 2006, 576) that characterizes prajnaparadha.

Depression as a physio-moral-cognitive problem

The Ayurvedic concept of depression and its correlates is multiplex. Based on what I have described so far and loosely building on Alter's notion of the "physiology of self-improvement" (Alter 1999), Ecks' concept of physiological self care (Ecks 2004), and Marriott's notion of bio-moral substances (Marriott 1976) I suggest that depression is understood and treated in Ayurvedic psychiatry as a physio-moral-cognitive problem.[82] The Ayurvedic notion of depression then cuts across local moral worlds and blurs Western notions of body and mind. It easily integrates physiological, psychological, moral and sometimes religious framings. Depression and other mental diseases are primarily conceived in terms of doshic or physiological imbalances and do not differ categorically from predominantly somatic diseases. In the context of institutional Ayurvedic psychiatry, depression is translated into three Ayurvedic categories that are all related to dosha vitiation. Ayurvedic psychiatrists describe vishadam as a symptom of vata vitiation and kaphonmada as a syndrome or illness category. Vishadam can be translated as the mild or neurotic form of depression or as reactive depression while kaphonmada is translated as endogenous or severe depression and adhijonmada is depression following a loss or depression due to stress and strain. The physiological notion of depression that transpires here is closely related to a physiological or embodied concept of the mind. Moreover, the three gunas play an important role in the Ayurvedic theory of depression. Sattva guna is equated to mental health, whereas rajas and tamas are understood to be potentially detrimental to mental health. In its gunic framing, mental health becomes related to Brahmanical notions of purity. Depression is then the result of a pathological excess of activity and ignorance. Most Ayurvedic psychiatrists describe depression as a preponderance of tamas or ignorance, but others mainly saw rajas (that they translated as over-ambition) as a key causative factor. Closely related is the notion of mental strength or will power as a synonym and a prerequisite to mental health, and mental weakness as a predisposition to depression and other mental illness. Inasmuch as gunas are physio-moral qualities or tendencies and sattvabalam is a physio-moral concept of mental health, depression, then, is understood as a physio-moral pathology. Using the notion of mental health expressed in terms of gunas and sattvabalam, Ayurvedic psychiatrists engage a Brahmanical, high-caste ideology of physio-moral purity and superiority that is also related to other areas of social life in Kerala. Depression framed as a physio-moral problem is closely associated and tied up with ideologies of normative "traditional" family life and habitual practice. But depression is also an emotional problem or rather a problem related to excessive emotions, passions, or emotional turmoil [*manovikara*] of any kind as either a cause for or an equivalent to mental ill health. In contrast to Western theories, negative and positive intense emotions, passions and desires that disturb the steadiness of the mind are considered to be causative factors of depression and other mental disorders. Recovery consists accordingly in purifying the mind by removing or replacing the passions and intense emotions rather than fathoming out their deeper meaning as manifestation of one's inner self.[83] Like manas, manovikaras are not expressions of a deeper self but epiphenomena, aberrations from a normative healthy physio-moral state (cf. Langford 2002). As a disruption of the chain of perception, finally, depression is also a problem of cognitive ignorance and of moral transgression.

This complex Ayurvedic notion of depression is, I argue, closely related to South Asian notions of the self that can be described, following Marriott's anthropological research (Marriott 1976), as bio-moral or physio-moral selves. In his ethnosociological attempt to understand India through Hindu categories, Marriott (1976) advocates giving up the Cartesian distinction between mind and body. This is exemplified in the concept of dharma, which is often conceptualized as a moral code of conduct, religious guideline or law. Dharma, however, is material *and* conceptual, and is made up of "substance codes" related to an "embodied morality", "a bio-physical as well as a socio-moral category" (Quack 2014). No action is purely "social" in India; there is always a substantial or biological implication for an actor's substance-code (Quack 2014). Likewise, the Ayurvedic physio-moral-cognitive framing of depression merges biology and morals; it is material and also incorporates an embodied morality. It is the physio-moral notion that is embodied in the coded substances of the doshas and the gunas. According to Ayurveda, "fluent bodies" (Langford 2002), "network bodies" (Zimmermann 1979) or "near-hegemonic bodies" (Osella and Osella 1996) in addition to embodied substantial minds and morals make up depressive patients. I suggest that the Ayurvedic physiological notion of depression is more compatible with the allopathic neurochemical conception of depression than with the biodynamic model, which never achieved a substantial foothold in India (Hartnack 2001). Yet, the neurochemical imbalance narrative is transcended by including morality in a model of depression that can best be described as physio-moral-cognitive.

4 The politics and pragmatics of nosologies and their translations: reconfiguration, translation and autonomy

Vaidyas [traditional Ayurveda practitioner] have always treated various forms of mental distress and illness, but the institutionalization of Ayurvedic psychiatry as a separate discipline and as a clinical and educational field of specialization is a recent phenomenon. This development, I argue, is closely related and responsive to recent global and national mental health agendas and policies. Yet, asymmetries with regard to knowledge, validity, evidence and research often make global and local mental health policy makers and mainstream psychiatrists "structurally blind" (Quack 2012; Sax 2014) to Ayurvedic psychiatry. Ayurvedic psychiatry's position within a hierarchical mental health field is characterized simultaneously by biopsychiatric hegemony and a persistent vernacular healing tradition. The Global Mental Health (GMH) movement, World Health Organization (WHO) policy on mental health (WHO 2001b; 2008) and India's recent National Mental Health Policy *New Pathways, New Hopes* (Ministry of Health & Family Welfare 2014) aim to close what is called the "treatment gap" by improving access to mental health care services and reducing inequalities in the provision of care mainly by integrating mental health within primary health care. These policies are based on the globalization of psychiatric discourse, the generation of scientific evidence through evidence-based medicine

(EBM) and randomized controlled trials (RCT), and human rights discourses. It was through a new form of metrics – the DALYs (disability adjusted life years) that provide a measure of overall disease burden expressed in terms of years lost due to ill health, disability or premature death (Bemme and D'Souza 2014) – along with the emergence of psychiatric epidemiology (Lovell 2014) that depression moved from a marginal to a central position in global and national health policies. However, the GMH movement and WHO policies do not mention indigenous mental health services as important actors in public and private mental health care. When ritual healing is mentioned, it is usually in a negative context and represented as superstitious or dangerous, something to be replaced by mental health literacy and overcome by scaling up psychiatric services. India's AYUSH[84] disciplines are not even alluded to in these documents. India's mental health policy (Ministry of Health & Family Welfare 2014) on the other hand does acknowledge Ayurveda and Yoga, noting that the policy includes "identification of effective treatments including those from indigenous systems of medicine which can increase the therapeutic choices for persons with mental health problems." The policy also acknowledges, "Practitioners of Ayurveda and Yoga systems are a resource who need to be included as activists for promotion of mental health."

In this subchapter, I analyse the reconfiguration of *bhutavidya* into Ayurvedic psychiatry, and the engagement between Ayurvedic and allopathic psychiatry and mental health policies in terms of translation and autonomy. Using a Latourian concept of translation, I argue that these processes of engagement serve to enrol Ayurveda into the network of global and local mental health care while at the same time maintaining its basic incompatibility. It is from this incompatibility that the possibility of the autonomy of Ayurvedic psychiatry arises, and also the possibility of recognition as an alternative or complementary medical discipline and legitimate player in public mental health. The engagement with allopathic psychiatry and mental health policies preserves difference through practices that appear to render diagnoses as compatible that at the same time maintain distance between the two approaches. It is translation in the Latourian sense of making incommensurable frames of reference commensurable that produces the (re)invented discipline of Ayurvedic psychiatry as both a credible actor and an autonomous actor in the glocal (global and local) network of mental health care. Incompatibility is what gives rise, in this situation, to the autonomy of specific discourses of distress that nonetheless must be articulated in terms of global categories because those are the classifications through which resources and treatment can be accessed and identified. At the same time, Ayurvedic psychiatrists are engaged in the double process of demarcating their field from the vernacular sector while also engaging in translation processes to make their practice legible to patients and wider discourses of mental health.

Translations have been a key concern of Ayurveda since the encounter with allopathic biomedicine began in the colonial period, right through to its post-colonial professionalization and institutionalization (Brass 1972; Leslie 1976;

Langford 2002) and emergence as a modern and global practice (Wujastyk and Smith 2008; Langford 2002). Scholars of Ayurveda address the translations of Ayurvedic into biomedical nosologies in the light of structural asymmetries between these two medical systems. In the context of the medical pluralism of South Asia, Leslie (1976; 1992) identified that there were contradictions and ambivalence in the modernization process and revivalism of Ayurveda. Leslie used the concept of "syncretisation" to describe the meeting and mixing of allopathic and indigenous medicine in South Asia, and scholars since have worked to understand this syncretisation in more detail and at multiple scales. For example, Naraindas (2014a) proposes the use of the concept of "creolization" to analyse what he calls "nosopolitics" in the context of asymmetries marked by colonialism. As in the linguistic process of creolization, where the superstrate language provides the lexicon and the subordinate language the grammar, in the translation from Ayurvedic into biomedical nosologies, the Ayurvedic pharmacopeia is used to address a biomedical nosology – that is, biomedicine furnishes the lexicon and Ayurveda the grammar. In this process a new Ayurvedic language or therapeutic protocol emerges to address a biomedical nosology (Naraindas 2014a). In a paper "Asymmetrical Translations in contemporary Ayurvedic nosology", Anand Chopra describes how he began with the hypothesis that contemporary Ayurvedic physicians treat on the basis of a modern nosology and that Sanskrit names are just traditional labels applied to allopathic nosologies when he undertook ethnographic research on translation processes with Ayurvedic physicians in Kerala.[85] However, this hypothesis proved "too simple if not wrong" (Chopra n.d.). From an emic perspective of contemporary Ayurvedic physicians, Chopra finds a "rather unexpected and different kind of asymmetry" in that they use translation in order to "assert the validity of their basic episteme in the face of biomedicine's dominance" (Chopra n.d.). This kind of "salvage translation" (Wolfgram 2009, 79) that attempts to recapture lost knowledge has been part of Ayurvedic revivalism since the early twentieth century. Ayurvedic physicians like P.S. Varier, one of the central figures of the reinvention and standardization of Ayurveda in Kerala, described the need to translate Ayurveda into allopathic medicine as a means of rediscovering knowledge lost through decline and disruption to revive a previously complete and comprehensive system (Wolfgram 2009). Through this kind of engagement, Ayurveda connects with other elements of the mental health care network such as diagnostic manuals, educational institutions, global and national policies, public health, media and the Global Mental Health movement. Ayurveda thus enters and joins the network of glocal mental health care while simultaneously maintaining its autonomy. In this way, Ayurvedic psychiatry shows itself to be both deeply modern and highly pragmatic.

The reconfiguration of bhutavidya as Ayurvedic psychiatry

Out of the eight branches of Ayurveda described in the classical texts Caraka Samhita, Sushruta Samhita, and Asthangahrdayam that are authoritative for

Ayurvedic teaching and practice there is no one branch that focuses explicitly on mental illness. Instead, the texts deal with the theory and treatment of mental health problems in the context of two branches of specialization: (1) *kaya chikitsa* [general medicine] and (2) *graha chikitsa* [treatment of grasping entities] or *bhutavidya* [knowledge of the *bhuta* – a being, but this also denotes a ghost, demon, spirit or simply the past tense]. These texts differentiate between physiologically endogenous *unmada*[86] [madness, mental illness] and exogenous *unmada*. While the former denotes "madness" due to an imbalance of one or more of the three *doshas* [humours or principles], the latter denotes "madness" with reference to external entities. Today, the theory and practice of Ayurvedic psychiatry mainly focuses on endogenous unmada and either discards or is ambiguous towards exogenous unmada. In contemporary Ayurvedic psychiatric clinical practice and teaching, but also in efforts to popularize Ayurvedic psychiatry, practitioners focus on endogenous dosha-based unmada largely to the exclusion of exogenous unmada. Most Ayurvedic psychiatrists do not discuss bhutas or *grahas* [grasping entities], and if they do they reinterpret them as mere metaphors for sudden changes in behaviour, as psychotic features or personality disorder. Indeed, the very notion of the existence of exogenous unmada and bhutavidya (or graha chikitsa) has given rise to a highly controversial debate among Ayurvedic psychiatrists.

The crux of the disagreement is the question of whether or not the bhutas or grahas are to be understood as possessing entities or as mere metaphors describing sudden changes in behaviour or character (Lang and Jansen 2013; Naraindas 2014a). According to college-trained Ayurvedic psychiatrists, the description of the grahas in the Ayurvedic classic texts [*samhitas*] is metaphorical but has been misinterpreted in recent decades in the context of possession. This interpretation is related to the narrative of an ancient scientism that morphed into medieval superstition and irrationality, the ghosts, esoterica and contradictions of which must be cleansed from modern Ayurveda (Langford 2002). The classical texts themselves are highly ambivalent on this point (Weiss 1977).[87] A related question, which presumes the ontological existence and agency of spirits, is whether the motivation for a bhuta or graha to possess a human being is located in the spirit itself, in the faulty behaviour of the afflicted person, or in a malevolent third person as in the practice of sorcery and counter-sorcery. Finally, the question of whether or not bhutavidya has ever been practised as a branch of Ayurveda is highly controversial.

Scholars of Indian medicine are likely to agree with a translation of bhutavidya as something like knowledge of existent beings "most of which are invisible or assumed to be inhabiting other beings [...] and are believed to cause various diseases, including certain forms of mental illness" (Smith 2006, 472). Alongside these ontological transfigurations of bhuta and graha, all Ayurvedic psychiatrists with whom I discussed this issue translated bhutavidya as "Ayurvedic psychiatry", despite the fact that, as noted above, the theory and treatment of mental disorders in Ayurveda draws on sections of the classical texts other than bhutavidya. The rhetorical manoeuvre of reconfiguring bhutavidya as

"Ayurvedic psychiatry" serves to join this newly created discipline to a reinterpreted past while at the same time rendering it commensurable with global and national mental health agendas.

Bhutavidya has been translated as "demonology" by some scholars; however some Ayurvedic practitioners interpreted bhuta as bacteria, viruses and fungi in a mid-twentieth century effort to biomedicalize Ayurvedic categories, and reconfigured bhutavidya as bacteriology (Langford 2002, 87; Lang and Jansen 2013; Naraindas 2014a). Later, the sections on bhutavidya in the samhitas were reinterpreted and integrated into what is today called Ayurvedic psychiatry by college-trained Ayurvedic practitioners, but not, of course, without purifying them of their reference to spirits. In their translation as bacteria, viruses or fungi, the externality and ontology of the bhutas are retained but the translation of bhutavidya into Ayurvedic psychiatry abolishes agency and ontology entirely. All Ayurvedic psychiatrists with whom I spoke distanced themselves from the understanding of bhuta (or graha) as spirits or demons. For example, in my first discussion with Dr Sundaran, he criticized the "misconceptions" about bhutavidya held by Ayurvedic practitioners themselves (who discard this branch because of this assumption) and by "society" at large:[88]

> Bhuta is ghost or devils; that is the image of every Indian. While hearing the word bhut, they immediately think it is some ghost or goblins or devils. Actually they don't know the meaning of the word bhuta, which is "living organism." For that you have to study Ayurveda for many years. The postgraduate teachers also don't know about this, so this is not too easy.

Other Ayurvedic psychiatrists repeatedly voiced this sentiment and, indicative of the importance of this issue, one of the topics of the first paper on the syllabus for the Ayurvedic psychiatry postgraduate course is "controversies, myths, and misconceptions regarding bhutavidya" as related to gods, spirits and demons. It was clear from interviews with patients and caregivers that many of them associated mental illness with possession or sorcery. This was the reason most had a long history of seeking diagnosis and treatment from astrologers, religious healers such as Hindu mantravadis, priests and thangals, or at religious healing centres, in addition to pursuing treatment with allopathic and Ayurvedic practitioners.

The elimination of spirits from Ayurvedic psychiatry is also evident in the context of Ayurvedic medication. In the classical texts, spirits and sorcery are among the indications for certain Ayurvedic medications. Although these medications are still widely used, contemporary practitioners no longer identify spirits or sorcery as indications. For example, a widely-used medication called Kalyanaka grtha is described in two of the classic texts as beneficial for warding off evil spirits, curing unmada, cough, epilepsy, diseases caused by sin, anaemia, itching, poison, *garavisha* [magic poisoning], fever, azoospermia and for persons with no offspring, low intelligence and poor digestive power. However, contemporary Ayurvedic psychiatrists use it only for certain forms of endogenous madness and ignore the other "indications." Moreover, the literal understanding of bhutas or grahas as spirits has been replaced by a mere metaphorical or descriptive understanding as "behavioral similarities" to certain spirits or other mythological figures. "Just like narcissism," Dr Sundaran stressed.[89] "Nobody says narcissism is an affliction of Narcissus or possession." For example, diagnosing a patient with *preta graha* does not mean that a person is actually possessed by a *preta* [dead person]. Rather, it means that the patient's "appearance and activities [...] resemble a cadaver or are like a person who is still as dead. Activities of the person are highly reduced, reduced body movements, slowed intellectual activities and reduced talk" (Anwar 2004). Graha then is reduced to mere descriptive categories like resemblance, without signifying etiology and is deprived of ontology. The etiological or ontological gap resulting from the expulsion or rationalization of bhuta and graha was exemplified in a classroom discussion between Dr Devdas, an instructor in a general medicine department, and his postgraduate students.[90] I asked if preta graha described either the symptom of being "like a cadaver" or the cause itself, and Dr Devdas and the students answered that it described the symptoms only, not the cause. According to the classical texts, the cause would be a spirit, but, as Dr Devdas maintained, "the cause you cannot tell." Without committing himself to a certain ontology of graha or, in other words, leaving ontology purposefully open, Dr Devdas excluded grasping spirits as a cause of *graha unmada* [madness of graha kind] but hinted at the spiritual implications of *karma* [actions in this life or in past lives] which, as opposed to spirit possession, he saw as compatible with modern scientific knowledge.

The ontological insecurity of grahas was also expressed by Dr Sarasvati.[91] She was talking about dissociative identity disorder and I asked whether patients came to GAMH with this problem. "Yes, some patients are there." Referring to an inpatient she continued:

> She was talking like her elder sister. This elder sister committed suicide, some years back. After the suicide she talked like her. Here we have done treatment and we did *dhupana*[92] [fumigation] two, three times a day. After some days she became normal. She was very attached to her sister. We cannot tell what is the correct reason. And they had done some religious therapies and after that they came here. She got relief. We cannot tell, is there any graha.

Dr Sarasvati was deliberately ambiguous regarding the grahas and left ontological space, I assume, for the spirit of this patient's sister to play a role in the affliction. In the next breath, however, she closed this space by relocating grahas into a psychological space.

> The reason might be that she is of *hina sattva* [deficient sattva quality; a predisposition for mental illness] and she was very attached to that sister. How can we diagnose it as graha? We cannot tell it correctly. Previously

> people believed in astrology, some astrologers were there, they diagnosed the grahas and sent them to some specialists. But nowadays, most of the astrologers are fakes.

In Ayurvedic psychiatry classes at the college, students and professors correlated graha unmada with psychotic disorders, in which graha are regarded as the proportion of psychotic features in a patient. Dr Sundaran, in his classic Malayalam-language work on Ayurvedic psychiatry, *Treatment of Mental Diseases in Ayurveda* (1993), translates *bhuta unmada* [madness of bhuta kind] or graha unmada[93] as "personality disorder". Thus, the graha unmada, which in the classical texts are only treatable by religious ritual remedial measures, are rendered medically "untreatable" (Sundaran 1993). Dr Joshua, a young Ayurvedic psychiatrist in private practice, provided a different interpretation.[94] He understood the different forms of graha unmada as an elaborate classification system of different forms of delusion. Dr Sarasvati told me that graha unmada[95] was purely psychological as compared to *dosha unmada* [madness of dosha kind], which was somatic:

> For all unmadas we can see graha symptoms, all are mixed. But we cannot tell it is pure graha. Because the cause of graha is guilty feeling for not going to the temple or not obeying the teachers. But we cannot say it is only because of this guilty feeling. Some other factors will be there. The graha is purely psychological, there is no dosha involvement. That is what is told in our texts. But how can we tell it's pure because of this guilty feeling and that no dosha involvement is there? We cannot tell. It is always both.

The understanding of bhuta or graha unmada as "psychotic features", as "delusions" or as "personality disorders" serves the same purpose: it transfers causality from exogenous causes to internal configurations that conform to a modern psychiatric understanding of mental disorders. These translations deprive bhutas and grahas of ontology by transposing them into the inner psyche.[96] I often asked practitioners and students at GAMH if they used graha diagnostics with patients. Most began their explanation by stating that grahas are not used for diagnosis since treatment is purely based on dosha diagnoses. A graha diagnosis is only considered when symptoms cannot be classified into either dosha unmada or *apasmara* [convulsion, epilepsy]. However, the former was never written in medical charts, nor were grahas used for explaining diagnoses to patients or families. Doctors argued that bhuta could potentially be "misunderstood" by people other than Ayurvedic psychiatrists as being "related to demons and exorcism," which would thereby discredit Ayurvedic psychiatry and mark it as unscientific, superstitious and antiquated. Although symptoms were listed in detail in the charts and a dosha-based diagnosis was usually recorded (though this field was sometimes left blank), I never saw a graha diagnosis in a patient chart.

In their efforts to establish Ayurvedic psychiatry as a distinct specialization, practitioners and students negotiate on two fronts. Vis-à-vis their Ayurvedic colleagues, they seek to justify the development and support of a distinct subfield that focuses exclusively on the mind. Ayurveda is a holistic system and instead of separating body and mind, Ayurvedic practitioners regard and treat them as coexisting parts of a resonating system, in which psychological problems resonate in the body and somatic problems resonate in the mind. Consequently, only recently has a separation arisen in Ayurveda between practitioners treating the body and those treating the mind. The (re)invention of Ayurvedic psychiatry as a separate theory, practice and academic discipline in Kerala, which is influenced by the ontological and institutional power of allopathic psychiatry, establishes a distinction between body and mind that did not exist before. My findings support an argument put forward by Naraindas et al. that "because biomedicine is so overwhelmingly dominant throughout the world, the many forms of 'alternative' medicines are compelled to position themselves in relation to this basic, structuring dualism" (Naraindas et al. 2014, 9). Ayurvedic psychiatry pursues this by redefining this structuring dualism and discovering it in its own past (reconfiguration of bhutavidya as Ayurvedic psychiatry) and by mimicking (Bhabha 1984; Langford 2002) allopathic division of medical fields of specialization. In establishing a distinct field of academic and clinical practice, Ayurvedic psychiatrists are building a niche for themselves by dividing up illness categories between illness of the body and those of the mind.

At the same time, vis-à-vis allopathic psychiatrists and other mental healthcare planners, Ayurvedic psychiatrists seek to legitimize their discipline as a distinct yet equally valid and reliable form of mental health care thereby constituting themselves as relevant actors in the network of mental health care in Kerala. For this latter project, clinicians and students navigate the simultaneous tasks of purifying theory and practice from allopathic psychiatry on the one hand and translating Ayurvedic concepts and treatments into allopathic ones on the other. Correspondingly, clinicians and students seek to rid Ayurvedic psychiatry from associations with spirit possession and occult violence, yet often draw upon these same ontologies in patient interactions. Through these practices of purification Ayurvedic psychiatrists contribute to the professionalization (Brass 1972; Leslie 1976; Langford 2002) of institutionalized Ayurvedic psychiatry centred on the Sanskrit classical body of knowledge to the exclusion of subaltern, non-textual knowledge and practice.

By the rhetorical manoeuvre of translating their field into psychiatry, Ayurvedic psychiatrists lay claim to the modern science of psychiatry that developed as a medical subject in Europe at the end of the eighteenth century under specific historical circumstances (Shorter 1997) as one of the classic fields of Ayurveda. By a second rhetorical manoeuvre, they include the treatment of dosha unmada and apasmara along with graha unmada under this (re)invented Ayurvedic field of bhutavidya or psychiatry. Although the theory and treatment of mental disorders in Ayurveda draws largely on the general medicine sections of the classical texts, it is bhutavidya (one of the eight branches of Ayurveda) that is translated into Ayurvedic psychiatry. Although spirits as etiologies of bhutavidya are discarded and the classifications reinterpreted as "personality disorders" or as "psychotic features" and rarely used in diagnosing mental disorders within Ayurvedic psychiatry, the whole project of reconfiguring bhutavidya as psychiatry serves to tie this newly-created discipline to a reinterpreted past.

Students and practitioners of Ayurveda start from the premise that the two knowledge systems or ontologies that define the body and mind, mental health and illness – Ayurvedic and allopathic – cannot be neatly mapped on to each other, and in principle are untranslatable. For example, when I asked Ayurvedic psychiatrists about Ayurvedic concepts that correlate with depression, Dr Rasheed explained:[97]

> You won't find categories such as depression, schizophrenia or mania in our texts as you find them in the ICD. What you will find are umbrella terms such as *vatonmada* [a state characterized by unsteadiness of thought and emotions and psychotic features], *pittonmada* [a state characterized by excessive emotions or passions], *kaphonmada* [a phlegmatic, despondent state], or *adhijonmada* [mental illness following a loss]. They can be correlated with some aspects of psychiatric diagnoses, but not with all.

Ayurvedic psychiatrists propagate a fundamentally different yet equally valid and reliable approach towards mental health. This basic untranslatability, "medical parallelism" (Wolfgram 2009), or "conceptual bilingualism" (Naraindas 2006), is obvious in the syllabus for the course Ayurvedic Psychology and Psychiatry, edited by the Central Council of Indian Medicine (CCIM).[98] This syllabus was written under the aegis of Dr Sharma, the former head of Department of Kaya Chikitsa at the Ayurveda College in Kottakkal and the architect of its *manasika* [psychiatry] postgraduate course. Although as a proponent of *suddha* [pure] Ayurveda[99] he wanted to craft a purely Ayurvedic syllabus, he had to make concessions. "The senior members of the commission told me that they wanted to have some modern[100] points also. These people, their thinking is modern now so they have added modern things in it," he told me. In the syllabus, "modern" and "Ayurvedic" etiologies and nosologies are merely juxtaposed without an attempt to relate them to one another. For example, postgraduate students of Ayurvedic psychiatry study the concept of the mind in different Indian *shastric* [scholastic] traditions, including the three Ayurvedic classics, as well as in modern psychology. They learn "psychological processes" like attention, perception, cognition and, as a separate field, the Ayurvedic theory of mental states, emotions and disturbances, their etiology and their treatment. They are taught the basics of neurophysiology and of the *manovahashrotas* [mind-carrying channels], *sattvabalam* [mental strength] and the three *gunas* [qualities]. They write papers on the classifications and types of mental disorders, their etiologies and diagnostic tools in Ayurvedic classics and allopathic textbooks. They study different forms of psychotherapy that are regarded as relevant to clinical practice such as transactional analysis, behavioural therapy and psychoanalysis alongside yoga and *sattvavajaya* [Ayurvedic psychotherapy]. They learn the importance of intellect, willpower, memory and self-knowledge for mental health. They are taught *dravyaguna* [Ayurvedic pharmacology] along with allopathic psychopharmacology and the three parts of Ayurvedic treatment *yuktivyapasraya chikitsa* [rational treatment], *daivavyapasraya chikitsa* [faith therapy] and sattvavajaya.

Students are introduced to allopathic concepts and the management of anxiety disorders, stress induced disorders, depression, somatoform and mood disorders, and psychosexual disorders. They are given an introduction to the threefold division of the Ayurvedic management of mental disorder into daivyavyapasraya, sattvavajaya and drugless treatment, and *medhya rasayana* [mind rejuvenating] in the management of mental diseases. Finally they receive an "introduction to bhutavidya with special reference to diagnosis and management of disorders in the field."[101] The parallel organization of knowledge becomes even more obvious when considering how the course is organized. A class on "Depression: The Modern View" might be followed by a session on "Depression: The Ayurvedic View" without any effort to develop an integrative model. Thus, students study both biomedical ("modern") and Ayurvedic nosologies, etiologies and therapies. However, they study them in parallel and juxtaposed to one another, without prioritizing one over the other, without relating them to each other, without reconciling their ontologies and without logically connecting them in one coherent model. The separation of Ayurveda and allopathy is also strictly maintained on institutional levels. For example, doctors working at GAMH emphasize that it is a "pure" Ayurvedic hospital. The mental state examinations and diagnoses are Ayurvedic, and the drugs and procedures prescribed are Ayurvedic. It took me quite some time, however, to understand that almost all patients at GAMH and the Ayurveda College continued the psychopharmaceuticals previously prescribed by allopathic psychiatrists. Indeed, GAMH doctors do not *prescribe* allopathic drugs; the parallel treatment approach is the result of legal regulations restricting Ayurvedic doctors from prescribing or stopping allopathic medication.

The main aim of policing the boundaries between Ayurvedic and allopathic psychiatry is, I argue, to establish and institutionalize a separate, distinct and autonomous yet equally valid alternative theory and practice of mental illness and mental health. In this way, doctors maintain a space for Ayurveda in a field dominated by allopathic psychiatry.

Translating diagnoses and physiologies

In order to become a relevant actor in public mental health in Kerala and to communicate effectively with allopathic practitioners, mental health planners, patients and caregivers, Ayurvedic psychiatrists not only reconfigure bhutavidya into Ayurvedic psychiatry but also engage global psychiatric nosologies. In a simplifying effort, the three main forms of unmada are correlated with the "big three" categories of modern psychiatry: vatonmada is roughly translated into schizophrenia; pittonmada into mania; and kaphonmada into depression.[102] They thus mimic mainstream psychiatric presumed disease entities and do so at a time when these disease entities are becoming less stable and bounded in the light of recent neuropsychiatric research (Insel 2014). However, Ayurvedic psychiatrists treat the DSM and the ICD in a similar way as they treat the classical texts: as eternal truths.

The asymmetrical relations between biomedicine and Ayurveda and the epistemological and ontological hegemony of biomedicine force practitioners and students to engage and appropriate mainstream psychiatric nosologies, to integrate them into Ayurvedic theories, and translate Ayurvedic knowledge into the language of mainstream psychiatry. Although practitioners of Ayurvedic psychiatry emphasize that Ayurvedic terms and concepts cannot be neatly translated into mainstream psychiatric ones, in their interaction with patients, in classroom debates, research, medical charts and the interviews I conducted, students and practitioners were constantly involved in translation processes in both the conventional and the Latourian sense. The question of how modern psychiatric classifications of mental disorders can and should be translated into Ayurvedic nosologies is a topic of continuing debate in academic and clinical contexts. Through simultaneous processes of translation and purification, Ayurvedic and biomedical bodies and minds are rendered commensurable while at the same time maintaining their respective autonomies. At the same time, Ayurvedic psychiatry is created and stabilized through Latourian translations. This kind of medical parallelism positions Ayurvedic psychiatry as an actor in the network of mental health in India while at the same time safeguards its autonomy as a distinct system.

But Ayurvedic psychiatrists do not only translate diagnoses, they also translate physiologies. I have shown the ubiquity of the neurochemical imbalance narrative of depression as an important element of what is regarded as mental health literacy in India that is propagated by psychiatrists and the mental health movement (Chapter 3). Consequently, the terms that signify a modern and scientific approach to mental health such as hormones, neurotransmitters, synapses and neuronal structures are translated into and made commensurable with Ayurvedic concepts. Dr Krishnan translated manovahashrotas [mind-carrying channels] into neuronal circuits and integrated Ayurvedic and allopathic knowledge in explaining the phenomenon of neuronal networks:[103]

> If I see something new for me for the first time it will make a circuit in me. After several years if I see the same thing I will get a memory. That means this circuit will again be channelized or synthesized. If these circuits are facilitated and repeatedly stimulated, they will remain and make a life-long memory in me. This only happens through these newly developed channels. These same channels we will call manovahashrotas. Allopathic people will speak about neuronal dendrites and axons. But if you ask about the anatomy of manovahasrotas we are not in a position to show that. Manovahashrotas is not a structural term, purely a functional one. You dissect and nothing

> will be seen. Dendrites and axons we can see. But you will never get to see our manovahashrotas. So I am telling, what happens in modern psychiatry, these channels and all, that is more or less the manovahasrotas in Ayurveda. But anatomically we can't identify these things.

Dr Nayar, a former student of Dr Krishnan, jumped in and continued the translation and assemblage of depression, neurons, neurotransmitters, kaphonmada, *vata* [wind, moving principle] and manovahashrotas:[104] "Depression," Dr Nayar began,

> is a process that causes the blockade of the transport of information from one neuron to the other. So that itself is happening in Ayurveda also. Manovahashrotas, there is some obstruction. Because of this obstruction the information cannot travel from one area to another.

"From the neuron comes the message," continued Dr Krishnan.

> The message has to jump from one neuron to the other. A lot of neurotransmitters are here at the junction. Only because of these elements the messages are transported to another synapse. This is the modern thing. In Ayurveda these are the manovahashrotas. And the message is conducted to other parts only because of vata.

"I touch you," explained Dr Nayar, "This touch reaches your brain through sensory nerves. Through the sensory nerves some electric current passes. The neuronal conduction, the sensory perception, our responses, everything comes under vata." Dr Krishnan continued:

> If *kapha* [phlegm, stabilizing principle] obstructs the channels vata cannot pass. Both are the same. The modern doctors say, because of serotonin this message is transported to here. If serotonin is decreased this message is not transported, it is blocked. So the patient develops depression. If acetylcholine, another neurotransmitter, is decreased, it will affect the memory. And melatonin is good for calmness and peace, sleep and all. If it is not transported, the patient becomes irritable in the night and develops sleeplessness, insomnia. So everything happens because of a block. A block because of the loss or decrease in quantity of the hormones. In Ayurveda we say that kapha is increased and blocks the channels and vata is not passing, being obstructed by kapha. That's all. So functionally, seen from outside, both are the same.

Dr Nayar concluded:

> There is a decrease in serotonin, it can cause depressive illness. This means some factor has gone down. If you analyse it in terms of modern science

> there is some chemical change that happens in your brain. That chemical change we are talking about here takes place in a very broad way. What is the function of serotonin? It carries information from one neuron to the other. If serotonin comes down there is a block in this connection and you don't get the proper meaning here. If we are telling in this way, you are telling in that way. We are finding symptoms of kapha here and we are treating against kapha. You try to increase serotonin by giving SSRI [selective serotonin reuptake inhibitor, a type of antidepressant], so you inhibit the reabsorption of serotonin. We try to reduce kapha.

These doctors described vata as responsible for transporting and transmitting information, but Dr Varghese translated vata somewhat differently[105]: "The motivating force is vata. In modern terminology, vata is the nervous system. Without this nervous system, the stimulation of nervous system, without motivation and moving up of the nervous system, nothing moves in our body." Both the nervous system and the transmission of messages were often framed as the activities of vata, however Ayurvedic physicians often translated the chemical activities of neurotransmitters or local hormones into activities of *pitta* [bile] and *agni* [digestive fire]. "Local hormones can create mood disorders," began Dr Nayar.[106]

> Hormones and neurotransmitters are the activity of agni and behind the curtain we can find pitta dosha. Hormones are always catalysts; they will accelerate a certain type of chemical reaction. Serotonin is a neurotransmitter and it acts like a local hormone. Serotonin and noradrenalin come under agni; they are a type of agni. As per our concept agni is the transforming agent. It can include all those factors that create the biocatalysists; it converts something. What is the function of a neurotransmitter? It carries the information from one neuron to another. So somehow it acts like a carriage.

"So it doesn't come under vata?" I asked. "It supports vata. The hormones support the activity of vata," he replied.

> The *kapha dosha* [kapha humour] has become so high in the body. And vata dosha has become very low. The increased kapha has deranged the pitta status also. It has also subdued pitta because kapha is a thing of a watery nature. So what will happen with fire [pitta][107] if water[108] comes? Fire will set down. So naturally all the metabolic processes will come down in our body. In that way pitta is subdued.

Dr Nayar's framing of the function of enzymes, hormones and neurotransmitters as pitta was a formation I heard frequently from other Ayurvedic physicians.

Most patients in Kerala are more familiar with notions such as depression, schizophrenia, or mania than with Ayurvedic concepts of (and terms for) mental illness.[109] Many come to Ayurvedic clinical encounters equipped with these terms, and doctors must therefore "pre-translate" (Wolfgram 2009) Ayurvedic categories. For example, in the experience of Dr Joseph John:[110]

> People are more scientific than us. They get onto the Internet and study all about the etiology of the disease, the process of the disease, and its treatment. All those [allopathic] things are well-studied and people come to us with this knowledge. The Internet is a way to enter into this kind of education themselves. But we Ayurveda doctors will speak another language, that of Ayurveda.

Dr Rasheed[111] connected these translations with psychiatric epidemiology:[112]

> The reason for this [translation] is if a patient is coming, we cannot get the data of how many kapha unmada persons are there in Kerala. But we can get the data of how many depression patients there are. So we have to look: what are the diseases currently, what diseases are prominent, what diseases cause problems in society? So by seeing and studying the disease we will compare it to Ayurvedic parlance. But we have to treat only on the basis of Ayurvedic categories. We correlate modern diagnoses to Ayurvedic parlance.

As these practitioners demonstrated, Ayurvedic psychiatrists engage allopathic psychiatric knowledge and terminology to make them understood, taken seriously and considered relevant by both patients and allopathic psychiatry more broadly. In this way, they "translate up" to establish Ayurvedic practitioners, knowledge and drugs as actors in mental healthcare. While doctors are convinced of the epistemological incompatibility of the two systems on the level of ideology which leads them to the construction of boundaries, in practice they are often involved in translation processes both for the sake of legitimacy and for patients' and their caretakers' understandings.

Ayurvedic psychiatrists usually do not use or explain Ayurvedic diagnoses in consultations with patients and their caregivers, nor do they mention graha diagnoses. In most cases, Ayurvedic psychiatrists focus their explanations on the correct mode of administering medicines. If they mention a diagnosis, it is always the allopathic one. What Dr Sarasvati told me was typical of most Ayurvedic psychiatrists.[113] "Outside people, they cannot understand what is kaphonmada or vatonmada." "So what do you say if you talk with the patients or with the families if they ask, 'what is wrong with me?'" I asked. The first thing, she said, was to avoid "shocking" the family with the diagnosis.

> For most patients we do not tell the diagnoses to them. Simply treat them. Otherwise they will ask about what is schizophrenia. It's a major disorder, it's very difficult to cure and the patient will get depressed after getting the diagnosis. The patient will be shocked after hearing the diagnosis. So for most people we do not tell the diagnoses to them.

Moreover, most patients or family members are not interested in the diagnosis. "The patients do not ask what is the name of the disease, they are not concerned about that. They want to cure the patient, the disease." "And what about families?" I insisted. "Only some people ask about the background and the treatment. Most of the people here are not asking about the diagnoses of the disease. They want a cure."

Refraining from informing patients and their family members about the disease – although contradictory to the politics and protocols of informed consent – is a form of "ethical pragmatism" (Sousa 2011) employed also by many mainstream psychiatrists. It is intended to prevent patients from the stigma of being labelled with a mental illness. I then asked Dr Sarasvati whether she would rather share the Ayurvedic or the allopathic diagnosis, particularly in the case of depression. "I think it's better to say depression," she replied.

> Otherwise it's very difficult to explain about kaphonmada to them. If we tell them that the patient has depression, they will know because they read it in the newspaper or heard it on the TV. But they don't know what kaphonmada is.

Similarly, Dr Mangalam used allopathic physiologies to explain the disease:[114]

> If the patient says, "I am always feeling sleepy the whole day", I will say, "You don't worry, your sleeping nature is only because you have some neuro-hormonal affliction along with the disease. Don't bother about it." I will also tell them, "in those who suffer from depression there is a tendency to develop hypothyroidism features along with that. Don't worry, it will be corrected." The disease status should be explained.

In the case of depression, it was always the allopathic terms and physiologies that doctors employed, never the Ayurvedic.

"We are damn sure about it": research and evidence in Ayurvedic psychiatry

The relationship between mainstream and Ayurvedic psychiatry is characterized by asymmetries with regard to both political influence and funding. A major objection to Ayurvedic psychiatry is the criticism by mental health planners and mainstream psychiatrists that its claims of efficacy are "not proven". That is, that the procedures and drug formulations of Ayurvedic psychiatry have not been adequately tested by randomized control trials (RCT) – the epitome of evidence-based medicine (EBM) – or other accepted forms of clinical research. In fact, Ayurvedic psychiatrists demand more research, recognizing it as a requirement for recognition and acceptance. But are clinical control trials as standards of EBM applicable to Ayurveda and specifically to Ayurvedic psychiatry? Even in mainstream psychiatry the question of whether EBM is applicable is highly contested (Gupta 2007), and this is true to an even greater extent for Ayurvedic psychiatry. "Scientific evidence is increasingly becoming a challenge for the integration of traditional medicine in health care", write Bode and Payyappallimana (2013). My findings confirm they are correct in their basic argument that the main reason for the lack of EBM and RCT in Ayurveda and other traditional medicines (apart from lack of financial resources) is that those processes were developed in and are centred on biomedicine whereas the medical and pharmacological logics of Ayurveda have a different basis (cf. also Naraindas 2014b). The "methodological monoculture" (Bode and Payyappallimana 2013, 5) of scientific medical research is characterized by asymmetrical translations of EBM in that it imposes biomedical nosologies – tools for measuring outcomes and research methods – on Ayurveda. Bode and Payyappallimana therefore suggest a host of methods for testing the efficacy of Ayurveda and other traditional medicines, some of which are already included in the WHO "General Guidelines for Methodologies on Research and Evaluation of Traditional Medicine" (2001). One example is the "black box design" in which the treatment is delivered as usual in the clinical settling and studied as a whole, and no element of treatment is isolated for independent study. Another example is observational studies or single case designs (World Health Organization 2001a). Although the problematic of isolating singular chemical ingredients can be partly addressed by these alternatives, asymmetrical relations between biomedicine and Ayurveda are not resolved by these methods as both the diagnoses on which the research is based and the outcome have to be framed using biomedical and not Ayurvedic categories.

How does this debate play out in the clinical and academic practice of Ayurvedic psychiatry in Kerala and what consequences does it have for academic research? How do clinicians and teachers of Ayurvedic psychiatry deal with this structural asymmetry? Their pragmatic solution lies, I argue, in the strategic combination of a systematic medical parallelism of biomedicine and Ayurveda based on the fundamental untranslatability of both systems on the one hand and the constant engagement in translation processes on the other that opens the field for Ayurvedic research to both acknowledge and question mainstream psychiatric authority.

When I talked with mainstream psychiatric mental health professionals and planners, they were either unaware of or "structurally blind" (Quack 2012; Sax 2014) to Ayurvedic psychiatry. One of the key reasons for this is that Ayurveda is not legible to mental health planners because its practitioners do not participate in practices of scientific truth making (Adams 2002) which is regarded as equivalent to research. Dr Lakshmi Nair, an allopathic psychiatrist working in the psychiatric unit of the Guruji Institute of Medical Sciences, criticized Ayurveda (as did many of her colleagues) for not producing research.[115]

> The problem is that they take their knowledge from very old texts. It's not translated into research. They need to do a lot of research. Where are the randomized controlled trials of Ayurvedic medicines testing their efficacy?[116] Without any research they cannot claim that it is effective. Ayurveda is

> basically a traditional kind of healing. The concepts are very different. It is talking about humours. That's not a scientific way. The concept of mental illness is totally different in Ayurveda. There is no concept of neurotransmitters. The latest developments that are happening in modern medicine, they should benefit by that and modify it, but that doesn't happen. Most modern doctors are convinced that it is all humbug. There isn't much to it. It wouldn't stand scientific scrutiny. That is what I think at least. I am being a little arrogant there. But will it stand up to scientific scrutiny? I don't think they want research. There will be some vague kind of so-called research. It won't be a rigorous randomized controlled trial.

Dr Nair's critique is harsh, and it is one Ayurvedic psychiatrists are not only familiar with but also endorse. As Dr Nair's explanation indicates, randomized controlled trials are considered the hallmark of evidence-based medicine (Lambert 2006; Ecks 2008). Whether designed to study psychiatric drugs, psychotherapeutic techniques or Ayurvedic medicines, they are expected from every credible actor that enters the mental health care network. Most of those people I interviewed who had completed the MD course in Ayurvedic psychiatry and/or worked at GAMH or another Ayurvedic institution explicitly called for research and accused the Central Council of Indian Medicine (CCIM) and the Directorate of Indian Systems of Medicines (ISM) of not supporting research in Ayurvedic psychiatry. In 2013, GAMH doctors drafted a report for the Kerala minister of health entitled *Vision 2020*, which recommended dividing the hospital into two wings, one for research and the other for treatment. Dr Shaila, a GAMH doctor and one of the authors of the report, elaborated:[117]

> This is considered a research institute actually. But it operates like a hospital. There is no research organization substructure here. There should be a principal investigator, researchers, research staff, some kind of scientific and ethical committee, some publication, communication. It doesn't operate here. According to our experience, 100% of [patients with] psychological and behavioural disorders benefit from Ayurvedic interventions. 60% can be managed by Ayurvedic interventions alone; 40% require modern psychiatric intervention. For this latter group, Ayurvedic interventions can be used as adjacent or to manage the side effects of the modern medicines; in this case, it improves quality-of-life. In long-term maintenance, modern medicines can be tapered, sometimes even replaced by Ayurvedic medicines. But whatever we say, the actual significance should be supported by actual research data. So for policy, recommendations based on research data are necessary.

Ayurvedic practitioners base their truth claims in three different sources: Ayurvedic *shastra* [the classical texts], *anubhava* [experience] and *yukti* [logical inference or reason] (cf. Wolfgram 2010). Thus, clinical experimentation, which Obeyesekere (1992) has called "samyogic experimentation", has always been part of the generation and enhancement of Ayurvedic knowledge (Trawick 1987) even though randomized controlled trials have not. Ayurvedic practitioners base their knowledge on textual, experiential and logical evidence whereas allopathic psychiatrists and mental health policymakers ground their knowledge and truth claims in clinical research and randomized controlled trials. As Dr Nair noted (above), randomized controlled trials are expected from every credible actor in the officially acknowledged mental health care network. Ayurvedic psychiatrists are also concerned about this problem. Research, therefore, is the conduit for several key processes: the legitimization of Ayurveda alongside biomedicine; the successful marketing of Ayurvedic pharmaceutical companies and medications; and the entry of Ayurvedic knowledge into broader psychiatric regimes of truth.

The translation process involved in this effort is twofold: Ayurvedic researchers integrate ICD nosologies into Ayurvedic terms and thus interpret classical texts into the framework of recent psychiatric classifications. At the same time, they confer authority to Ayurvedic texts and clinical practice "to speak on behalf of" (Callon & Latour 1981, p. 279) allopathic psychiatry, thereby integrating themselves into a mental health care network dominated by allopathic actors. In stark contrast to biomedical research, however, the aim of Ayurvedic research is not the development of new knowledge but rather to prove the efficacy of already existing knowledge, medicines and procedures as laid out in the classical texts. Ayurvedic research thus explicitly addresses and aims to convince non-Ayurvedic health planners and policy makers, not Ayurvedic practitioners.

Dr Krishnan, one of the teachers in the manasika postgraduate course at the Ayurveda College, explained the intent and scope of research in Ayurvedic psychiatry:[118]

> We are doing research for other people, not for Ayurvedic people, for other scientists apart from Ayurveda, to convince them there is something in Ayurveda. That is the purpose. So in that respect, when we discuss it, it has to be dealt in their language. If we say this particular drug is effective in unmada or apasmara, nobody cares about it. They want to know very specifically, for example, what is the role of Ayurveda in depressive disorders? Depression is a term coined by ICD. According to their nomenclature, their diagnostic and assessment criteria, we have to do something. Otherwise it won't be recognized in scientific parameters.

"So you are forced to use allopathic terms?" I asked. "Forced only in order to convey the results to other people, not for us people," he replied.

> For us people [Ayurvedic practitioners] it is better to use categories such as unmada or apasmara. That is better for us. But research is for them only, not for us. Because we are very damn sure about the effect of a drug. No research is needed. We practise daily. That empirical experience is there. For us research is not needed. Mainly to convince other people it has to be tested, toxicity, safety measures, all these stages we have to pass. Otherwise

> nobody will accept it. Even at a national level also. In institutions it is OK, you can do a lot of things, keeping Ayurveda terms and all. But the outcome will be worthless; it can be kept on the shelves only.

Having stated the need for research in order to achieve scientific recognition of Ayurveda, Dr Krishnan clearly separated academic research from "real research" and emphasized that "real research" in Ayurvedic psychiatry does not take place, either at the College or at the Government Ayurveda Research Institute for Mental Diseases. "Real research" would include all five stages of clinical trials, double-blinded and with large numbers of participants lasting over several years.[119] The research at the colleges does not fulfil either of these criteria, he said.

> Here we are not doing research. What you have seen in the theses of our students, that is not research, that is dissertation only. That is just for getting a degree, that's all. First and second stage is pharmacological studies and testing on healthy people. Our students do the third stage only, clinical efficacy. And their sample size is just around ten patients only. That will never be accepted. [...] Research is a very long-term process; it will take years and years to come out with a new drug. But nobody is doing that in Ayurveda, that is the problem. [...] Research is not for the sake of people, not for the sake of science. It is for the sake of the government or the sake of the research. Research is for the sake of research only. [...]. Real Ayurvedic research is happening nowhere in India.

Dr Krishnan envisioned the establishment of public research institutions for Ayurvedic psychiatry. Another possibility Dr Krishnan imagined was the creation of a national institute of Ayurvedic psychiatry with a similar form and scope to the National Institute of Mental Health and Neurosciences (NIMHANS) in Bangalore.[120]

He did not preclude collaborative research involving the assessment of Ayurvedic treatment using allopathic tools, in accordance with the WHO black box design where treatment as a whole is evaluated:

> We will do our treatment protocol according to our freedom, let them look from outside and evaluate. Let them tell the society. If they claim our treatment is efficient that will be useful. If we [Ayurveda] people make claims, nobody will accept it. Our government supports collaborative works only. So we have to associate with some allopathic people and come out with the outcome. I am not against allopathic doctors, they have to be with us. All contemporary knowledge we have to accept, then only the science will develop. So when we do *vamana* [therapeutic vomiting] let them do their scan, look into what happens in the brain. That they can do only, I can't do, I have not studied that. That collaboration is needed.

In an institution of that kind, Dr Krishnan said, real research could take place. The problem of the incompatibility of concepts of the body and mind, health and disease, and efficacy and effectiveness, as noted by Bode and Payyappallimana (2013), is undeniable. But Dr Krishnan believed these problems could be overcome by engaging in collaborative and rigorous research.

Broadly speaking, there are four kinds of contemporary institutional research in Ayurveda based on biomedical guidelines of scientific truth. The first is postgraduate research in Ayurveda educational institutions consisting of both textual and clinical research; however this is rarely published or peer-reviewed. The second is that conducted by the Central Council for Research in Ayurvedic Sciences (CCRAS) that has units across the country and is run by the Government of India. Although the Council produces publications, their impact on clinical practice is slight. The third type of institutional research is conducted by the research and development units of the larger, private Ayurveda pharmaceutical companies. The fourth kind is research conducted in non-governmental Ayurvedic research institutions such as the Integrative Institute of Ayurveda (IIA), Bangalore funded both by the government and private industry (Ganguly 2014).

Research undertaken by postgraduates – the first of the four kinds of contemporary institutional research in Ayurveda – involves two steps. First, in a kind of hermeneutic exegesis of the ancient Ayurvedic texts in light of modern nosologies and etiologies, students comb through the classic texts to correlate modern diagnoses to Ayurvedic ones. Second, on the basis of the latter, they find treatment protocols described in the classical texts and conduct small-scale clinical studies comparing the effect of Ayurvedic treatment with its allopathic counterpart, sometimes blinded and sometimes not. For their postgraduate research, students choose a special field of interest such as schizophrenia, depression, alcohol dependence or attention deficit hyperactivity disorder (ADHD). The theses begin with conceptual groundwork in which "modern" and "Ayurvedic" conceptions, nosologies and etiologies are presented in parallel, often without synthesis. Research subjects are selected from among GAMH inpatients and college outpatients. When patients first arrive at these institutions most are seen by the head of department, then closer examination and treatment is delegated to a student specializing in their particular complaint or illness. The student's work with the patients assigned to them constitutes a key part of their research. Because this form of research is the most prevalent, it is important to examine in greater detail how research in Ayurvedic psychiatry is conducted at the college. To do so, I examine three cases – two clinical studies and one hermeneutic project.

For his MD thesis, Hamid Mevekari (2003) tested the effect of passive and active smoke inhalation on kaphonmada. The classic texts describe inhalation of smoke [*dhumapana*] with the help of a pipe as a measure against mental illness due to an imbalance of the doshas [*dosha unmada*] and other diseases of the head and neck. Passive inhalation of smoke is described as a measure against *agantu unmada* [mental illness caused by external agents] and is often used in ritual healing. As Mevekari explains, doctors explain to patients that the smoke treatment is a religious treatment to improve their compliance. In the first chapters of his thesis, Mevekari describes the modern and Ayurvedic concepts of normal and abnormal *manas* [mind and emotions] and of mental illness and mood disorders, followed by a short comparison of kaphonmada and depression, and a general discussion of the treatment methods outlined for mental disorders in the classic texts. His "drug study" describes the "pharmacodynamics" of the two drugs used in his clinical trial, *shankhapusphpyadi churna*[121] and *brahmyadi varti*, both a mixture of several ingredients, in which pharmacodynamics is used as a direct translation of the Ayurvedic terms guna and karma.[122] For each ingredient, names (including the botanical) are given, and their "pharmacodynamics" described in Ayurvedic and biomedical terms. Shankhapushpyadi churna comprises three and brahmyadi varti twenty-one ingredients, out of which Mevekari chose nine for his clinical study. He prominently justifies the need for research in Ayurveda in his project construction:

> In the present era, there is no place for blind faith in tradition and authority of the shastras. Faith has been replaced by scepticism and scientific inquiry even for the truths traditionally established. Only the facts established by proofs derived after careful investigations, observations and experiments and supported by accurate clinical data and convincing reasoning can convince today's science about the validity of any hypothesis. [...] A clinical study will be required to support the literary findings about the role of dhupana and dhumapana in the management of kaphonmada.
>
> (Mevekari 2003, 126–127)

This emphasis on the importance of textual and clinical evidence in Ayurvedic psychiatric research and training is echoed in most of the theses I read. For Mevekari's study, twenty patients attending the OPDs of the Kaya Chikitsa Department of the Ayurveda College and GAMH were selected on the basis of DSM-IV criteria for major depressive disorder (not according to the criteria for kaphonmada although this Ayurvedic classification appears in the title of the thesis) and divided randomly into a treatment group who were given *shankhapusphpyadi churna* and *brahmyadi varti*, and a control group who received only two herbs. Both groups were treated for one month. For assessment, the author used both Ayurvedic[123] and mainstream psychiatric scales. Though details such as the sex, age, religion and socio-economic status are carefully noted for the subject group, these are only listed, not correlated with certain results or observations. In terms of analysis, the effect of therapy and the difference between the treatment and the control group are identified with relation to the symptoms of kaphonmada. The same process is repeated for the symptoms of major depressive disorder. Mevekari found that a high percentage of patients in the treatment group experienced significant improvement, whereas the majority of the control group experienced mild to moderate improvement. Mevekari's findings are twofold: (1) the symptomatology of kaphonmada and depression are approximately the same; and (2) dhupana and dhumapana used in conjunction with the described drugs are effective in *kaphonmada* [depression].

In the second case, Dawn Abraham conducted a comparative study on the effects of an Ayurvedic medication and antidepressants on moderate depression for her postgraduate thesis in the manasika course at the Ayurveda College, Kottakkal (Abraham 2009). Abraham begins with a conceptual study dealing with the "modern view" of depression including the neurobiology, clinical features and management followed by separate consideration of the "Ayurvedic view". Here, Abraham distinguishes between *nija* [internal] and *agantu* [external] mental disorders, and stresses the role of "intellectual errors" [*prajnaparadha*] with regard to supernatural entities and living persons that makes a person prone to graha unmada. In her analysis, for grahas, "the actual cause is the sinful act due to *prajnaparadha*[124] that causes worry, fear and guilty consciousness about that act". *Manovikaras*[125] [abnormal emotional conditions, overflowing emotions or passions] such as lust, greed, and grief are identified as the main causes for unmada which Abraham translates as "unsoundness of mind" (Abraham 2009, 42) and which is characterized by "dysfunction of mind, intellect, consciousness memory, desire, manners, behavior, and conduct" (Abraham 2009, 42ff). Abraham also addresses the issue of biomedical and Ayurvedic translation: "In Ayurveda we cannot directly correlate depression to a particular disease entity. Anyway some of the features of depression can be seen in many of the diseases mentioned in Ayurveda" (Abraham 2009, 47). She argues that neurotic depression cannot be included under unmada since it affects only the mind and not the other functions above while psychotic depression falls under unmada because it affects these functions. Psychotic depression as a form of unmada requires *shodana* [purifying] and *samana* [pacifying] treatments, whereas in neurotic depression psychotherapy and the use of medhya rasayana drugs may be sufficient (Abraham 2009, 51). Abraham correlates kaphonmada to a more severe and psychotic form of depression, and *vishada* to minor depression. Kaphonmada arises due to a causative factor (she does not specify what this was in the research subjects) that affects the body including agni and kapha dosha, and the mind including *rajas* [activity] and *tamas* [ignorance] gunas. These affect the heart and lead to a disturbance of manas that might again manifest somatically or mentally and lead to dysfunction of the mental faculties or to decreased psychomotor activity and increased fatigue. Both are symptoms of the diagnosis kaphonmada (Abraham 2009, 52). Vishada also identifies the role of a causative factor that leads to a rise of rajas and tamas, and somatically, to a rise in vata and kapha. In this case, manas is again disturbed which can result in prajnaparadha and associated mental dysfunction and physical debilitation. Both are indicators for vishada.

Abraham then describes the pharmacodynamics and effects of an Ayurvedic drug comprised of *jatamamsi* (Nardostachys jatamansi) and *jyothishmati* (Celastrus paniculata) (known as the "JJ tablet"), and SSRI antidepressants. Fifteen outpatients from the Ayurveda College and GAMH received the JJ tablet; fifteen outpatients from Calicut Medical College received fluoxetine, sertraline and/or citalopram. The diagnostic criteria were based in the ICD-10 diagnosis of moderate depression, and for assessment frameworks Abraham employed the Hamilton Depression Rating Scale (HDRS), the Tamas and Rajas Rating Scales (two Ayurvedic rating scales developed by students of the Ayurveda College, Kottakkal, described further below) and the Mental State Examination (an assessment developed by the Ayurveda Research Centre, NIMHANS). Abraham found that both the JJ tablet and the SSRIs were highly significant in reducing the symptoms of moderate depression, and that the difference between their effectiveness was statistically insignificant. The SSRI group of drugs was more effective in treating insomnia, suicidal tendencies and symptoms of anxiety. The JJ tablet was more effective in cases of agitation, somatic symptoms, paranoid symptoms and obsessions.

Particularly notable in Abraham's study are the assessment frameworks she employed. The appropriation of depression also involves the creative integration and transformation of instruments to quantitatively measure the degree to which the disorder is affecting an individual. In an effort to mimic mainstream psychiatric rating scales such as the Hamilton Rating Scale for Depression or the Beck Depression Inventory, and to develop quantitative tools for the evaluation of Ayurvedic psychiatry in terms of what is regarded as evidence-based medicine, students of Ayurvedic psychiatry in Kottakkal use the two Ayurvedic rating scales developed by former students of the college and based on the descriptions of the three gunas.[126] In the rating scales, rajas and tamas as predispositions to mental disorder become measurable indices of the degree of mental health or disorder in a patient. The Tamas Rating Scale (TRS) encompasses nine items and Rajas Rating Scale (RRS) thirteen, and are rated from zero (indicating an absence of symptoms) to three (indicating severe presence of symptoms). TRS employs Sanskrit terms to enquire about the patient's depressive states such as belief in God and the degree of nihilism, guilty conscience, communication and understanding of the disease. Further, inquiries are made regarding retardation of speech, decreased interest in activities, disturbed sleep and deviant opinions. Items in RRS relevant to depression are the perception that life is miserable, disturbed relationships with family members and colleagues due to *ahamkara* [ego], and anger. TRS in particular resembles mainstream psychiatric rating scales due to shared items such as depressed mood, feelings of guilt, self-reflection, work and activities. However, students emphasized that the Ayurvedic scales were not developed in concordance with allopathic tools, but are purely Ayurvedic and based on short verses in Ayurvedic classic texts that describe the features of the three gunas. Although some professors criticized Ayurvedic rating scales as superficial and not scientifically validated they are nonetheless regarded as important tools that depict the complexity of the Ayurvedic approach much more effectively than allopathic rating scales and instruments (for a detailed description of these rating scales, see Lang & Jansen 2013).

The third, more conceptual thesis has been quite influential for the pedagogics of Ayurveda psychiatry at the College. Anwar (2004) focused on depressive disorders and carried out a hermeneutic exegesis of the classical texts in light of the ICD-based classification of disorders. His aim is "to examine the scientific basis of the correlation of kaphonmada with depressive disorder".[127] For this purpose he compares depressive disorders with all information available in Ayurvedic texts on kaphonmada and other forms of graha unmada. Additionally, a clinical study of thirty patients who met the criteria for depressive disorders of the ICD-10 was used to test the conceptual work and Anwar collected information on "treatment packages" for mental disorders, including kaphonmada, from twenty traditional religious practitioners. Early on he highlights general untranslatability of the Ayurvedic categories and classification of unmada:

> The most important thing is that Ayurvedic psychological diseases are classified according to specificities or similarities shown by speech character and activities of the abnormal person. But in modern psychiatry each disease has its own specific psychopathology. In Ayurveda no specific psychopathology is explained for each disease. So it is difficult to explain the psychopathology of Ayurvedic diseases on [a] modern basis. So correlation of Ayurvedic mental disorders to modern psychiatric disorders has a lot of limitations. Still for explaining different Ayurvedic psychological disorder[s] to the public some knowledge about modern psychiatric disease and their psychopathology and its apparent correlations in Ayurveda is necessary. [...] Though Ayurveda has a rich description of mental disorders they are rarely in practice today. Now it is high time to explore the real sense of Ayurvedic psychiatry and to remove the misconception about it in the society.
>
> (Anwar 2004, 5–7)

Anwar explains, "Most of the Ayurvedic psychiatry is dealt in one of the eight branches of Ayurveda called bhutavidya." Although bhutavidya has been "misunderstood as demonology and related to possession", compared to "treatments similar to black magic or exorcism", and discredited by most contemporary Ayurvedic practitioners as unscientific, "the real sense of the science is entirely different" (Anwar 2004). In the context of Ayurvedic psychiatry, the term bhuta means "being like or similar" denoting similarities in behaviour, speech or character of patients to a particular mythological being. "So in short bhutavidya deals with abnormal behavior of a person and has nothing to do with demonology" (Anwar 2004, 10–11). Anwar goes on to describe the development of Ayurvedic psychiatry in terms of a narrative of decline from a "science" that was "highly developed" in the classical period into demonology and "something like exorcism". After its decline, Ayurvedic psychiatry was "rediscovered" by Indian psychiatrists interested in "Indian concepts of mental illness" from the 1960s and institutionalized through the addition of papers on psychiatry to the BAMS curriculum, the founding of a research centre for Ayurveda attached to NIMHANS, the development of postgraduate courses and the establishment of GAMH.[128]

Anwar then provides a detailed symptomatology of kaphonmada and various forms of depressive disorders that form the basis of comparison between the two concepts, in which he finds that 88 per cent of the symptoms of depressive disorders are common to kaphonmada. In order to examine the possibility of correlating depressive disorders with some forms of graha unmada, he examines *preta* [spirit of a dead person] and *pitre* [ancestral spirit] graha unmada and concludes that, in these cases, the correlation was much lower.[129] He determines that depressive disorder is most appropriately correlated to kaphonmada, and emphasizes the importance of conceptual study:

> On the basis of modern terminologies and signs and symptoms the real concepts of Ayurvedic disease and its naming techniques can be explained in a more transparent manner. Conceptual studies will help us to get better understanding of these disorders and its corresponding modern parlance and they will pave the way for newer correlations.
>
> (Anwar 2004, 138)

So do the findings of postgraduate theses in Ayurvedic psychiatry have practical consequences for treatment and practices? In large part, it depends on the nature of the research. Some students test drugs and procedures already in use at GAMH or the Arya Vaidy Sala, and this research contributes little-by-little to supporting experience-based and text-based knowledge through evidence-based knowledge Others test drugs and formulations found in the texts but currently not in use, and according to Dr Kumar, some of these rediscovered or newly arranged formulations are integrated into treatment protocols.[130] In the main, the small-scale clinical trials conducted by the postgraduate students reinforce Ayurveda's functioning as shastra (Ganguly 2012).

As in many other disciplines of Ayurveda, postgraduate students of Ayurvedic psychiatry are involved in these small-scale clinical trials of Ayurvedic single drugs, *yogams* [compounds, formulations] and procedures key to scientific truth making and creating evidence for this (re)invented academic and clinical discipline. By these practices, modes of evidence which are specific to Ayurveda such as textual evidence [*shastra*], experiential evidence [*anubhava*] and reasoning [*yukti*] are replaced by allopathic modes of evidence making. These latter are epitomized in biomedicine's randomized controlled trials while shastric knowledge is confirmed by clinical research. By bringing together shastra and science, students not only demonstrate their scientific expertise and academic credentials but also lend legitimacy to Ayurvedic knowledge and clinical practice in the field of mental health. Research is regarded by both allopathic and Ayurvedic health professionals as essential to scientific credibility. Mainstream psychiatric research is designed to make discoveries, but research in Ayurvedic psychiatry aims to prove and confirm knowledge of the classic texts and the experience of Ayurvedic practitioners over the centuries, and in so doing to legitimize Ayurvedic psychiatry as a credible actor in mental health care. This is related not only to the inferior position of Ayurveda vis-à-vis allopathy with regard to power, truth claims and financial resources, but also to a different understanding of science. Ayurvedic shastra and Western science fundamentally differ in their conceptions of time. Most doctors of Ayurveda engage a narrative of decline with regard to Ayurvedic knowledge. In Ayurveda, science was pure and complete in the past and degenerated over time; hence it is only partial in the present. In biomedicine, by contrast, more complete knowledge is located in the future and theory and practice progress from discovery to discovery. Ayurvedic shastras transmit knowledge that has been complete and primordial, and scientific progress is more a kind of "regress" understood as a rediscovery of the lost parts of the shastra (Pollock 1985; Wolfgram 2009). For many Ayurvedic doctors it is a sign of the superiority of Ayurveda over allopathy that allopathic knowledge keeps changing and is involved in constant correction, while Ayurvedic knowledge is constant (or at least supposed to be) over the centuries and therefore comprises eternal and universal truth (Pollock 1985; Trawick 1987; Langford 2002). Ayurvedic psychiatrists concede that mainstream psychiatric systems of classification are more detailed and fine-tuned than Ayurvedic categories and that many find it easier to think in mainstream psychiatric terms; however students are taught that the Ayurvedic shastric knowledge they study not only anticipated but also transcends modern psychiatric categories, knowledge and treatment. Science and research are appropriated and retooled in Ayurvedic psychiatry – as in other branches of Ayurveda and in Indian shastric knowledge more broadly – and used to legitimate truth claims, negotiate the ontological basis of Ayurveda and create an alternate science based in biomedical epistemology. They thus perpetuate contradiction *and* ambiguity: seeking to rid Ayurvedic psychiatry of Western influence while at the same time relying heavily on Western scientific methods and language to authenticate Ayurveda's scientific status (Leslie 1992; Prakash 1999; Wolfgram 2010; Ganguly 2014).

Clinical trials and research in Ayurvedic psychiatry thus contribute to a project that the former superintendent of GAMH, Dr Sundaran, highlights in the introduction to his comprehensive Malayalam-language *Treatment of Mental Diseases in Ayurveda* (Sundaran 1993). He explicitly calls for the inclusion of bhutavidya as Ayurvedic psychiatry into the canon of medical science as a branch of Ayurveda instead of regarding it as historical. He argues that bhutavidya merits the interest of the scientific medical community instead of the attention of historians of Indian medicines. In this regard, an important tool is the pedagogical and clinical institutionalization of Ayurvedic psychiatry and research. Sundaran writes: "Indian psychiatry also has been a separate entity like kaya chikitsa and *shalya chikitsa* [surgery]. *Bhuta chikitsa* [treatment of bhutas] became an antiquity due to the lack of proper research and development after some time." He goes on to deplore that "those who searched for Indian psychiatry ended up with Bhagavad Gita, the Upanishads and the Smritis" rather than with the rich literature on Ayurvedic psychiatry. The renewed interest of Western scholars in what has been considered "Indian psychology" has not helped, Sundaran notes, to develop Indian psychiatry into a full-fledged science. But he sees progress in the form of the establishment of GAMH and postgraduate courses, the inclusion of psychiatry in the BAMS syllabus, public interest in Ayurvedic intelligence-enhancing products and, last but not least, in the writing of dozens of "scientific dissertation theses" by MD students of Ayurvedic psychiatry. Finally, he calls for rediscovery of the depths of Ayurvedic shastras for distributed parts of Ayurvedic knowledge on mental health in order to feed the (re)invented field of Ayurvedic psychiatry and make it a scientific, credible, reliable and legible actor by translating the shastras into research: "Let's collect those little drops of knowledge and compile the whole to make it a comprehensive science. Let's liberate the indigenous knowledge from collecting dust in some corners of an archeological museum" (Sundaran 1993, 2).

Research is regarded as the hallmark of scientific credibility. What is practised as research in Ayurvedic psychiatry can be conceived of as "mimetic acts" (Bhabha 1984, 40) that bestow legitimacy on this (re)invented branch of Ayurveda and make their knowledge and practices based on shastra, experience and logic legible to the scientific community. In spite of claims of the superiority of Ayurvedic psychiatric knowledge, the project of scientization is related to asymmetric power relations and hierarchies between the systems with regard to knowledge, financial resources and status. The research activities in Ayurvedic psychiatry conform to what Banerjee (2008) terms the "pharmaceuticalization of Ayurveda" or the "pharmaceutic episteme" (Banerjee 2002) that reduces it to a mere supplier of pharmaceutical products. According to Banerjee, the application of biomedical standards to evaluate the efficacy of Ayurvedic drugs substantially changes the character of these medicines and renders them indistinguishable from allopathic pharmaceuticals. Taking a piece of Ayurvedic knowledge and evaluating it using "modern" methods, evidence-based clinical research dismisses Ayurveda's theoretical foundations and disregards its context. With the (re)invention of Ayurvedic psychiatry and its scientific legitimization, its proponents are establishing a psychiatry that mimics mainstream psychiatry and runs both in parallel and at cross-purposes to it.[131]

Medical charts and diagnosing in clinical practice

The Ayurvedic questionnaires and forms for assessing mental illness are complex elaborations of notions of health and illness, healthy and pathological behaviour and development, and etiologies and symptomatologies. They are also mimicries (Bhabha 1984) of mainstream psychiatric mental health examination questionnaires and part of the translation processes by which Ayurvedic psychiatry aims to become recognized as scientific and as an important part of the network of mental health care in India. In this section, I use the examination of the outpatient ticket (the form for outpatients at the Ayurveda College, Kottakkal), the case record (the form for inpatients at GAMH) and the mental state examination (the patient notes for those treated by Dr Joseph John at his private clinic) to show how such questionnaires are tools that render Ayurvedic psychiatry both compatible with mainstream psychiatry and autonomous from it as a parallel and equally scientific approach to mental health.

After personal details including the name of the "informant" (this might be "self" but more often a spouse, parent or sibling), under "present history" the college's OP ticket requires completion of information on complaints, mode of onset, precipitating life events, progress of the disease, present (allopathic) treatment, physical illness and personal and family history. The "complaints" field in the OP ticket for a patient diagnosed with depression might look like this:

> burning sensations of abdomen, crying spells, palpitation, dryness of mouth, tremors, fatigue, decreased attention and concentration, feeling that neighbours are against her and discussing about her, feeling that she is alone and she doesn't have the ability to do anything, increased anger, irritability, 15 days, total duration 15 years.[132]

The "personal history" section calls for information on birth order, education, occupation, social background, marital status, children, personal habits, development and premorbid personality. The "mental state examination" focuses on appearance, rapport, eye-to-eye contact, psychomotor activities, speech, thought disorders, subjective mood (entries include "depressive", "sad" and "no one is there to help me"), objective mood (for example "depressive", "sad"), delusions, hallucinations, sleep, consciousness, attention, concentration, memory, orientation, judgement, intelligence, insight and risk of suicide. In the field "diagnosis", students recorded mainstream psychiatric diagnoses such as "mild depression", "moderate depression" or simply "depression" – I never saw an Ayurvedic diagnosis in this field on the college's OP tickets. The last element is a field for "treatment". Diagnosis and treatment are also noted on the outpatient department sheet the patients bring to each visit.

The GAMH case record includes more detailed personal information including religion, nationality, mother tongue and whether the patient is literate or illiterate and comes from an urban or rural area. Details such as date, time and type of admission (observation, regular, voluntary, civil, criminal) are recorded, as are tendencies (suicidal, homicidal, epileptic, dangerous, destructive or escaping, for example) and administrative particulars (income and status as paying or non-paying). After "presenting complaints" and "history of the present illness", the questionnaire moves to the treatment history. This includes "present medicines" and the options Ayurveda, allopathy, homeopathy or other. In nearly all the case records I saw, almost all were marked "allopathy". It is notable that, although the questionnaire includes both allopathy and the AYUSH disciplines under the treatment history, there is no field for religious treatment or, in Ayurvedic terms, daivavyapasraya chikitsa – this despite most patients having a long treatment history of religious healing and daivavyapasraya chikitsa being one of the three kinds of treatment described in Ayurvedic classic texts. In the field "provisional diagnosis", an Ayurvedic diagnosis such as kaphonmada, vatonmada, pittonmada or sometimes also *vishadam* [sadness, confusion], *gatodvegam* [hypochondriasis] or *chitotvega* [anxiety] is noted. The field "final diagnosis" is almost always left empty. It follows the section on family history including "home atmosphere", sex and marital history, menstrual history (in women) and childhood history as well as the educational and occupational history and a physical examination.

The GAMH case record differs from the college's OP ticket in that in addition to a daily detailed treatment report, it includes an "Ayurvedic assessment". This includes the Sanskrit notions (and their English translations as provided to students): *manas* (mind), *buddhi* (intellectual capacity with options such as immature behaviour, inappropriate crying, insight and others), *samjnajnana* (orientation), *smrti* (memory), *bhakti* (devotion), *shila* (habits, temperaments), *chesta* (psychomotor activity) and *acarah* (personal and social standards). It follows a "diagnostic summary" with the points "in modern psychiatry" and "in Ayurveda". The field for the diagnosis "in modern psychiatry" is a recent addition as in 2010 there was only one field (for the Ayurvedic diagnosis). The reason doctors and students should note only the Ayurvedic diagnosis, doctors explained to me, was that GAMH was under the department of Indian Systems of Medicine and guided by the ideology of suddha Ayurveda. Second, as Dr Kumar told me, doctors and students are not qualified to diagnose in modern terms:[133] "Officially they are allowed to write in Ayurvedic terms only." The recent addition of a mainstream psychiatric diagnosis is another example of efforts to achieve recognition of Ayurveda as an actor in the provision of mental health, which in Kerala is dominated by mainstream psychiatric discourse. Finally the mental status examination has a field for "etiological factors" where doctors note details on the patient's doshic constitution with the options vata, pitta or kapha; mental constitution which may be satvikam, rajasikam or tamasikam; and sattvabalam with the option *pravaram* [strong], *madhyam* [middle] or *hina* [weak].

The mental status examination of Dr Joseph John included personal histories similar to the OP ticket and case record and also a "mental status examination" consisting of the evaluation of appearance, talk, thought, affect and perception and a field for the "higher mental functions" (attention and concentration, orientation, memory, intelligence, judgement and insight – all given in English terms). The field "provisional diagnosis" is always completed with an allopathic psychiatric diagnosis such as "depression".[134] While the OP ticket of the Ayurveda College, Kottakkal and Dr John's mental status examination rely upon mainstream psychiatric mental health examinations and diagnoses – more elaborate in the former and less detailed in the latter – the GAMH case record includes detailed Ayurvedic assessment categories. Administrative and legal requirements and AYUSH policies lead to a strong emphasis at the GAMH on institutional Ayurvedic psychiatric discourse which again stabilizes their professional authority as Ayurvedic psychiatrists. The College OP ticket is probably less elaborate with regard to Ayurvedic assessment because students find it easier to think "in modern terms". Dr John's mental status examination finally is less restricted and guided by administrative, legal or training requirements but rather serves his own record keeping.

Ayurvedic psychiatrists differentiate between endogenous or doshic forms of mental illness or madness and exogenous, graha-based ones. Though the graha diagnoses are part of the syllabus of the manasika postgraduate course and students sometimes try to understand the patients in these terms, grahas have – with some very rare exceptions – no clinical relevance to diagnosis and treatment which, as doctors stressed, were "purely based on the doshic assessment". Ayurvedic psychiatrists then either use Ayurvedic doshic disease categories or allopathic ones to note the diagnosis in patient charts. In the following section, I examine more closely the notions that are used to diagnose patients and what relevance they have for treatment choice.

Earlier, I showed how spirits are expurgated in Ayurvedic psychiatry by translating grahas [grasping entities] into metaphors, psychotic elements or personality disorder. In this section I deal with the question of whether Ayurvedic psychiatrists at GAMH used graha diagnoses to diagnose their patients. I never heard doctors using grahas in patient diagnosis at the College OPD. Dr Joseph John represents a special case because of bringing spirits back into his clinical practice (Chapter 5). Every time I brought up the subject of graha or agantu [external] unmada [mental illness] in clinical contexts, practitioners and manasika students displayed the same kind of evasive smile. After observing this for a while I asked the reason. What follows here is an effort to explain that smile.

GAMH doctors were not unanimous when I asked about cases of graha unmada. Most started by telling me that they rarely saw patients suffering from graha unmada and explained this as due to early intervention in cases of mental illness that headed off graha unmada. "Nowadays," Dr Kumar observed, "graha unmada can rarely be found."[135] He speculated: "Maybe, because of all this awareness about mental health and because people get help rather soon, they don't develop graha unmada." Other doctors and especially the students of Ayurvedic psychiatry considered graha unmada difficult to identify. "It is told in our classics, but it is very difficult to diagnose", one postgraduate student summed up.[136] Dr Kumar said, "A graha diagnosis is rare. We can't say it is not relevant; it is relevant in certain cases. If we are not able to diagnose on any other basis and if we find it fits into the criteria of graha we can go for that."

Often, after a bit of my probing about graha, a doctor would concede that graha were involved in almost every patient. They recognize them if the symptoms correspond to the graha symptomatology of the canonical texts, if they do not follow a typical doshic course, or if they do not improve with the purifying and pacifying treatment that targets doshic imbalances. "Actually," Dr Rasheed said,

> in every mental disease there will be some graha and dosha mixing. But sometimes the predominance will be graha, sometimes the predominance will be dosha. We start suspecting graha in cases if in spite of our purifying and pacifying treatment the disease will aggravate. However, the basic logic principles of Ayurveda will not apply for graha.[137]

In other words, as often stressed by other Ayurvedic doctors and students, there is no Ayurvedic medical treatment for graha unmada apart from daivavyapasraya chikitsa, which is not offered in the clinical practice of institutionalized Ayurvedic psychiatry.

Doctors were always hesitant to talk about patients they had diagnosed with graha unmada. A notable exception was Dr Vidya who told me about a female patient she had diagnosed with *pisachu graha* [madness related to a specific kind of ghost]:[138]

> Lastly one lady was there and we diagnosed her as pisachu graha, we have written the diagnoses as such.[139] Dosha involvement was not correlated and also we didn't get any results with our treatments. She is very chronic, she is now sixty years. Immediately after their marriage her husband noticed such symptoms like she was always dancing, singing songs without dress and she was very dirty but there was no hallucination. She cannot keep her kitchen clean, everything she keeps untidy and eats old food items. Such symptoms we cannot correlate to any doshas. She does not take a bath, for days together she will be closed in one room. She will not take care of her children. Three children are there. They don't have any problem; they are all well settled, highly educated. And later she got this skin disease (vitiligo). Her body colour started changing. No effects of any medicine. After one month we found there was no change. She even took allopathic medicines for over thirty years without improvement. So we just left her like that. Relatives were also not ready for staying with her here. They were saying, "we didn't get any results after thirty years, so why should we do any treatment?" Even in the ward the husband did not at all take care of her. He doesn't believe in the treatment. He is fed up. So sometimes there is no treatment. Family members can just take care of patients so that no other extra symptoms will come and that the patient doesn't harm him or herself.

In those rare cases in which graha unmada is diagnosed because the symptoms are not compatible with any dosha involvement but instead fit well with the description of graha unmada in the canonical texts, medical treatment is barely possible. The symptoms of this patient corresponded with the features of pisachu graha[140] as described in the canonical texts. The most elaborate description of pisachu graha can be found in Asthangahrdaya 6.4.30a–34b:

> One whose thoughts are unhealthy, who runs around, not remaining in one place, who is fond of leftovers, dancing, gandharvas [male nature spirits and exceptional singers], laughter, wine, and meat, who becomes depressed when rebuked, who cries without reason, who scratches himself with his nails, whose body is rough and voice trails off, who trumpets his many miseries, whose speech freely associates what is relevant and irrelevant, who suffers from memory loss, who enjoys nothing, who is fickle and goes around desolate and dirty, wearing clothes meant for the road, adorned with a garland of grass, who climbs on piles of sticks and rocks as well as

> one top of rubbish heaps, and who eats a lot is understood to be inhabited by [a pisachu].
>
> (translated in Smith 2006, 496)

Once, I talked to Dr Sundaran about pisachu.[141] In his typical manner he tried to find European equivalents for Indian spirits and engaged Euro-American filmic representations of the uncanny to explain the Indian (and Ayurvedic) notion of pisachu:

> The literal meaning of pisachu is cat. In every Indian language, general people believe that the word meaning of pisachu is ghost, Dracula. Now please remember when you see a movie like Dracula or a horror movie, in all horror movies a ghost is there and a black coloured cat is also there, whether it is produced in Germany, England, India, or America, especially in India, the black cat is there. So why it happens we don't know. The literal meaning of the word pisachu is cat. What is the nature of a cat? It is very shy and fearful. And every time meow, crying for fear of others attacking it. The cat collects the waste, rummages in ugly substances outside. If a patient collects dirty substances from the street and collects them in his bag or in his room, if he is of a frightful disposition, if he has unnecessary crying with the fear of others attacking him and if his food habits are very ugly, not good, vulgar, then we diagnose pisachu graha.

Dr Sundaran then compared these features of picachu graha to depression and concluded: "If we compare the symptoms of depression one by one we will get a maximal correlation with [the symptoms of] kaphonmada. But in pisachu graha also, many symptoms resemble depression."

Whether doctors diagnose graha, translate grahas into personality disorders or psychosis, or do not consider grahas at all, I have never seen graha diagnoses written in the case records, the hospital registers or any other official documents. The most important reason is that grahas as spirits are considered superstitious not scientific. "We will not write the grahas in the reports," said Dr Rasheed.[142]

> Even though the grahas are there, we will think twice before writing graha. Because the problem is, if we write grahas in our certificates, others will think that this is some possession state. Modern psychiatrists will not know this concept of graha. They will associate it with exorcism. In one psychiatric conference I heard a psychiatrist saying that Ayurveda takes people with mental illness back to prehistoric times by writing *deva* [deity] *graha*, pisachu [ghost] graha, *gandharva* [celestial musician] *graha* and so on. They have in mind that graha means possession, something like that. They don't know the actual meaning of this word graha. Such a misinterpretation will be there. So to avoid this we will not use the nomenclature of grahas in our files.

A related reason is that as a government institution GAMH is supposed to be a secular institution. In order to avoid "misconceptions" and "confusion in the society" about Ayurvedic psychiatry being an unscientific endeavour related to superstition and to become a legitimate actor in the mental health care of Kerala, Ayurvedic psychiatrists not only avoid noting graha diagnoses in their documents but focus treatments explicitly on the doshas (vata, pitta and kapha). "Even if it is a graha," one student told me,

> we can't plan a treatment protocol according to it. We have to relate to dosha only because medicines are related to dosha principles only. We diagnose according to the symptom similarity of the doshas only, not on the basis of graha and we go for treatment on the basis of dosha. Whatever is the case, whatever is the graha, we need to find out whether there is any dosha basis.[143]

Although most doctors rejected the ontology of spirits, several of them brought up the topic of *daivavyapasraya chikitsa* [spiritual treatment] described in the canonical texts as one of the three treatments in Ayurveda. Although doctors would not refer their patients explicitly to a ritual healer they nonetheless were tolerant if families sought their help before, after or parallel to Ayurvedic treatment.[144] Although the canonical texts of Ayurveda include daivavyapasraya chikitsa, Ayurvedic psychiatrists in institutional settings do not practise it. Ayurvedic professionals were careful not to reject religious treatment altogether and preferred to stress that they were not trained to do it and that patients expected medical and not spiritual treatment from them. Dr Sarasvati explained:[145]

> Some authorities are there for this daivavyapasraya chikitsa. If I tell them to tie a string on their hand, they will not believe us. But if a priest in a temple or some other religious practitioner gives it, they will believe. That's why we cannot give these types of daivavyapasray chikitsa. Patients come for medical treatment. Otherwise they will go to some temples or churches.

In sum, though used in rare cases in internal diagnostics, graha unmada is never used in official documents or in medical consultations with patients and families. Doctors suspected that the graha diagnoses could be "misunderstood" by people other than Ayurvedic psychiatrists as being related to demons and exorcism thereby discrediting Ayurvedic psychiatry as an unscientific, superstitious and antiquated endeavour. Thus, the more universal and "context-free" (Halliburton 2005) dosha-based and mainstream psychiatric categories that are regarded as more scientific are used in official documents.

Doctors at GAMH noted Ayurvedic Sanskrit terms such as kaphonmada along with a diagnosis "in modern psychiatry" such as depressive disorder in their case records and their registers, and used a combination like "depression (kaphonmada)" for patient certificates. Doctors told me that since the institution is run by the Directorate of Indian Systems of Medicine, government administrative requirements govern their practices. In the Ayurveda College and in the private clinic of Dr Joseph John, only mainstream psychiatric terms such as "depression", "mild depression" or "moderate depression" were written on patient charts. Although teachers at the Ayurveda College told me that the aim is that students learn to diagnose in purely Ayurvedic terms, students usually write the allopathic diagnosis on the OP ticket and into their register. In communication with patients and families, doctors in all three institutions exclusively used allopathic psychiatric terms (if they conveyed a diagnosis).

When diagnosing, Ayurvedic psychiatrists often think both in allopathic and in Ayurvedic terms. This bilingualism holds not only for those who write allopathic diagnoses but probably also for most who are guided by institutional requirements to diagnose in Ayurvedic terms. Dr Shankaran, a general clinician and college teacher from another Ayurveda college who also treated patients with mental illness, was particularly open about the appropriateness of mainstream psychiatric terms as compared to Ayurvedic ones.[146] Since he worked in the context of an Ayurvedic governmental institution he was held to writing Ayurvedic diagnoses in the records.

> Though we write kaphonmada or vatonmada, our mind will think in modern terms. To speak frankly, when we see the patients, the modern symptomatology is more effective to categorize them. When we see a patient we can say the patient has depression or the patient is manic. We can easily identify the patient. But in Ayurveda psychiatry it is difficult. We are not writing the modern diagnosis. We are writing kaphonmada, vatonmada, like that only. But our mind will think that this symptomatology is more correlated with this depression. But as a style we are writing our Ayurvedic diagnosis and assessment.

What contributes to this "thinking in modern terms" is the practice of almost all Ayurvedic psychiatrists I observed to use prescriptions of mainstream psychiatrists for reverse diagnosis. Although mainstream psychiatrists prescribe psychopharmaceuticals based less on disease categories and more on symptoms, Ayurvedic psychiatrists find it easy to gather a provisional diagnosis from the prescriptions of their allopathic colleagues. As Dr Sarasvati demonstrated, doctors typically switched easily between and combined the languages of allopathic and Ayurvedic psychiatry.[147] We were talking about a female inpatient: "She is a typical vatonmada. Also kapha involvement is there. That's why depression and mania, mood is fluctuating. Some months ago, it was depression." I asked whether they were at present treating her for vata. "We have to give medicine for stabilizing the mood," Dr Sarasvati replied. "So you have mood stabilizers in Ayurveda?" I asked the question because doctors had told that there were no mood stabilizers in the allopathic sense in Ayurveda, only medicines related to vata and others related to kapha. "Ah, *pancagavya ghrta* [ghee made of the five products of the cow], *mahapancagavya ghrta* [another ghee made of the five products of the cow] we have to give as mood stabilizers." Dr Sarasvati's translation of these two *ghrta* [medicated ghee] as mood stabilizers is an example of the appropriation of the diagnostic entity bipolar disorder into the Ayurvedic diagnostic canon. Other doctors told me they could only diagnose either vatonmada or kaphonmada and did not see one single disease encompassing both in Ayurveda.

Translations undercover: Ayurvedic psychiatry and occult violence

In vernacular theories in Kerala, a sudden change of character and behaviour is often understood as a symptom of *kaivisham,* a form of occult violence that is specific to the local context of Kerala. Originally, kaivisham denoted two types of sorcery, the first involving intentional poisoning by means of a substance absorbed or taken into the body intended to cause *dosham* [mental, somatic, familial or economic difficulties]. The second involves love magic, and can cause the victim to fall in love with the poisoner. Sometimes the two meanings converge. Today, kaivisham is either understood as occult violence or it is rationalized and medicalized to mean poisoning through toxins in food (particularly industrially produced and processed foods), incompatible foods or alcohol abuse. Kaivisham is primarily mediated by astrology (Smith 2006) and is identified in Prashnamarga, the most influential and widely used astrological text in Kerala, as one of eleven possible sources of occult violence (cf. Tarabout 2003; Smith 2006). Accordingly, an astrologer refers patients either to a ritual kaivisham specialist or to an Ayurvedic doctor for treatment. A detailed astrological analysis can determine both the cause and perpetrator of the kaivisham, often in a somewhat cryptic manner that leaves ample room for the afflicted family to debate disturbed social relations with relatives, neighbours or colleagues. Thus, it is often astrologers who invoke the idiom of occult violence and frame social conflict as spirituo-physiological affliction. In Kerala, kaivisham treatment is undertaken in the well-known Tiruvizha Temple or in smaller treatment centres, and consists of intense vomiting brought about by the consumption of ritually charged herbs. Ritual specialists in treatment centres have observed an enormous increase in people seeking treatment for kaivisham over the last ten years. Various explanations have been offered: social conflict due to increasing competition and social inequality, declining moral standards related to the decreasing value placed on joint families and decreasing influence of elder family members on younger ones, increasing mental health problems and changing diets. One of the reasons the notion of kaivisham is so persistent is because its ontology is flexible, liquid and mobile on the one hand and deeply rooted in Kerala's vernacular and folk-Ayurvedic notions of body and mind on the other. It integrates ideas of occult violence, envy, jealousy, ideas of external substances that can be removed as being the cause for mental health problems, a sudden character changes or failures in life, and ideas of impurity and purification. Moreover, it can serve as a critique of the modern diet when kaivisham is conceptualized as toxins introduced by the consumption of processed, non-organic or genetically modified food. Finally, it addresses the widespread problem of alcohol consumption in Kerala.

Several Ayurvedic doctors at the Ayurveda College in Kottakkal equated kaivisham with the Ayurvedic notion of garavisha. According to them, Ayurvedic sources differentiate between two kinds of poison: natural poison and garavisha [poison administered with the intention of destroying or attracting]. They explained that garavisha could be understood as a low-potency poison that the body cannot fully digest, metabolize or expel, so it accumulates and slowly becomes toxic, leading to digestive impairment. These substances can take the form of toxic chemicals in one's daily food, alcohol, Ayurvedically "incompatible food" or substances purposefully (and maliciously) administered like insect faeces, hair, nails, metals or glass powder. It affects the whole system, including the mind, and can provoke personality changes and mental disorders such as depression or psychotic symptoms. In her MD thesis, Swayamprava (2009) analysed the concept and treatment of *garavisha* as described by Ayurvedic texts and its contemporary conceptualization as kaivisham in Kerala. Apart from vomiting as a first line of treatment, Ayurvedic classics describe the chanting of mantras as a quick and effective way to eliminate garavisha from the body, because mantras are light and pure in nature and thus opposite to garavisham. Typical of college-trained Ayurvedic practitioners, Swayamprava reinterprets Ayurvedic spiritual treatment in a neurochemical way in the sense that the sound of chanted mantras is explained as creating chemical changes in the brain or, in Ayurvedic terms, it "cleans the channels" through which the mind moves. Swayamprava correlates garavisha with toxic chemicals found in fertilizers or pesticides, adulterated food and water, incompatible food, and alcohol, and thus offers a "scientific view" that excludes both the intentionality of the act and its potentially occult aspects.

In Ayurvedic psychiatry, *vamana* [therapeutic vomiting], which is similar to but not the same as the vomiting in the treatment of kaivisham, is an important treatment for kapha unmada. Induced by consuming liquorice and large quantities of milk, vamana is used to eliminate aggravated kapha from the body's channels, including its mind-carrying channels. After having been lubricated and transported into the gastrointestinal tract, the phlegm is vomited out, thereby purifying the mind (understood as a physiological substance). In contrast to the use of vomiting in the treatment of kaivisham, vomiting in Ayurvedic psychiatry is negotiated as a scientific treatment, a status reinforced in clinical practice by the use of biomedical devices during treatment such as stethoscopes or sphygmomanometers.

But doctors at GAMH do not only prescribe vamana for kaphonmada. They also prescribe it for other patients with, as they express it, "a strong belief in kaivisham". Dr Vidya explained,[148]

> Here most patients or their bystanders want vamana. If we give vamana to one patient, definitely the other patients or their bystanders also want it. It is a difficult procedure but still they want it. It is a placebo effect only. They suspect kaivisham.

"In the society there is a belief in kaivisham," Dr Sarasvati clarified:[149]

> Patients believe in that. In such conditions we cannot tell them it's only a belief. We have to give medicine to remove that. What they vomit, the pitta [bile] is a colourful vomit. They and their bystanders think that the kaivisham is gone out. They believe there are some enemies. They think some daiva-vyapasraya chikitsa should be done. We cannot convince them that it is a belief, it is a concept; it is not real. We cannot say that. They will not believe us, because the astrologer told them there is kaivisham inside them and that they should come to us to for expelling it. If we tell them it's only a belief, it's not real, then they go for another religious therapy after the treatment. And there they will be charged much. Here they have to buy only two litres of milk and some medicine. And the charge is below hundred rupees [approximately $1 USD]. For a puja [prayer, ritual] they have to pay thousands.

And, Dr Sundaran writes:

> The relief of vamana is because of the belief of the patient that the poisonous substance that somehow got into his/her body is being vomited out and is removed completely from his body. So if not made to vomit he may believe that the causative poison still remains inside the body. This belief may cause problems.
>
> (Sundaran 1993, 58)

In contrast to the Ayurvedic medical framing many patients and their relatives at GAMH or in the private clinics of Ayurvedic psychiatrists understood vamana as a treatment for kaivisham, which they perceived as the cause of their problems. Some astrologers support this perception when they send their clients diagnosed with kaivisham to Ayurveda clinics rather than to dedicated kaivisham treatment centres. For these patients and their families, the vomit is regarded as a sign that kaivisham has been expelled.

All the Ayurvedic psychiatrists with whom I discussed this issue rejected the ontic reality of kaivisham and regarded it as a superstitious and unscientific concept. This denunciation contributes to purifying Ayurvedic psychiatric clinical practice of its "backwards" connotations and implications. Yet, at the same time these clinicians engaged and made use of patients' understanding of vomiting as a treatment for kaivisham in order to improve their compliance with therapeutic vomiting as part of Ayurvedic procedures. Since many patients and their caregivers understood vomiting as a treatment for kaivisham, many explicitly asked for it. The Ayurvedic practitioners at GAMH and elsewhere do not challenge this interpretation, but use it in patient interactions to facilitate Ayurvedic treatment. For example, in exchanges that I observed, psychiatrists explained that vomiting helps treat kaivisham and that the prescribed medications protect against this and other kinds of occult violence. Although strictly speaking this treatment is only indicated for kaphonmada (a despondent phlegmatic state, often translated into severe endogenous depression), doctors prescribe it for other patients in order to "satisfy their belief", as several doctors expressed it. This explanation is further reinforced when GAMH doctors and some astrologers prescribed an expensive pill with the telling name *Kaivisham Padihara Gulika* [kaivisham relief pill] which is purported to remove kaivisham. Ayurvedic psychiatrists emphasize the mentally strengthening and anxiolytic effects of the pill, but many patients and their families, supported by astrologers, regard it as a kaivisham antidote. One astrologer explained that the pill "absorbs all the poison from the body and nullifies its harmful effects. Then the poison will be expelled through the faeces or urine."[150]

Therapeutic vomiting for the purification of the mind and body is a procedure in which Ayurvedic psychiatry, Ayurvedic notions of garavisham and vernacular ideas of kaivisham are intertwined. Common to both Ayurvedic psychiatric and vernacular framings is the notion that mental health problems are caused by impurities or pollution that block the unhindered flow of substances, thus creating dosham. This pollution and blockage can be treated by a one-time vomiting procedure that cleanses mind and body. For kaphonmada and for auditory hallucinations, doctors at GAMH also prescribe *dhupanam* [fumigation] for inpatients and outpatients, a procedure in which the patient inhales medicated smoke. A powder made from *vacha* (Acorus calamus), *jatamamsi* (Nardostachys jatamansi) and other ingredients is sprinkled onto a burning ember. The patient is asked to inhale the smoke and apply it all over the head. Mevekari describes the action of this treatment:

> When *dhuma* [smoke, fumes] is inhaled it spreads out very fast all over the head which is the site for all the sense organs. It travels through all *shrotas* [channels]. It eliminates kapha and pacifies vata. It leads to a clarity of mind, throat and sense organs, a lightness of the head and elimination of doshas.
> (Mevekari 2003, 128)

Dr Paul Thomas, a BAMS intern at GAMH, explained to me that "the irritating medicine used for dhupanam stimulates and actives the nervous system."[151] According to Dr Sundaran, this smoke is "very useful in kaphonmada and in the symptomatic treatment of graha unmada [...] With dhupanam soul, mind, (perception), speech, and the sense organs become purified" (Sundaran 1993, 66). Dhupanam is mentioned in the classic texts as effective treatment not only for endogenous dosha unmada but also to cast out bhutas in graha unmada. Dhupanam therefore is described in the textual corpus of institutional Ayurveda both as part of yuktivyapasraya (rational, medical) and of daivavyapasraya (spiritual) treatment, and fumigation is part of many Hindu religious practices. Additionally the Namboodiri religious practitioners of Poonkudil Mana and Kattumadam Mana and other religious healers use and prescribe spiritually charged smoke for treating mental diseases and behavioural disorders and for warding off spirits (Smith 2006; Sax 2014).

The use of dhupanam at GAMH is characterized by ontological ambiguity. The use of smoke is deeply rooted in religious practice for dealing with afflictions of spirit possession and occult violence, and some of those seeking medical help at GAMH understand and practise dhupanam to ward off spirits and occult violence. In this way, the same procedure that doctors prescribe and practise as a medical treatment is transferred into another ontological context and reconfigured as a treatment addressing the spirits. As with vamanam, GAMH doctors harness the ontologies of their patients and present dhupanam as a spiritual treatment in order to improve patient compliance with the Ayurvedic psychiatric treatment. Dr Sarasvati told me of a female patient who suspected the family of her husband of using occult violence against her.[152] The patient felt completely controlled by them and demanded something to grant her immunity from their malicious intentions. In response, Dr Sarasvati prescribed dhupanam in order to protect the patient from the occult violence. "After three weeks," Dr Sarasvati concluded, "she got good relief from this delusion of control." Whether doctors reframe vernacular cosmologies of possession and sorcery as hallucinations or delusion, reconfigure medical treatments as spiritual ones or deliberately deploy ontological ambiguity depends from the context in which they speak and act and contradictions are not necessarily resolved. This kind of ontological reconfiguration is a process I observed in various contexts in Kerala. Psychologists or psychiatrists presented pharmaceuticals as protection against occult violence in order to ensure patients completed their course of treatment for mental health problems or to calm a patient by making them feel secure against occult violence. Religious practitioners psychologized spiritual treatments as psychotherapy (Tarabout 1999) or applied therapeutic techniques to remove occult violence thus leaving the question of ontology deliberately unresolved (Lang 2014). This kind of "pragmatic realism", "ontological pragmatism" or "ontological ambiguity" helps practitioners to negotiate religion and science by simultaneously engaging vernacular and scientific ontologies. Langwick (2011) argues that ontologies are created through therapeutic practice, and what happens in these cases is that multiple coexisting ontologies are created through one and the same therapeutic practice. Further, there are several local phenomenologies of recovery associated with that practice. When patients feel purified of kaivisham through vamanam or relieved of *badha* [spirits, a spiritual affliction] or occult violence following dhupanam, this indicates an embodied relief from spirits and occult violence even at an institution that does not specifically "ask for" (Basu 2014) or suggest these ontologies and phenomenologies.

In this subchapter I described parallel processes of translations and purifications in the Latourian sense. While the "work of purification" (Latour 1991) is an effort to maintain separation and distinction between mainstream psychiatry, Ayurvedic psychiatry and occult violence, the "work of translation" (Latour 1991) creates hybrids of allopathic and Ayurvedic psychiatry on the one hand and of Ayurvedic psychiatry and spirits and sorcery on the other. These processes serve different purposes. First, the purification of allopathy and Ayurveda establishes Ayurvedic psychiatry as a distinct and parallel mental health approach, and similarly, the policing of the boundary between the world of spirits and sorcery demarcates Ayurvedic psychiatry from "superstition" and "backwardness." At the same time, while Ayurvedic psychiatrists use translations between Ayurvedic and allopathic nosologies and etiologies to support scientific recognition of Ayurvedic psychiatry and its establishment as a recognized actor in the mental health network, they use translations into the world of occult violence to increase patient compliance. Just as the doshas flow between bodies, minds and ecologies, the complex and subtle translations that I have discussed flow between diverse ideas, entities, agents and practices and form Kerala's network of mental health care. These practices of translation and purification are important strategies for the invention and legitimization of Ayurvedic psychiatry. Thrown into the bargain is a vernacularization of (re)invented Ayurvedic psychiatry through engagement with mainstream psychiatric categories which have become more vernacularized than Ayurvedic psychiatry. Practitioners use biomedicine as a culturally familiar safeguard to popularize and vernacularize the new field of Ayurvedic psychiatry. Ayurvedic psychiatrists translate Ayurvedic knowledge and practice into the field of mental health while at the same time producing this discipline as an autonomous actor.

Most Ayurveda scholars have interpreted the transformation of Ayurveda following its colonial encounter with Western medicine as a victory for proponents of *mishra* [integrated] Ayurveda – an approach integrating Ayurveda and allopathy – over proponents of *suddha* [pure] Ayurveda. While from late colonial times onwards the proponents of mishra Ayurveda tried to develop an integrated system of medicine including Ayurveda and biomedical knowledge and practices, the proponents of suddha Ayurveda wanted to develop Ayurveda as a parallel medical system (Brass 1972; Leslie 1976; Wujastyk 2008; Langford 2002). To capture what Ayurvedic practitioners themselves have depicted as mishra Ayurveda in pedagogics and clinical practice, scholars have proposed terms such as syncretism (Leslie 1976), hybridization, "epistemological carnival" (Cohen, 1995), appropriation (Lang 2013) and most recently "creolization" (Naraindas 2014a). Other scholars (Wolfgram 2009) stress the victory of suddha Ayurveda in Ayurvedic education, at least on the level of ideology since Ayurveda and biomedicine are taught parallel to each other and no one etiological or nosological system that integrates both had been established. I argue that it is possible to reconcile these two positions by recognizing, as I have shown, that processes of both integration and purification are present on the ideological and institutional level and in clinical and pedagogical practice. Considering processes of purification and translation simultaneously allows not only for the recognition that "integrative" and "pure" Ayurveda are both at work in the pedagogics and clinical practice of Ayurvedic psychiatry, it enables the analysis of relations between Ayurveda and vernacular epistemologies and ontologies in addition to those between Ayurveda and allopathy.

5 Purifying the body, controlling the mind and excising the spirits: negotiating medical treatment, sattvavajaya and "spiritual therapy" of depression

In the last three subchapters, I described the education and practice of Ayurvedic psychiatry, the physio-moral-cognitive conceptualization of depression and the translations of diagnoses and etiologies as important processes for establishing Ayurvedic psychiatry as a recognized actor in the local network of depression specifically, and in mental health care more generally. In this subchapter I investigate the Ayurvedic treatment of *kaphonmada*, and other states of mind and body that are negotiated as the Ayurvedic correlates of depression. How are embodied depressed minds treated at GAMH and the Ayurveda College? What is the rationale behind the therapeutic procedures, the Ayurvedic drugs and yogams and how do Ayurvedic psychiatrists translate these into biomedical terms? How is *sattvavajaya* reconstructed and practised as Ayurvedic psychotherapy? And finally, how do Ayurvedic psychiatrists struggle with the meaning and the ontology of daivavyapasraya chikitsa or what is framed as "spiritual therapy" of depression and other mental health problems?

A poster designed by students of Ayurvedic psychiatry at the Ayurveda College, Kottakkal depicts the ideology of the Ayurvedic treatment triad of mental illness and behavioural disorders consisting of *yuktivyapasraya chikitsa* [rational treatment], *sattvavjaya chikitsa* [Ayurvedic psychotherapy] and *daivavyapasraya chikitsa* [spiritual therapy]. According to the poster's graphic representation, the rational treatment includes both medicine and *pathyam* [diet] with medicine being either *shodana* [purifying] or *samana* [dosha pacifying]. Sattvavajaya includes both cognitive and behavioural modifications, while the spiritual treatment consists of Hindu religious practices such as mantra, *bali* [sacrifice, offering] and *homam* [fire sacrifices]. It is this model of a threefold approach that Ayurvedic psychiatry students are taught in their classes at the college and in their clinical work at GAMH and that all Ayurvedic psychiatrists I spoke with drew upon to describe the theory of Ayurvedic "management" of mental diseases. They referenced this threefold approach in spite of a discrepancy between this ideology and actual clinical practice, which focuses almost exclusively on the rational treatment, only rarely includes sattvavajaya and – at least in institutional Ayurvedic psychiatry – discards daivavyapasraya chikitsa. In this subchapter, I begin with a description of the theory and practice of this rational treatment [*yuktivyapasraya*] as it is practised at GAMH and the Ayurveda College Manasika outpatient department (OPD). Then I turn to sattvavajaya and its problematic translation as "psychotherapy" and investigate the marginalization of daivavyapasraya chikitsa and its reinterpretation as psychological therapy in institutionalized Ayurvedic psychiatry.

Yuktiyapasraya chikitsa: purifying the mind by purifying the body

The Ayurvedic approach to treating the mind, all Ayurvedic psychiatrists I spoke with agreed, is through treating the body. "By treating the body, the mind also gets cured", Dr Rasheed said.[153] And Dr Sarasvati explained, "After purifying the body the mind also becomes purified. We are purifying the body, not the mind. After the purification of the body, the mind also becomes purified."[154] A common metaphor used to explain the relationship of mind and body was water in a vessel. "If the water is hot, the vessel also gets hot. If the vessel is heated, the water also gets hot, if it is cooled, also the water gets cool," Dr Ganapati told me.[155] Before medicines and sattvavajaya, psychotherapy or counselling can have an effect, doctors maintained, the body must be purified. "If we give food on a polluted plate, the food given will not be good. Likewise if we apply medicines in a polluted body the medicines will not have good effects," Dr Paul Thomas explained.[156] The aim of medical treatment is first and foremost to make the mind clear. Dr Sundaran writes:

> In the shodana treatments, the body gets cleansed of unwanted materials. When the body becomes pure the mind also becomes pure. That is the peculiarity of Ayurvedic treatment. The body can be considered as an association of the organs mind and soul. These cleansing activities will brighten all the organs, and lighten up the mind. The very essential purpose of the purifying procedures is to brighten up the organs and mind. This condition is akin to the condition that prevails after the mental disease is cured.
>
> (Sundaran 1993, 58)

A healthy mind always involves the smooth connection of sense objects, sense organs, mind and intellect, and a healthy body, as Anwar writes in his MD thesis:

> Good intellect and healthy senses are said as the benefits of shodana therapy and purity of sense organs, their objects, intellect, soul and mind and normalcy of the tissues of the body are the features of a person relieved form insanity. From this it is clear that these purificatory measures [...] have high importance in the treatment of doshonmada.
>
> (Anwar 2004)

The Ayurvedic psychiatrists with whom I spoke often used "clarity" and "coolness" synonymously: A clear mind is a cool mind, and the pacifying treatments have cooling effects on the body and the mind. The equation of clarity, coolness and mental health is a notion Ayurvedic practitioners share with vernacular Malayali concepts. For instance, Xavier Francis, a man in his sixties and a relative of Dr Joseph John, once told me when we were discussing people affected by depression and the potential of Ayurveda to treat it,

> Mentally they need some maturity. They have little mental strength. They are thinking only worst things, unnecessary feelings, hopeless. They are thinking all the time. Their mind is very hot. It needs some cooling. Some treatment is there in Ayurveda for cooling the mind. After that, doctors' counselling will have more results.[157]

This clarity or purity of the mind is again meant in a physio-moral sense which becomes obvious, for instance, when Dr Sundaran writes, "There are many treatments which help the patient to inculcate healthy thoughts in his mind by bringing in an improved awareness of social norms, cultural values and ethos, manners and good demeanor principles, and principles of societal accuracies" (Sundaran 1993, 68). At a press conference, Dr Joshua explained how physiological purification affects the distressed mind:[158] "Good thoughts come into a mind that has been cleansed. That is healing." The aim of the treatment is not autonomy of the self but rather thinking, behaving and developing a physio-moral-social self in accordance with one's place in the social and cosmological order.

Shodana treatment

The yuktivyapasraya chikitsa consists of medical management including purifying and pacifying procedures and medications on the one hand, and pathyam[159] consisting of *aharam* [diet][160] and *viharam* [daily activities] on the other. Whatever food and activities are good for maintaining mental health can be used for treating mental disorders. In the case of kaphonmada, food items that increase *kapha* [phlegm, stabilizing principle] like heavy and oily food or activities like sleep during the daytime are to be avoided and physical activities like walking or yoga are recommended.

In what is today called "Kerala Ayurveda", a typical shodana or *panchakarma* [literally the five treatments, consisting classically of the purifying procedures vomiting, enema, purgation, nasal purification and blood letting, and certain pre- and additional procedures] treatment for non-psychiatric disorders starts with a sequence of *snehapanam* [drinking of medicated ghee in large quantities] to lubricate the body, soaking out toxic materials and the vitiated *doshas* [humours or principles] and bringing them into the gastro-intestinal tract to then be eliminated by *svedana* [steam therapy], *vamana* [therapeutic vomiting], *virechanam* [purging] and vasti. For a patient suffering from mental illness, however, these therapies are often not an option when patients begin their treatment as GAMH doctors explained. Patients often arrive in a state of severe distress and disorientation and are therefore not prepared or able to comply with the difficult and unpleasant snehapanam. Instead, doctors usually begin treatment with virechanam and *talapodichil* [medicated mudpack for the head made with Indian gooseberry and other ingredients] to reduce symptoms, induce good sleep, improve calmness and to make the patient more compliant. After being admitted to GAMH, a patient diagnosed with kaphonmada is given virechanam with *avipathi churnam*, a digestive powder with *tikshna* [penetrating] qualities to reduce the heat in the body. This powder is mixed with hot water and taken a few times every half an hour on two alternate days, with each treatment day followed by a day of observation. According to Ayurvedic theory, virechanam – a treatment intended to dry up the body and to pacify *pitta* [bile, transforming principle] – is the treatment of choice for pitta-related problems.[161] Like vomiting and emesis, it leads to dehydration that in turn causes calmness and coolness in patients, with the effect of brightening up the organs and the mind. Yet doctors at GAMH also prescribed it for kapha-related psychopathologies because pitta plays a vital role in every form of mental disease.

After virechanam, patients usually receive tapalodichil for fourteen days. Talapodichil (literally "covering the head") is a medicated "mudpack" (Halliburton 2009) of Indian gooseberry (described as *rasayana*[162] in the canonical texts) ground into a fine paste and soaked in whey or buttermilk overnight. It is applied to the patient's head between the forehead and the top of the head, covered with banana leaves and left for forty-five minutes. It is then removed and replaced by fresh paste and new leaves and kept in place for another forty-five minutes. Finally, the paste is removed and the patient bathes and washes the head with cold water. The treatment of talapodichil, Dr Sundaran told me, is not described in any of the canonical texts.[163] Rather, it seems to be a part of folk medicine [*nadu marunnu*] in Kerala for "problems of the head" incorporated into the Ayurvedic treatment for mental diseases. My research assistant Neena told me that there is a common joke in Kerala when somebody displays strange behaviour. People say: "It's time for *nellika thalam* [head application of Indian gooseberry]!"[164] Talapodichil, doctors at GAMH told me, is good for cooling the mind, calming restless and irritated patients, and improving their sleep. Dr Kumar told me that this procedure "cleans the brain" and is "good for thought disorders and wrong thoughts" of any kind and relieves patients of psychotic features.[165] It is cooling applications such as talapodichil that lead Halliburton (2009) to argue that the Ayurvedic treatment for psychopathologies is perceived by patients as much more pleasant than mainstream psychiatric treatment with its side-effect heavy psychopharmaceuticals and unpleasant electro convulsive therapy.

GAMH doctors explained that, according to Ayurvedic theory, talapodichil would not be given to patients with kaphonmada. However, therapeutic pragmatism led them to apply talapodichil to all patients since it helps them maintain good hygiene because the procedure requires patients to wash their head and body daily. This in turn helps patients, they argue, to feel somewhat better. In this sense, doctors understand talapodichil as a form of behavioural therapy. "It changes the behavioural pattern of the patients," Dr Vidya said.[166] One of the other benefits of talapodichil is that family members can apply it at home. This means that patients who come to GAMH for regular treatment once a year or so can skip the two weeks of talapodichil if they have already been using the treatment at home. It also means that talapodichil can be used for relief and management even after a patient leaves the hospital.

In terms of therapeutic effect, doctors told me, talapodichil is not markedly different from *shirodhara* [pouring medicated oil onto the forehead] and *thakradhara* [pouring medicated buttermilk on the forehead], procedures that are successfully applied in cases of mood and behavioural disorders in other Ayurveda settings (Langford 2002). However, these procedures are not in use at GAMH. There are several reasons for using talapodichil instead of shirodhara and thakradhara in this context. First, shirodhara requires around three litres of medicated oil, which most patients cannot afford; second, the preparation of medicated buttermilk for thakradhara is rather time-consuming for caregivers who are responsible for preparing this; third, shirodhara and thakradhara take half an hour and requires several staff members, time and people the hospital is unable to provide for every patient (and in the hospital there is little privacy, so privileging some patients would lead to quarrelling and problems); and fourth, psychotic patients find it difficult to lie down calmly for the time required for the treatment. For reasons of cost, time and practicality, these treatments are only used in exceptional cases where an illness has proved resistant to other treatments at GAMH. For outpatients, doctors usually prescribe *ksheerabala thailam*, an oil that pacifies *vata* [wind, moving principle] and thus reduces worrying thoughts, anxiety and crying spells and improves sleep, to be applied to the head in the same manner as talapodichil.

Following the talapodichil treatment, all patients are given snehapanam, a preparatory procedure for further purification procedures. Patients drink daily doses of *ghrtam* [medicated ghee] starting with 60 mL and increasing daily by 60 mL[167] up to a maximum of 300 mL per day. Doctors frame the effect of snehapanam in physiological terms as lubricating the doshas and toxins in the body in order to transport them into the gastro-intestinal tract. Using the metaphor of crusted dirt in a pot that has to be soaked before cleaning it, Dr Sarasvati explained the effect of snehapanam as soaking the body.[168] The ghee used for this procedure is chosen according to the symptoms, based on the descriptions in the sections of endogenous and exogenous *unmada* [madness, mental illness] in the canonical texts. In patients diagnosed with severe depression or kaphonmada, doctors told me, either *panchagavya ghrtam* or *mahapanchagavya ghrtam*[169] that contain the "five products of the cow," with their penetrating and rough qualities, are used.[170] Alternatively the ghrtams made of *brahmi* (Bacopa monniera and other ingredients) or *hingu* (Asafoetida and other ingredients) may be taken. Ghrtam preparations, apart from alleviating doshic debilitations, are described in the canonical texts as remedies for externally caused madness to destroy all sorts of *bhutas* [living beings, spirits][171] as well as the effects of occult violence[172] (Smith 2006, 539). Nonetheless, no doctor I spoke with described the effects of ghrtam in terms of spirit possession or sorcery.

Ghee preparations are important elements in Hindu religious healing centres such as Poonkudil Mana, Kattumadam Mana and Chottanikkara. In treating patients with mental health problems, religious healers use the same kinds of ghees that are used by Ayurvedic practitioners at GAMH for snehapanam. Religious practitioners at Poonkudil Mana and Kattumadam Mana use ghee preparations empowered by mantras for internal use and for ritual purposes (Smith 2006; Sax and Bhaskaran Nair 2014). Krishnakumar, a Namboodiri Brahmin at Kattumadam Mana, explained the use of ghee in homam to dispel evil spirits and drew parallels to Ayurveda[173]: "Here the ghee is bespoken with some special mantras, put into the homam that we use for *avahana* [removal of spirits]. But eating ghee in the form of snehapanam is also an important part of professional Ayurvedic treatment. However for snehapanam, there is an own theory about the efficacy of the ghee in Ayurveda." In the discourse of institutionalized Ayurvedic psychiatry, the effect of ghee on bhutas has completely disappeared while doctors highlight its lubricating and intelligence-boosting [*medhya*] qualities.

Apart from lubrication, the effect of ghee is described in terms of mental rejuvenation, intelligence boosting, memory improvement, and increased mental clarity. Dr Sundaran (1993) also translates its effect into biomedical terms such as "insulin shock,"[174] "stimulating the endocrine system", or "providing nourishment to the cells".

> How snehapanam helps a patient cannot be explained accurately. Whether like the insulin shock of the modern treatment, by stimulating the endocrine system, or by providing nourishment to each and every cell and system, it is sure that in some mental conditions, snehapanam alone produces satisfactory results. In almost every patient this treatment helps to reduce the seriousness of the condition.
>
> (Sundaran 1993, 58)

Dr Joshua explained the effect of ghee in terms of neuronal connections:[175] "Ghee is important nourishment for the brain and helps to develop new neuronal circles. As such it is supportive in psychotherapy. Many parents told me that their children understand much more after taking ghrtam." Dr Mary said:[176] "Ghrtam is the most powerful medicine in unmada treatment. The unmada chapters in the texts are full of ghrtas. Ghrta has effects on *dhi* [short form of buddhi, intellect, sharp thinking], *dhairya* [courage], and *smrti* [memory]. They nourish the brain." Yet, many patients find it unpleasant to take ghrtam and often discontinue the medicine. The effect of ghee as promoting intelligence is deeply rooted in local knowledge, as evidenced in the oft-quoted intelligence of the Namboodiri Brahmins (presumably, as I often heard, due to the prominence of ghee in their diet). By promoting intelligence, GAMH doctors emphasized, ghee helps to reduce fear and irritation in patients, and to clear their minds or increase their mental capacity thereby making the patient more receptive to counselling and sattvavajaya. It is for this reason that ghee is not only used in snehapanam but also given to in- and outpatients for regular use.

Dr Narayanan, an Ayurvedic physician from one of the Asthavaidya families in Thrissur, stressed the psychotherapeutic qualities of ghee.[177] "If a person has a lot of anger and family quarrels, this ghee is very effective. It brings down the anger and helps the person to develop insight and to solve the problem." Similarly Dr Sarasvati stressed the importance of ghrtam.[178] "If the quarrels in a family are the reason for the depression of a patient, counselling is not enough. You need some way of solving the problem in a pacifying way," she said referring not to psychotherapy or family counselling but to snehapanam. Rather than solving the problem in a purely psychological way, her approach favoured addressing psychological and social problems on a physiological level. Echoing the "somato-psychic approach" (Obeyesekere 1977) of Ayurveda and in stark contrast to Western psychotherapies, social conflicts are thus medicalized, embodied and treated with ghee and other mind-strengthening preparations.

Snehapanam addresses several key aspects of mental illness: embodied minds, social relations and supernatural agents. It is interesting therefore to relate the Ayurvedic practice of snehapanam to a discussion of the Malayalam term *sneham* [care, affection, grease, unctuousness]. Osella and Osella (1996) use sneham to demonstrate how bodies and morals are intertwined in Kerala. Sneham denotes both a cooling lubricating fluid within the body and love and care for others. It can therefore be understood as a "bio-moral substance" (Osella and Osella 1996, 46), a quality both physiological and moral that is the prerequisite of somato-psychic and social action and well-being. In both physiological and social contexts, a lack of sneham leads to *dosham* [problem, blockage] such as mental health problems, behavioural problems, lack of success in one's endeavours, or generally a difficult and frustrating life (Osella and Osella 1996). Although doctors did not talk explicitly about snehapanam in relation to this physiomoral notion of sneham, they might be related and further studies are needed to explore the relationship of snehapanam to Malayali concepts of bodies, morals, care and wellbeing. The consumption of large quantities of ghrtam is difficult, and I suggest that these shared cultural assumptions of the beneficial effects of ghee and sneham for alleviating mental problems are what help patients to comply with this procedure.

After a day of rest and another day of svedana to make the patient sweat and further lubricate the channels, patients with severe depression or a correlated Ayurvedic diagnosis undergo vamana. According to Ayurvedic theory, vamana is the purifying treatment of choice in all diseases related to kapha including kaphonmada. Patients are given large quantities of milk and water or sometimes sugarcane juice along with medicine, liquorice and *vacha* (Acorus calamus) to induce intense vomiting. It is applied to eliminate aggravated kapha from the body's channels, including its mind-carrying channels. Doctors describe the effect of vamana as bringing clarity and calmness to the mind, brightening up the mind and cleansing the channels. Another effect is that vamana usually improves patient compliance for further treatment.[179]

After vamana and possibly another virechanam procedure, patients are given medicated vasti for further purification. Patients receive *snehavasti* [enema with oil[180] or ghee][181] or *kashaya vasti* [enema with fermented decoction] alternating for several days. According to Ayurvedic theory, vasti is the key purifying treatment for vata related diseases. Since vata is affected in all kinds of mental diseases due to its essential role in mental processes, doctors at GAMH apply vasti to almost all patients. "The procedure vasti itself is vata pacifying," explained Dr Shaila.[182]

> Vasti is an important treatment for all types of mental disorders. In all types of mental disorders, there will be vata involvement because of its chronicity, because of its relapse, recurrence, vata involvement is there. There will definitely be mood and cognitive disturbances in all types of

> psychiatric disorders. Along with it we use kapha samana drugs for the *thailavasti* [oil enemas] and kashayavasti in kaphonmada. So this treatment will alleviate vata as well as kapha. But we have no special anti-vata drugs, like anti-depressants or anti-serotonin reuptake drugs, that kind we don't use.

"Vasti applications," writes Dr Sundaran,

> can be administered in all types of *dosha unmada* [mental illness due to an imbalance of the doshas]. In *bhuta unmada* [bhuta-related mental illness], it can also be administered towards the end of the treatment. Though vasti is advised in *vata dosha* [wind, moving principle] problems mainly, also in other doshas it is important. Since many types of medicinal substances are included in the *vasti* procedure it is found to be useful in most of the diseases. Mental disease [*unmadam*] is one of the 80 *vata rogangal* [diseases due to *vata*]. That simply suggests that vasti is ideal in those types of diseases.
>
> (Sundaran 1993, 59)

In Kerala, procedures such as purgation, enema and vomiting are generally perceived to have a purifying effect on bodies and minds. These are thought to wash the viscera and to remove toxins from the body, including in some cases the poisons of occult violence. Several of my Malayali friends regularly practise these detoxifying forms of purgation for prophylactic reasons. The purifying effect of these procedures on bodies and minds is thus part of the shared knowledge of Ayurvedic doctors and their patients.

For the purpose of further purification and to evacuate the kapha of the head, patients with kaphonmada are given *nasyam*, the application of medicinal drops via the nose.[183] Nasyam targets head- and mind-related diseases and purifies the different parts of the head. This procedure is described as treatment both for dosha unmada and for *graha unmada* [mental illness caused by grasping entities]. It is used for symptoms like auditory illusions, the perception of receiving divine advice, and in patients who cry unnecessarily, Dr Sundaran told me.[184] In patients with kaphonmada, a paste made of *hingu* [Asafoetida], *vacha* [Acorus calamus] or *anuthailam* or *vilwadi gulika* [two classic yogams of different ingredients] are used for nasyam. Alternatively, Dr Sarasvati explained, doctors also use irritating powders for nasyam in patients with severe depression.[185] Dr Sundaran told me,[186]

> If a normal person gets this experience, she would not be able to sit still, would wander around as if mad. In patients with severe depression it will provoke a slight response only. It is really getting into the brain itself, from the nose it is directly entering into the brain.[187]

He suggested that further research is needed to identify other effective herbs for nasyam to address different symptoms of mental diseases. Dr Sundaran also explained that nasyam especially affects the smooth functioning of the senses and mental faculties. Nasyam, he continued, directly addresses the *shrunga-taka marma*[188] [vital spot] in the head that is the confluence and centre of the sense organs (eyes, ears and nose) and the epicentre of the intellectual or analytical ability of the brain. In this way, he concluded, nasyam immediately affects the brain.

I have already mentioned the procedure of talapodichil as a pacifying procedure usually given at the beginning of a course of Ayurvedic psychiatric treatment. Other pacifying procedures patients are given in the further course of treatment at GAMH are *anjanam* [medicated eyewash], fumigation and *picchu* [oil application with a cloth on the head]. Especially in the case of kaphonmada in which a patient is constantly lying down, cannot work, is fearful and does not interact with others, doctors prescribe anjanam with medicated eye drops that are applied to the eyelids. The medicine that is most frequently used for this procedure is *vilvadi gulika*, hand rolled pills consisting of different ingredients including *pippali* (Piper longum), ginger and turmeric mixed with goat urine. Another pacifying treatment similar to talapodichil that all patients undergo on a daily basis is picchu in which two cloths are tied around the top of the head and medicated oil is poured into a hole at the *simanta marma* [the vital spot where the sutures of the skull meet]. As during talapodichil, patients can move freely during the picchu application. The oil is chosen according to the condition: in kaphonmada, *shankhupushpa* [Clitoria ternatta] oil that is medhya in quality would be the best, although this oil is rarely produced nowadays. Most of the other oils that are used are described as sleep inducing. Doctors emphasize that the effect of picchu is the same as shirodhara, where medicated oil is slowly dripped onto a point on the forehead (Langford 2002). Doctors stressed that picchu has both tranquilizing and brain stimulating effects; it cools and calms the patient and is effective in insomnia. The Ayurvedic notion of applying oil to the head to improve any kind of health problem related to the head including mental health is in concordance with vernacular notions of how to treat ear, nose and throat (ENT) and mental health problems. Malayalis often apply oils and powders for prevention and treatment of illnesses of the head.

For kaphonmada and for auditory hallucinations doctors at GAMH also prescribe *dhupanam* [medical smoking] in which a powder of ground *vacha* [Acorus calamus], *jatamamsi* [Nardostachys jatamansi] and other ingredients is put onto embers. Dhupanam purifies the head and leads to a clarity of mind. It is also said to stimulate the nervous system.[189] The use of dhupanam at GAMH is characterized by ontological ambiguity. The use of smoke is deeply rooted in religious practice dealing with afflictions of spirit possession and occult violence. So much so that some GAMH patients prescribed dhupanam to treat mental diseases understood and practised the procedure as a technique for warding off spirits and occult violence. In this way, the same procedure employed by doctors as medical treatments is transferred into another ontological context and reconfigured as a treatment addressing the spirits. Like in vamanam, GAMH doctors engage what they understand as the "belief" of their patients and present dhupanam in these cases as a spiritual treatment in order to improve compliance with the treatment.[190]

Nutrition is an important element in the Ayurvedic treatment of mental diseases. Yet, apart from some exceptions, the diet patients receive at GAMH is not governed by therapeutic reasoning but by pragmatic adjustment to financial considerations, personal preferences and government supplies for the general ward. Patients on the general ward (apart from the ones undergoing snehapanam and vasti) get slices of bread and a glass of milk in the morning. For lunch and dinner they receive rice along with two or three vegetarian curries. Since meat, fish and eggs are not recommended during treatment for mental diseases due their *rajas* [the quality of activity] and *tamas* [the quality of ignorance] qualities, the diet at GAMH is fully vegetarian and doctors recommend outpatients refrain from non-vegetarian food as much as possible. They should also avoid spicy and oily modes of food preparation. Their food should be as *sattvik* [the quality of purity] as possible in order to increase sattvik qualities in them and decrease rajas and tamas. Inpatients are also restricted from eating fruit, especially during snehapanam, since most fruits are cooling and might induce loose stools and thus counteract the effect of the sneham. During snehapanam, patients usually eat only *kanji*, a soup made of broken rice that is regarded as a light food that is easy to digest.

Many of the Ayurvedic drugs doctors prescribe at GAMH are medhya[191] or mind-strengthening in quality. They address depression as impaired functioning of the mental faculties, related to a physio-moral-cognitive concept of depression and to mental health as mental strength and purity (cf. "The physiology and morals of depression", this chapter, subchapter 3). The medhya drugs, or "mind boosters" or "brain tonics" as they are often translated and promoted, strengthen intelligence and memory, rejuvenate the brain and renew the intellect thereby leading to insight and behaviour corresponding to social and cosmological norms. Many Ayurvedic psychiatrists emphasized that there are no equivalents in mainstream psychiatry to these intellect and memory rejuvenating drugs, which are understood as brain nourishing and beneficial both for the healthy and the mentally ill. One might be inclined to interpret the importance of mind-strengthening drugs and formulations in Ayurveda as a way to make the patient "better than well" (Alter 1999) or to encourage development of an "enhanced mental state" (Langford 2002, 240). However, as discussed previously, my interviews with Ayurvedic psychiatrists do not support this argument. What Ayurvedic psychiatrists in their clinical practice aim to achieve is the restoration of a normal mental state or rather a normal functioning of the patient in the society and not a kind of "hyper fitness" as Alter (1999) suggests. Nevertheless, there is a booming Ayurvedic pharmaceuticals industry promoting medhya drugs as "mind boosters" especially for improving concentration, intelligence and school performance for the children of Kerala's ambitious parents. The renewal of intelligence and memory is an important part of the Ayurvedic treatment of depression and other mental disorders. Though most Ayurvedic psychiatrists divided the medical treatment into shodana and samana procedures and drugs, some students of Ayurvedic psychiatry declared medhya rasayana [mind rejuvenation] as a third pillar of the medical treatment.

Ayurvedic medications in depression and kaphonmada at GAMH

Apart from the purifying and pacifying therapeutic procedures, patients with kaphonmada at GAMH are usually given a variety of Ayurvedic medications. Like most patients they receive "special powder" daily. This powder is a mixture of *sarpagandha* (Rauwolfia serpentina), *shankhupushpa* (Clitoria ternata) and *gokshura* (Tribulus terrestris). Ayurvedic practitioners describe sarpagandha as a sedative effective "against anger" and sleep inducing; shankapushpa is medhya rasayana, often given to children; and gokshura is also medhya rasayana and a diuretic and that purifies the body of toxins. Sarpagandha is closely associated with the development of mainstream psychiatric treatment for psychosis after the psychiatrist Nathan Kline tested the alkaloid "serpentine" (the active ingredient of sarpagandha) on patients at a hospital in the US, and several research papers were published by different authors about the treatment in the 1950s (Halliburton 2009). Patients with kaphonmada who have suicidal tendencies cannot be given sarpagandha since it might lead to suicide. Instead they receive shankhupuspha powder that includes also *ashvagandha* (Withania somnifera) and *vacha* (Acorus calamus). Moreover *manasamitram vatakam* pills, a yogam used mainly for restlessness and specific oils[192] for cooling and inducing sleep to be applied on the head while in the bath are prescribed. To a small extent, doctors prescribe patent and proprietary drugs although doctors disagree on the degree of their potency. Most branded drugs that were prescribed at GAMH were prescribed as "sleeping tablets".

Medical therapy in the Manasika OPD of the Ayurveda College in Kottakkal offers similar drugs and formulations as GAMH. Dr Joshua, a former MD student of the manasika course, once said that the Ayurvedic psychiatric treatment teachers and students try to develop at the college is based *only* on the canonical texts that they analyse for traces of what they call today Ayurvedic psychiatry.[193] In contrast, he asserted, the treatment at GAMH followed the family tradition of the first superintendent with only minor changes. However, a conflicting view can be found among the doctors at GAMH. For example, Dr Sundaran held that treatment at the hospital exclusively followed what is described in the classical texts.[194] Dr Joshua's criticism bears witness to the self-image of the manasika postgraduate course as developing what those involved term "scientific" Ayurvedic psychiatry. This is based on the two pillars of Ayurvedic research and exegesis of the canonical texts in the light of the invented tradition of Ayurvedic psychiatry. It further testifies to the contested nature of authenticity and scienticity in the context of this (re)invented tradition. Teachers and students at the college's kaya chikitsa department developed medicines out of recipes identified in the canonical texts that are now being produced by the Arya Vaidya Sala pharmacy for the use at the college. In what Obeyesekere (1992) has called "samyogic experimentation," through the interplay of Ayurvedic texts, experience and logical inference, the list of formulations prescribed at the college manasika OPD keeps changing and reflects new experience, new experimentation and new "research" at the college. However, the ingredients of the new compounds are basically the same as those prescribed by doctors at GAMH. One powder's name is *adhinasakan*, an acronym for ashavagandha, vacha and shankupushpa. Another powder, *ankusha*, consists of asvangandha, *kushtha* (Saussurea lappa) and shankhupuspa. Apart from these self-developed powders, doctors at the manasika OPD prescribe Ayurvedic single drugs, yogams, ghrtams, oils, and patent and proprietary medicines that are also basically the same as those in use at GAMH for ingestion, smoking and external application. Thus, treatment for "depression" is largely consistent apart from minor deviations: according to my observations, minor variations in prescriptions for depression were the result of differences in the salience of symptoms, preferences of the respective guide of the OPD and activities of pharmaceutical representatives rather than resulting from fundamentally different perspectives on knowledge and medicine.

Most GAMH doctors told me that branded products are not as effective as classical yogams. An exception was Dr Vidya who held that patent and proprietary medicines were more potent than classical formulations due to their modern manufacturing.[195] Nonetheless all doctors at GAMH prescribed certain selected patent and proprietary pills to their patients, especially what they called "sleeping pills" with telling names such as Relaxat or Tab Sleepin (both are indicative pseudonyms) and ingredients including sarpagandha, vacha or shankushpa that are also ingredients of many powders and oils that patients are given. "Some patients complain that they do not get sound sleep. Many patients believe that after taking some sleeping pills they will get good sleep," explained Dr Sarasvati.[196] Moreover, she told me, patients expect more drugs. This is true for mainstream psychiatric practice (Nunley 1996) as it is for Ayurvedic psychiatry. Patients and their caregivers regard more drugs to be more effective and quicker in effect. The use of a large number of drugs is understood as a form of pharmaceutical care, and makes patients feel they and their problems are being taken seriously. Doctors at GAMH meet these expectations and use the subjective sense of improvement by giving either samples of or prescriptions for some patent and proprietary medicine. Asked about how they choose among the myriad products on the market, doctors told me that their choice was based primarily on their experience and if it is a new product, on the comprehensive transparency of indicated properties and ingredients. It is not my intention here to describe in full the Ayurvedic psychopharmacoepia. Instead, I investigate more closely the narratives of two patients and what they reveal about medical regimes and medications.

Disobedience and anger

I met twenty-year-old Pradeep, a Hindu man from a middle class family who had achieved his plus two standard, when he had already been at GAMH for three weeks. He had been diagnosed with kaphonmadam and had undergone the typical treatment of two alternate days of virechanam [purging] with *avipathi churnam* [a powder used as a purgative to induce a bowel cleaning motion], fifteen days of talapodichil (medicated mudpacks), one more day of virechanam, and he had just started snehapanam (drinking medicated ghee). He took special powder and also shankhupushpa churnam (for its medhya/mind boosting properties), ashvagandha (effective for depression and weakness) and vacha (for its medhya, calming and "antidepressant" properties).[197] He also received dhupanam (medicated smoking) daily. The interview was conducted in Malayalam with the help of an Ayurvedic house surgeon and translated later with the help of one of my research assistants.[198] Pradeep's father Manikandan, a cement fixture designer, recounted much of the narrative spontaneously without much prompting from our side. As such, I attempt here to reproduce his story following his own narrative structure.

> First of all, the boy started with disobedience. I was inquiring to all other parents if their children are also the same. At first we thought all children are like this, during adolescence. But later we found that compared to other children he is more irritated.

When he was in sixth standard, he was angry with his mother and was scared of his father, Manikandan began. "He was afraid that I would beat him that is why he wore two pairs of jeans. He felt a type of guilt after making some mistake," he continued.

> But he was very obedient to his tuition teacher. He explained all his difficulties to her. The teacher gave him a cross and a rosary. After receiving this, he deviated from Hinduism. He would not come to temples even if we invited him to do so. He started closing the door and reading something. When he was doing his pre-degree (twelfth class) I asked my wife to investigate what he was reading all the time. He was reading the Bible and other scripts of the Christian religion. Then we found that all the students of this tuition teacher were carrying Bibles and these photos.

Without prompting, Manikandan invoked inheritance as an initial explanation for his son's problems, something I encountered often when talking with people in Kerala about depression.

> Two of my brothers-in-law were suffering from this kind of disease, and I did not know. Only after my marriage I came to know that. They were suffering from mental difficulties from the age of eighteen [...] Both underwent treatment. Now they are all right. I believe that this disease is inherited. This brother-in-law after matriculation didn't want to mingle with others. This boy [Pradeep] also is introvert. He never goes out. When he went to college, he just sat at home, never mingled with friends or relatives.

Instead, he preferred to be on his own and indulge in reading, mainly travelogues.

> I had a talk with his friends. Pradeep used to go to the library and read books. One day, one of his teachers saw him sitting alone in the classroom bending his head. The teacher asked him, "why you are sitting alone?" He said "I have headache". He was reading S.K. Pottakkad [a famous Malayali travelogue author]. If he asked me for money it was for travelogues, nothing else.

Although all parents in Kerala want their children to be cogitating over books, these should be schoolbooks and not novels or travelogues or anything not directly related to school that might distract students from studying. A passion for reading and writing poems – apart from the occasions where they win students first prize at one of the many school competitions – is often perceived to be detrimental to children's mental health.

> I thought there is some problem with him. I wanted to take him to the doctor but he was not ready to come. So I forcefully took him to Hassan Hospital [an allopathic multispecialty Muslim hospital with a psychiatric unit] where he was hospitalized for twelve days. He was friendly with the doctor. The doctor said, "I will give you a small tablet then you go can to school again." My son said, "I will not take medicine." Then the doctor said, "I will have my lunch, after that you make your decision and tell me." Then he closed the gate. My son thought if he didn't agree to take the tablet the doctor would admit him. When people in the hospital asked who is the patient, the boy said "The father". At last he agreed with the doctor to take the tablets. But at home he was not ready to take them continuously. Sometimes he took them, but there was no change [*mattam*]. By this time he would not go to college and if he did, they had to take him by vehicle. He would not walk. He would not go out of the house, not even for cutting his hair. He said, "why can't you tell the barber to come here?" I told him "if the barber comes here he will spread the news and that would be a shame for you and the family." Whenever we wanted to go somewhere he never went by bus, we had to take auto [rickshaws]. When he saw his villagers he felt some inferiority complex. That is why he was not ready to go by bus. When his friends came to his house, we gave them tea. But he never agreed and told his mother to send them away. Then his friends would invite him to college but he would not come. He didn't want to see his friends or to hear from them. When he recognized their number on the phone, he cut the phone. Then friends would contact us. We said he has some difficulties.

Some months later, the family took Pradeep to a homeopathic clinic. There he agreed to take medicine only after the doctor threatened to admit him. He took it irregularly for around nine months but without any improvement. During this time, Pradeep invented strategies to escape hospitalization. He started demanding things as simple as *biriyani* [a fried rice dish] or as expensive as a computer without actually having much interest in them. Later in our interview, Pradeep spoke of an incident, a time while hospitalized that he demanded biriyani:

> Actually I didn't need it but I wanted to disturb you [his father]. I did it because I thought if I asked costly things from there you would lose all your money. Then you wouldn't have the money to pay for the hospital and would bring me home. I would ask for biryani and fresh juice and all but I never intended to eat and drink it.

Now, Manikandan continued, his son has come to understand that he has a sickness. After coming to this realization, Pradeep thought only about hospitals and religious places where he could get better treatment. He preferred Ayurveda to allopathic medicine and eighteen months previously had been taken to Kattumadam Mana, a Namboodiri Brahmin house specializing in *mantravadam* [magic, sorcery] for mental health problems and other spiritual afflictions. Manikadan explained:

> There they gave him some *neyy* [ghee, clarified butter]. He was happy with the *mantravadi* [Hindu healer] and he took the neyy. The man at Kattumadam was a colleague of mine. That is why he gave special attention to my son.

After that treatment Pradeep was taken to the Ayurveda College in Kottakkal where he was given "one tablet and some powder".

> He took it for a few days but after that he was not willing to come back to Kottakkal. After that, he said he wanted to go to the Ashram of Amma Amruthanandamayi that had an Ayurveda hospital in Kollam but we didn't go there. Then he read an article in *Matrubhumi* [a Malayalam newspaper] about a Poonkudil Mana and wanted to go there but was afraid to be admitted there. Finally we took him here [GAMH].

According to his father, fear was always with Pradeep. When he talked about this fear with his Christian tuition teacher in whom he trusted, she suggested he read the Bible and pray to Jesus. He used to stay awake at night to read the Bible. Later, when the students at Hassan hospital asked him about his problem, he said that he was scared because he had read the Bible. Christian students there consoled him, telling him there was nothing to fear from reading the Bible. At a later point in the narrative, Manikandan came back to his son's interest in Christian practices. Pradeep used to attend Saturday Christian prayers. Once he asked to go to Potta, a famous Charismatic Christian retreat centre located in Chalakudy near Thrissur (Jansen and Lang 2012).

> We suspected the tuition teacher. We asked her whether she had asked the boy to convert to Christianity. She said "I never did that. I only asked him to pray well." We scolded her. From his childhood onwards the boy was very curious to learn new things. Maybe because of that he was attracted to Christianity. It is not nice to manipulate children at that age because we can really modify them.

For Manikandan, Pradeep's deviance from Hindu religious practices was a further sign of his son's mental health problems:

> He wanted to come with us to Sabarimala [a famous Hindu pilgrimage place dedicated to Lord Ayyappan; cf. Osella and Osella 2008]. He was under ritual fasting also. He thought of coming, but in between he ate chicken. Then he told us that he would not come with us to Sabarimala since he had eaten chicken. I told him "You can come, it was only once." Then he said, "It's not OK; I have eaten chicken." He didn't come. And he never accompanies us when we regularly go to the temple where we use to do puja [prayers, rituals] for him every month.

Several times in his narrative, Manikadan returned to the strong influence of the Christian tuition teacher on Pradeep and his son's uptake of Christian practices. This indicates his own deep insecurity about this religious transgression as a possible cause of his son's mental health problems. Pradeep behaved violently and used to break things in the household. Before he came to GAMH, he had been forcefully taken to a *shanti* [priest] at a temple. The priest said that there were some problems with Pradeep's horoscope. When he returned from the shanti, his father remembered, Pradeep was even more violent and disobedient.

> Once we had a plumber in the house. When I was chatting with the plumber this boy walked in front of us few times. Then he came to me, held my neck and said, "You are talking about me." When the plumber later was sent home the boy started beating me. But I didn't do anything back. That was the only incident that he got violent. We brought him to a hospital at 10 p.m. The doctor gave him one injection and some tablets. He slept for two hours, started walking here and there, beating the walls.

The next morning, Pradeep was discharged. After that, he decided that if anything happened to him again, he wanted to be brought to the mental hospital in Kottakkal.

Manikadan identified one other possible cause for his son's violent behaviour: sibling rivalry.

> I think that he has become violent because his sister was taken to a college in Bangalore to study for her BDM [Bachelor of Dental Medicine] and he also wanted to be taken there. We contacted the principal of that college

> where his sister studied and inquired about different courses there. "Now nearly twelve lakhs[199] rupees you spent for the daughter,' he says. 'You should spend the money for me also."

I asked the father: "Have you taken your son for further religious treatment?" Manikadan replied that after his son had become violent, Pradeep had consulted an astrologer. He went alone because he did not want to be accompanied. As prescribed by the astrologer, he did remedial *karmas* [actions] at a Namboodiri mana for his *kantaka shani* [a difficult phase in his life due to the influence of Saturn]. The mantravadi there also made a *thakkidu* [protective amulet] for Pradeep but he refused to tie it onto his body.

> The astrologer said that he is a person who has got the brain to teach others and he has to do it but because of kantaka shani his intelligence had been damaged. "But everything will be all right," the astrologer said. "Perhaps he may become smarter than you think of him. But the present condition is like that and it will continue till a certain age." He has mentioned an age also but I forgot.

Later Manikandan consulted a *vastu* [Indian architecture] specialist. He gave him the plan of the house into which the family had moved twenty years ago. The vastu specialist told him that his son's problems might have arisen because the toilet was located in the wrong part of the house. He suggested demolishing the toilet and calling a Namboodiri to do *punyaham* [a cleaning ritual]. Although Manikandan had considered doing this, he had not yet rebuilt the toilet for financial reasons. Now at GAMH, Pradeep did not trust the treatment. "In his mind he does not accept the treatment, he is just following it", his father said. "And he still does not listen to others. I told him, 'If you get married and you behave like that it will be a problem.' I beat him. After that he started obeying, started taking everything." "Did the doctors tell you any diagnosis or give you any explanation?" I asked. Irrespective of his continuous enquiries, doctors did not explain Pradeep's problem or give any detail, Manikandan complained. "Doctors told us that his problem is only a minor one, it will be alright. That is what we heard from the doctors."

When I later talked to Pradeep, I asked him about his problems. Like his father, he framed the issue mainly in terms of anger: "I used to get angry very soon, I thought everyone is trying to go with me to some places. Even for silly reasons I used to get annoyed." He quarrelled frequently with his parents. "I wanted to go up in life, reading things and getting knowledge and so on, but no one else thought like this. This caused problems for me", he explained. Later in the interview he added, "Most of the time I get immersed in thoughts, thoughts that cannot be told outside." Prompted, he continued, "Some desires pop up, some wants. If I want to possess something, my mind troubles me. If I can't accomplish those desires I will be irritated." "Such feelings were cured once by an *ustad* [Muslim scholar]", he continued, "He can cure my thoughts, he has this ability. He told me, 'you should not take allopathic medicines. It can be cured otherwise, with certain natural measures.'" This was the ustad who was a vastu specialist and suggested changing the position of the bathroom. Pradeep wanted to seek Ayurvedic treatment at the Ayurveda hospital of the famous guru Amma Amrthanandamayi:

> I would like to stay there for some time, away from my house, do a bit of meditation and things like that, and come back. That was my strong-felt desire. As part of the treatment I came here [GAMH]. But I don't consider the treatment I get from here of any use to me. I may not get a proper relief from this treatment here.

When I asked him why he was gloomy and unconvinced about the benefits of treatment at the hospital, his answer seemed shaky: "If you ask like that, what the reason for me becoming moody is, it's so, you will become moody in certain ways. You know it's said that we have to understand certain things".

Depression, failed medical treatment in infancy, mantravadam and badhas

Madhavan had already been at GAMH for more than two weeks when I met him and his mother Punam.[200] They had just returned from the Ayurveda College where he had been sent by Dr Upadya for a scan to identify the cause of his persistent lower back pain. Madhavan was still unmarried at the age of thirty-six, educated up to tenth class and hailed from an economically poor Hindu family in a rural area not too far from Kottakkal. He was diagnosed with *vishada*m and *gatodvegam* [hypochondriasis]. When I met them, Madhavan had already undergone virechanam (purging) and a two-week course of talapodichil (medicated mudpacks). Moreover he had received special powder with hot water, powdered sarpagandha, vacha, ashvagandha with milk, dhumapanam (medicated smoking) and *thalam* [oil applications on the head] daily. Asked about what brought him to GAMH, Madhavan mentioned shivering all over the body, having no interest in anything, and an unspecific, total fear. These problems started, Punam continued, after an incident around fifteen years ago. Madhavan had seen a child from their neighbourhood fall into a pond. Madhavan dived down and rescued the child, but soon after, the child died. "When he got to know of the death, it affected him badly. He had a shock when he realized that the child had died", Punam said. Her son specified: "I had a twitching sensation inside my stomach when I touched the body of the child. It was after that I started having this shivering." As in so many cases, Madhavan's narrative located the beginning of a mental illness with a shock or peti experience.

Despite these problems, Madhavan went to work. However, his condition worsened seven years ago following the death of his father due to a stroke, and he stopped working after that. He was so weak that he could not perform the *kriyas* [death ceremonies] for his father. "My body doesn't have strength", Madhavan explained. His mother added:

> He shivers. When he stands he has a bent back. And he has pain in his bones. [...] Now, for seven years, he has been sitting like this. He is tired and unable to do anything. Earlier he used to go for work regardless of tiredness.

For his constant headaches Madhavan was taken to an allopathic ENT physician who told the family that it is "because of some problem with the mind" and referred him to a "manasika doctor" [mainstream psychiatrist]. "That doctor said, 'this is only a small problem. It has something to do with *vishada rogam* [depression]" and asked Madhavan to continue the medicine for some time. He took the medicine "for the headache" for eight months, Punam said, but stopped it due to financial difficulties and because his friends teased him. "Medicine was expensive", Punam said.

> Yet, the medicine could have been bought some way or other. But then his friends said something. They asked if he was mad. They said it was the mad who take these medicines. Then he didn't want to continue the medicine. Otherwise we would have bought the medicine even by borrowing some money. There was no point in buying the medicine if he wouldn't take it.

Then his mother spoke of another possible explanation for her son's problems: "His delivery was a bit complicated. Labour pains lasted for about three days. The baby was silent after the delivery. He didn't cry." Newborn Madhavan turned blue and he was given oxygen for two or three days. Asked by my research assistant Neena, Punam confirmed that her son had reached all the developmental milestones. But she remembered that a doctor had prescribed some drops before he was a year old:

> I don't know what it was for. The doctor said that there was a slight problem in the brain, only very slight. Nothing to fear, he said. But this medicine was not available anywhere. His father went up to Kozhikode but even there he couldn't get it. So we couldn't give that medicine to him. Sometimes I feel these problems are because we did not give him these drops. I think this way because the doctor was close to us. If he was not close then I may not have thought that way.

Neena asked if any scans had been done at that time, and Punam replied that no, the doctor had said there was no need. "He said it was due to the delay in delivering the baby. If you ask more," she said apologetically, "I don't know." I continued with my routine questions and asked whether she thought other factors such as *abhicharam* [a form of occult violence] or *dur mantravadam* [black magic] might have played a role.

> If you ask me this, I don't know. Sometimes I think so. It was said that something was done against him. It was when Madhavan had no sleep and

> when he started plucking his hair that some people advised us to find out what the problem was. So we went to a *panikkar* [astrologer]. The panikkar told us that he must have gotten peti by seeing a *brahmarakshas* [spirit of a dead Brahmin]. Then we remembered it. While studying in the fourth class he had gone to the school compound at around noontime and told us later that he had a fall and a run in with a brahmarakshas. The ground on which had fallen was the domain of this brahmarakshas. Four teeth were damaged. People brought him home and we immediately took him to a dentist. After this, he developed an intermittent fever. Symptoms of epilepsy that he had from the age of three years onwards were also seen along with this fever.

The astrologer who suggested brahmarakshas as the cause for Madhavan's problems suggested remedial pujas. "We went to Namboodiris at Narippatta Mana, had done some pujas and were given neyy." "This neyy", Punam explained,

> had to be taken after a bath for twenty-one days. One spoonful of ghee had to be taken with utmost cleanliness one should take a bath before taking the neyy. And no consumption of fish or meat during the period when this neyy was being taken.

I asked her about the costs of the treatment.

> It cost more than three thousand rupees [about $45 USD]. At that time his father was still alive. He gave the money. Three thousand rupees for puja alone. Then the other expenses. Three *paras*[201] of *thechippoo* [a flower used for puja]. This we had to get and give to them.

As was the same in many other cases, Madhavan's family was ready to spend a large amount of money on ritual treatment – much more than they would on medical treatment – even through they were of low financial status. I asked Punam if she suspected any kind of dur mantravadam. "My son suspects mantravadam", she replied, "Two days ago he told me so". He wanted to "stop the mantravadam" after successful treatment at GAMH. "Is there any person whom you suspect of having done mantravadam against him?" Punam replied that it could be somebody from her deceased husband's family.

> When my husband became ill we sold our property there and came to Thalassery. It was a small plot that could fetch a good price. However, they [some members of her husband's family] turned away all people who came to buy it. Then we had to sell it at a throw away price. What had been offered eight lakhs rupees [around $12,000 USD] had to be sold for one and a half lakhs [about $2,250 USD]. These people told me that nobody would buy the land at more than that price and asked us to sell it

> at that price and leave. I told them that I didn't want anything and took him [Madhavan] along with me to my house because of his disease. They [her husband's sister's family] didn't like my husband but they wanted his wealth. They didn't tell me this. But someone near them told me they were saying this.

"Did you get any indication that they were doing mantravadam?" I asked. "He [Madhavan] had a job and was living well. We feel that it was because of their jealousy. We cannot see anything but other people are saying so. They were jealous because he was hard working and had a good job", Punam reasoned. In this narrative, as in many others I heard, only scant attention was paid to inner psychology, and more attention was paid to larger family and social problems. In this way, mental ill health in Kerala is understood as an indicator not so much of unresolved inner psychological conflicts but of interpersonal and micropolitical conflicts.

At this point in the narrative, Madhavan's mother was deeply involved in what Good (1994) calls "subjective mood". Without a clear idea of which factors might have actually played a role in Madhavan's present problems, which did not, and what the causes and effects were of particular incidents, Punam recounted many and diverse events and aspects of her son's life. They came to know about the college psychiatric OPD after a neighbour told them about it. Punam was immediately inclined to seek help there because she connected the college to the Arya Vaidya Sala hospital and pharmacy in Kottakkal of which she had a good opinion. With the financial support of a wealthy neighbour, Madhavan was taken to the college OPD. There he received medicine but stopped it for reasons similar to the reasons he stopped taking allopathic psychopharmaceuticals: he did not want to be seen taking the manasika medicine out of the fear that his friends might call him *branthan* [mad]. He was prescribed Manasamitra vatakam, a popular and well-known Ayurvedic medicine produced according to a traditional formula by several Ayurvedic drug companies. "Everybody knows that Manasamitra vatakam is for mental", Punam said, "so Madhavan didn't want to take it." Now, two weeks later, she observed a slight change in him: "Before he withdrew into himself as if he was not interested in anything. Now he comes out occasionally but is unable to hear anything that causes tension." But Punam was optimistic about Madhavan's recovery: "He has a strong desire to get cured. Because of the stress and agony I am going through, he is sad and he wishes to get it cured. Now he also takes the neyy and the other medicines."

Although Pradeep and Madhavan had different diagnoses – Pradeep was diagnosed with kaphonmadam, Madhavan with vishadam and gatotvegam – these cases illustrate a typical pattern at GAMH, namely that the treatment follows a similar treatment plan almost irrespective of diagnosis. Other than in general Ayurvedic practice, in which patients are prescribed medical procedures according to their doshic diagnosis, inpatient treatment at GAMH is to a large extent standardized and guided by pragmatic considerations. Both got virechanam, talapodichil and special powder though the internal medicine of both slightly differed according to a difference in salience of symptoms. Madhavan did not get snehapanam as he was not ready to drink this high amount of ghee.

These two narratives further show what is "at stake" (Kleinman, Das and Lock 1997) for caretakers of patients being diagnosed with depression. They demonstrate that it is mainly behaviour that deviates from the social norms that initially concerns caretakers. Seeking help leads them to a host of different therapeutic practitioners and practices. As medical anthropologists of South Asia have shown, this help-seeking behavior is motivated more by pragmatic concerns such as affordability, accessibility and reputation, the aesthetics of treatments (Halliburton 2009), the "social network" (Sébastia 2009) or the "strong desire to get well, in any way possible" (Quack 2013), than by the congruence of explanatory models as Kleinman (1980) and others have suggested. Medical and religious practitioners and therapeutic institutions do not only ask for a certain behaviour or provide orientations to selves (Basu 2014). They also "shape the objects of therapy" (Langwick 2011) and create ontologies. Through their help-seeking, patients and their families traverse multiple therapeutic spaces, epistemologies and ontologies which leads to narratives that are shaped more by "subjunctivity" (Good 1994) uncertainty and slippery ontologies, rather than by coherent explanatory models and framings. In this itinerary, depression gets reconfigured and transfigured as patients are busy swallowing pills, endure medical and religious procedures, or have parts of their house reconstructed. These therapeutic practices do not only address the individual *per se,* but also configure depression as a moving target perceived through complex social configurations as a neurochemical, doshic, spirit or occult violence problem.

Ayurvedic pills against depression

The indications and modes of actions of Ayurvedic drugs, originally tailored to the individual constitution of the patient and expressed in terms of Ayurvedic pharmaceutical logics, have been adapted to popular psychological or psychiatric, universal and context-free idioms (Ramanujan 1989; Halliburton 2005) such as depression, stress or anxiety. There is a mutual relationship between the "reformulation" (Pordié 2014) of Ayurvedic pharmaceuticals and the appropriation of mainstream psychiatric categories. Standardized branded medicines matched to mainstream psychiatric categories led Ayurvedic doctors to increasingly diagnose disease entities instead of specific complaints. At the same time, the representation of emotional and behavioural problems as depression spurred the production of a market-tailored supply of Ayurvedic pharmaceuticals. Stabilizing depression as a disease category is closely related to psychopharmaceuticals designed to target depression – allopathic and Ayurvedic. All these shifts are part of a glocal network that aims to stabilize depression as a mental health category as one of the main health problems not just in Kerala, but worldwide. Although many authors have described the complex interrelations between the marketing of antidepressants and the introduction of depression as a common mental disorder from the 1980s, the implications of the stabilization of depression for the development of Ayurvedic branded drugs targeting depression have to date not been explored.

Since the beginning of the twentieth century Ayurvedic drug production has changed from pharmaceuticals prepared by the vaidyas themselves and tailored to a patient's individual constitution towards standardization and mass production, and finally industrial production. Consequently, the market for Ayurvedic pharmaceuticals has developed and become a competitive alternative to the allopathic pharmaceutical market (Harilal 2009). The trend is towards preparations in the forms of pills and capsules (borrowed from biopharmaceuticals), although in Kerala especially, classical preparations such as fermented decoctions [*aristham*], cooked decoctions [*kashayam*], ghees, oils [*thailam*] and hand rolled pills [*gulika*] continue to play a significant role. Kerala has the second highest number of Ayurvedic pharmaceutical production units in India after Uttar Pradesh (Harilal 2009). P.S. Varier and his pharmacy, Arya Vaidya Sala in Kottakkal, were particularly influential in the standardization and mass production of Ayurvedic pharmaceuticals at the beginning of the twentieth century, and the pharmacy accounts for the largest proportion of sales of Ayurvedic pharmaceuticals in Kerala (Cleetus 2007). Other important manufacturers are the publicly owned company Oushadhi, Kerala Ayurveda Ltd. and many smaller companies that differ in the proportion of classical and branded products they offer. The Arya Vaidya Sala pharmacy, for example, does not produce any branded medicines but relies completely on classical single herbs and yogams, while the bulk of the sales of companies like Dabur or Himalaya are made up of patent and proprietary products (Bode 2006). Although the pharmaceuticalization of Ayurvedic treatment increasingly leads to a decoupling from associated Ayurvedic diet and lifestyle practices, because the treatment comes in the same form as biomedical treatments (i.e., pills and capsules) and is marketed as holistic and traditional, they are perfectly adapted to the tastes and the needs of the Indian middle class (Banerjee 2002; Bode 2006; Nisula 2006). These companies sell Indian culture, tradition and nature with modern manufacturing and pharmaceutical research (Bode 2006) in an easy-to-swallow (both literally and figuratively) format. Since they address biomedical rather than Ayurvedic nosologies these products contribute to the increasingly common practice of Ayurvedic physicians diagnosing disease entities such as depression or anxiety according to a mainstream psychiatric model.

The market for Ayurvedic pharmaceuticals is growing constantly. Particularly with the rise of the Indian middle and upper-middle class since the 1990s, there has been increasing demand for Ayurvedic products of three general kinds: first, classical single herbs and, second, yogams [compounds] – both of which are usually prescribed by Ayurvedic physicians – and third, patented and proprietary medicines that are either sold over-the-counter directly to the customer or as prescriptions "ethical proprietary products". The classical herbs and yogams are based, in terms of their ingredients and production, exactly on the recipes of the approximately sixty *shastric* [scholastic] texts. These texts are codified in the standard Ayurvedic compilations of 1978 and 1998 and the two Ayurvedic Pharmacopoeias of 1990 and 2003, marking the parameters of legitimate and classical Ayurveda including drug manufacture (Naraindas 2014b). The yogams described in these canonical texts are characterized by an internal "compound formulary logic" and synergy (Naraindas 2014b), with some of the ingredients designed to mitigate the side effects or amplify the beneficial effects of others. Ayurvedic patent and proprietary or branded medicines, in contrast, combine ingredients from different yogams scattered throughout the canonical texts. However, ingredients for patent and proprietary medicines – both single and compound formulations – are limited to those drugs mentioned in the compilations of canonical texts (Bode 2006; Naraindas 2014b).

Biomedical pharmaceuticals are based on isolated active ingredients and their physiological effects. Conversely, Ayurvedic drugs are based on the whole plant or parts of it, harvested at the right time and in the right place, and prepared in a certain manner, and also on their combination and the resulting specific effects on individual constitution and physiology. In the compound drugs [yogams] that make up the majority of classical Ayurvedic drugs, it is the mixture of active and inactive ingredients and their synergy that accounts for the effect of a medicine (Banerjee 2008; Halliburton 2011; Naraindas 2014b). The guidelines for evidence-based biomedical research are therefore only applicable to a limited extent in the case of Ayurvedic compound drugs. Nevertheless, there is a great deal of research undertaken on pharmaceutically active agents of Ayurvedic preparations in research institutions promoted by the Department of AYUSH (Ayurveda, Yoga and Naturopathy, Unani, Siddha and Homeopathy) or the Central Council of Research in Ayurveda and Siddha (CCRAS), in the research and development (R&D) departments of the Ayurvedic pharmaceutical companies and, on a small scale, in Ayurveda colleges.

Ayurvedic patent and proprietary medicines that reformulate and simplify Ayurvedic medicinal compositions in order to create new "traditional drugs" are an example of what Pordié and Gaudillère (2014) term the "reformulation regime" in Ayurvedic drug discovery. This also includes certification and validation determined by external parameters and protocols instead of according to Ayurvedic standards of quality (Banerjee 2002; Nisula 2006; Sujatha 2011; Naraindas 2014b; Pordié 2014). Reformulation is based on shastric yogams and Ayurvedic pharmacodynamics and on multiple translations, epistemic interstices (Naraindas 2014b) and disconnectivities (Banerjee 2002) to create new Ayurvedic formulations to treat biomedically defined diseases and disorders. This reformulation regime of pharmaceutical innovation stands in contrast to the molecular paradigm of allopathic pharmaceutical innovation in which local resources are mined to identify active molecules which then can be mass produced through chemical synthesis (Pordié 2014). Single drugs and compound patent and proprietary medicines always address an allopathic nosology or pharmacology that is the result of multiple translations in pedagogics, the clinic and the lab. Naraindas (2014a) speaks of a "creolization" of Ayurvedic pharmaceuticals on par with similar transformations of pedagogy, diagnoses and prescriptions in Ayurvedic clinical practice and research. Naraindas argues that these creolized Ayurvedic compound formulations no longer address an Ayurvedic nosology, but rather speak to an allopathic nosology, and are similar to Western polyherbal formulas made according to an additive logic contrary to the synergistic logic of Ayurvedic yogams.[202]

Creating and promoting an Ayurvedic branded medicine involves "simplifying a complex grammar (Ayurvedic therapeutics) to address a lexicon (disease category) that is from the superstrate language, namely biomedicine" (Naraindas 2014b, 125). Ayurvedic pharmaceutical research on compounds developed to address a biomedical nosology is characterized, Naraindas argues, by "exogenous innovation", in which drugs and formulations are cherry picked from the Ayurveda pharmacopoeia and matched to allopathic frameworks and biomedical categories (Naraindas 2014b). The pedagogics, research, clinical practice and pharmaceuticals of modern Ayurveda are characterized by syncretism, hybridization or creolization of Ayurvedic and biomedical nosological and physiological epistemes and ontologies. Most students, practitioners and pharmaceutical developers do not see cognitive, ontic or epistemic dissonance between these two logics but instead conceive of them as two parallel approaches to what is basically the same reality. As I have shown earlier in this chapter ("Translating diagnoses and physiologies", subchapter 4), Ayurvedic nosologies such as *kaphonmada* [a phlegmatic, despondent state] or *adhijonmada* [mental illness following a loss], symptoms such as vishadam [sadness, confusion] and physiologies such as the doshas and *manovahashrotas* [mind-carrying channels] are smoothly translated into mainstream psychiatric diagnoses such as depression and related (neuro)physiologies. The nosological translations and correlations that are the result of mining the classical texts for symptoms similar to those described in the DSM and ICD then become the precondition for what is called Ayurvedic research and the development of Ayurvedic patent and proprietary medicines.

The bestselling Ayurvedic medications are patented and proprietary or branded drugs. These sell for a much higher price than classical preparations, and as such represent much higher profit margins for manufacturers. About ninety per cent of Ayurvedic products sold worldwide (Bode 2006) are patent and proprietary drugs, most of these sold at over-the-counter pharmacies in drug stores, food stores, supermarkets or beauty parlours (Bode 2002). The extremely high proportion of branded drug sales has developed since the 1990s as a result of the rise of a wealthy urban middle class, the growing significance of the global market and the aggressive marketing strategies of the Ayurvedic pharmaceutical industry. It is mainly, but not exclusively, through patent and proprietary drugs that Ayurvedic pharmaceutical companies enter the mental health care market. Through a focus on problems related to a lack of mental wellbeing, stress and tension, rather than those related to psychiatric disorders, they cover a wide range of minor problems of everyday distress especially in relation to what are perceived to be the exigencies of modern life. In the following pages, I describe examples of Ayurvedic patient and proprietary medicine, both single drugs and polyherbals, that address depression (though not exclusively).

One of the herbs widely marketed and prescribed for depression is *ashvagandha* (Withania somnifera). Ashvagandha is one of the plants of the Ayurvedic category of *rasayana* [rejuvenating] drugs aiming at nourishing and rejuvenating the mind and the tissues of the body. The Ayurvedic branch of rasayana is often translated as either geriatrics or psychiatry (Cohen 1998). Although only rarely do doctors go so far as to speak of "hyperfitness" or even "immortality" as Alter (1999) suggested, much promotion material for mind-rejuvenating drugs speak of their beneficial effects on the memory and intellect. Rasayana drugs are often linked in research papers with the antioxidant effects and biochemistry of secondary metabolites and promoted as preventing aging, improving vitality, and strengthening brainpower (Gaudillière 2014). In Ayurveda, medicinal substances are characterized by five properties *rasa* [taste], *guna* [properties], *vieerya* [potency], *vipak* [post-metabolic effect] and *prabhāva* [specific effect]. Ashvagandha is one of the prototypical rasayana drugs, and the properties of the roots of ashvagandha, according the logic of *dravya guna* [Ayurvedic pharmacology], are as follows: the taste is bitter, pungent and sweet; it has light and oily properties; the potency is hot; its post-digestive taste is sweet; and its mode of action is kapha and vata balancing. Much promotion material expresses its indications in biomedical terms ranging from anxiety, depression and stress to cardio-vascular diseases, asthma and constipation, as well as problems of reproductive health. Although its classical preparation is mainly *aristham* [fermented decoction], most ashvagandha prescribed and sold today comes in form of tablets. Of particular note is the patent and proprietary drug Stresscom by Dabur. The name alone implies associations with a modern, urban, middle class consumer life. On the package, the text reads, "Stresscom Ashvagandha Capsules combat stress, strain, fatigue." English text on the package describes how the fast and competitive modern lifestyle leads to physical and mental stress and disrupts the psychosomatic balance of the body, in turn leading to a loss of energy, vitality and immunity. Ashvagandha is praised as the "wonder herb of India" and "one of the most highly valuable herbs in Ayurveda", in use since the time of "the ancient rishis [seer]". More recent research is also quoted, describing the efficacy of ashvagandha in clinical trials as an antidepressant, anxiolytic, antistressor and adaptogenic. Several studies describe the effect in terms of ashvagandha's active chemical agents (withanoloides). Indications are "physical and mental stress, anxiety neurosis, general debility, depression".[203] Different Ayurvedic handbooks used by Ayurvedic psychiatrists that include classical and branded medicines describe Stresscom as being suitable for use in treating depression, anxiety, insomnia and other conditions.

Another herb that plays a vital role in the Ayurvedic treatment of psychopathology is *brahmi* [Bacopa moneri], a medhya drug used to treat all kinds of mental conditions and brain disorders. Used as a whole plant, Brahmi has a "cooling effect" on the mind that helps to relax the patient and calm persistent mental agitation – a major problem experienced by the depressed and anxious. Moreover, it is widely used to improve memory and learning ability for students and in cases of age-related mental deterioration. Depression is conceptualized and treated as a physio-moral-cognitive problem and drugs that target impaired memory are important agents for treating depression. Several studies have been conducted based on the claims in various Ayurveda texts that brahmi plays a role in relieving anxiety and depression especially in aggressive states of depression and anxiety given its pitta pacifying effects. Brahmi is also marketed as a rich antioxidant with specific action on brain cells, which has proven to be helpful in maintaining long-term memory and preventing age related mental deterioration, including symptoms of Alzheimer's disease. As an "antistressor", brahmi promises to help manage the pressures that come with a modern lifestyle. According to Ayurvedic logics, its taste [*rasa*] is described as bitter and *kashaya* [fermented decoction], its properties as light and bitter, its potency as cooling, its post-digestive taste as sweet and its specific effect as medhya. As classical medicine brahmi is sold in form of ghee, powder, oil, powder and tablets. As a patent and proprietary medicine, it is marketed as single herb by various companies under different names. It is also an ingredient in many branded Ayurvedic polyherbals.

Alert by Vasu Healthcare is another example of a branded polyherbal widely prescribed and sold for depression. Like all patent and proprietary medicines, Vasu declares the composition of the capsules on the package.[204] It contains the oil of *jyotishmati* (Celastrus paniculatu) and ghrtam, processed with *vacha* (Acorus calamus), shankhpushpa (Convolvulus pluricaulis) and *jatamansi* (Nardostachys jatamasni), three herbs widely used in Ayurvedic psychiatry, and *Bhringrai* (Eclipta alba). According to Ayurvedic theory, jyotishmati seeds are bitter and pungent in taste, oily and mobile in property, hot in potency, pungent in post-digestive taste and their specific action is *bhutas* [a being, but also denoting a ghost, demon, spirit or simply the past tense]-destroying. It is further described as being vata and kapha pacifying and medhya in effect. In several research papers, jyotishmati is described as acting on the central nervous system and having tranquilizing properties. The package announces Alert as effective for "stress management" and lists the indications: "anti-stress, useful in mental fatigue". Further indications mentioned on promotional pamphlets and online descriptions are depression, anxiety, stress and improving learning capacity in children. On several websites[205] Alert is announced as a "natural stress reliever", "a safe alternative to modern therapies" and "a natural tranquilizer with anti-depressant properties". As in all patent and proprietary polyherbals there are multiple translations and epistemic jumps involved in producing, marketing and prescribing Alert for depression. Different Ayurvedic handbooks describe depression, tension, anxiety, agitation and stress as the indications of Alert. In the case of the main therapeutic agent, jyotishmati, there is one additional delicate epistemic and ontic gap involved: in the canonical texts, the specific action of jyotishmati is described as destroying bhutas, as mind-strengthening and as dosha balancing of which only the latter two remain as legitimate modes of action. The therapeutic mode of action then shifts from destroying bhutas to strengthening the mind and finally to a treatment for stress and depression. This move distances Ayurvedic pharmaceuticals from bhutas and occult violence, and characterizes not only the marketing and prescribing of Ayurvedic medicine for mental health problems but also the reconfiguration of *bhutavidya* [knowledge of the bhutas] as Ayurveda psychiatry as a whole.

Another branded medicine marketed and prescribed for depression is Nubex by Trio Healthcare. Like most patent and proprietary medicine, Nubex is sold as capsules. This form is well adapted to the taste and preferences of Indian urban middle class customers: Nubex capsules resemble allopathic pharmaceuticals, are easy and quick to take and do not have the sometimes-unpleasant tastes and textures of classic Ayurvedic preparations. The package of a Nubex drug sample reads "Converts stress into smile, naturally". The slogan "The truly smile formula" on an older package was replaced on a newer one with "Convert negative to positive". Nubex contains ashvagandha, brahmi and shankhupushpa, which are widely used in Ayurvedic psychiatry, plus two other ingredients. The indications listed include, amongst others, stress, anxiety, nervous exhaustion, insomnia, behavioural disorders and, interestingly enough, "brain fag".[206]

Another example of a drug widely prescribed for depression is the polyherbal Mentat made by the Himalaya Drug Company. In contrast to the polyherbals above that contain not more than five ingredients and are thus perfectly adjusted to the global market (Naraindas, 2014b), the Mentat package lists around thirty ingredients, and as such more closely resembles a classic yogam. Its name suggests connections with allopathic psychopharmaceuticals in part because the name derives from the Latin term *mens* [mind].[207] Mentat includes many of the herbs also used in other single drug or formulation medicines, but there are no indications noted on the package. As for their other products, Himalaya provides detailed research for Mentat. One research paper (Sharma 1990) describes a placebo-controlled small-scale study of around seventy patients with depression or anxiety disorder identified according to the Hamilton rating scale for depression and anxiety. All participants received no treatment for two weeks, followed by a three-week course of treatment with Mentat. The study found significant improvement in both kinds of patients although patients with anxiety benefited slightly more than those with depression.

As a final example, the patent and proprietary Manomitram is produced by AVN Ayurveda formulations. With a name resembling "manasamitravatakam" (a classical yogam widely prescribed by Ayurvedic psychiatrists for depression and other psychiatric ailments), and the product name appearing in both Sanskrit and English on the package, Manomitram deliberately provokes associations with classical Ayurvedic medicine. At the same time, its Sanskrit name, which translates as "friend of the mind", carries comforting connotations of tradition and suggests the product supports and eases the mind. The company promises that Manomitram reduces depression and anxiety and increases concentration, retention and memory.

The other aspect of these modern branded medications is that the dosage is standardized, also making for easy use and fitting well with the allopathically informed preferences of India's modern urban middle class, and also the international market for alternative and complementary medicines. This mimicry facilitates the association between Ayurvedic pharmaceuticals, Western science and allopathic medicine. Ayurvedic branded medicines for depression promise natural, holistic, gentle and genuine Indian healing and wellness and the enhancement of mental capacities with the help of traditional Indian wisdom. The commodification and pharmaceuticalization of Ayurveda in this form assures the patient of the ability to maintain a modern lifestyle with the support of ancient authentic Ayurvedic knowledge of holistic wellness, free of side effects. Single Ayurvedic herbs such as ashvagandha or brahmi, or patent and proprietary drugs such as Alert, Nubex, Mentat, Manomitram and many others designed to address depression, anxiety and stress and that promise improvement to mental strength and mental rejuvenation and intelligence, are creolized or hybrid agents. They easily cross the "epistemic gaps" (Naraindas 2014b) between Ayurvedic theory and its logics of dravya guna on the one hand and mainstream psychiatric and popular psychological notions of depression, stress and anxiety on the other. They are "pervious drugs" in that they are porous, unstable, transient and circumstantial (Pordié 2014). Their objectness flows from acting as an antidote to occult violence or a dosha balancing agent with therapeutic proprieties defined according to taste, property, potency in terms of heat or cold, post-digestive taste and specific mode of action as a kind of Ayurvedic "antidepressant", "anti-stress remedy" or intelligence-booster. Yet, unlike mainstream psychiatrist antidepressants, they do not primarily claim to correct an imbalance of neurotransmitters (for a critique, see Moncrieff 2008) but rather promise wellness and the enhancement of the mental faculties through traditional wisdom. They are the result of the increasing prevalence and appropriation of depression in India as an idiom of distress and of translation processes in Ayurvedic psychiatry in the same way that they lead to further stabilizing the diagnosis of depression in Ayurveda.

Ayurvedic practitioners at the Government Ayurveda Mental Hospital (GAMH) and Ayurveda College in Kottakkal, North Kerala, as well as private Ayurvedic practitioners, use and prescribe different kinds of drugs and formulations for treating mental suffering, as I have shown here. They consist of: different modes of preparations of classical yogams (and single herbs); preparations, especially powders [*churnams*], developed by doctors and students, based on ingredients described in the canonical texts and produced for this use only by the pharmacy attached to these institutions (Oushadhi in the case of GAMH, Arya Vaidya Sala in the case of the college); and patent and proprietary medicine.[208] These are the three kinds of Ayurvedic medicines that Ayurvedic psychiatrists and other Ayurvedic physicians prescribe for depression and other problems of mental health and wellbeing. Moreover, it is not uncommon for astrologers and ritual healers to prescribe some of these Ayurvedic medicines to their clients and many Ayurvedic medicines are sold over-the-counter. It is mainly (though not exclusively) through patent and proprietary drugs that Ayurvedic pharmaceutical companies enter the mental health care market. Through a focus on problems related to a lack of mental well-being, stress and tension rather than mental disorders they cover a wide range of minor problems, everyday distress and stress, especially in relation to what are perceived to be the exigencies of modern life.

The reconfiguration of sattvavajaya as Ayurvedic psychotherapy

After the body is purified, the doshas pacified, and the mind clear, cool and rejuvenated, the patient suffering from depression is ready for sattvavajaya, a non-formalized part of the Ayurvedic treatment of depression and other psychopathologies. I argue that the way sattvavajaya is understood and practised by Ayurvedic psychiatrists in Kerala can best be described as a moral-physiological technology of the self with transformative power for both body and mind. Foucault (1988) describes three ways in which individuals relate to the self. These "self steering mechanisms" can be epistemological (knowing yourself), despotic (mastering yourself) or caring (caring for yourself). In this sense, sattvavajaya as a self-disciplining technique aligns with Foucault's despotic relationship to the self. Sattvavajaya, however, is a form of power relying not on brute coercion but on moral reconfiguration of the self, streamlining inner processes and moral norms, and seeking to promote wellbeing through the "management and surveillance of one's personal conduct" (Clarke et al. 2010).

The reconfiguration of sattvavajaya as Ayurvedic psychotherapy as one part of (re)invented Ayurvedic psychiatry next to yuktivyapasraya chikitsa (rational treatment) but excluding daivavyapasraya chikitsa (spiritual therapy) aims to correspond to the bifurcation of treatment in pharmacological therapy and psychotherapy in mainstream psychiatry. Through complex processes of translation in the Latourian sense, sattvavajaya is established as a parallel yet autonomous approach to Western psychotherapy. In this section, I describe the conceptualization of sattvavajaya and its problematic reframing as psychotherapy in the context of Ayurvedic psychiatry and the treatment of depression in Kerala.

In sattvavajaya, as Langford pointedly notes, "not only is an entire field of specialization elaborated from one verse, but this field is also found to correspond to and anticipate a modern therapeutic technique" (Langford 2002, 244). The reconstruction of Ayurvedic sattvavajaya as psychotherapy began in the 1980s and has found its way into the conceptualization and practice of Ayurvedic psychiatry in Kerala. In institutionalized Ayurvedic psychiatry at the Ayurveda College, sattvavajaya is taught as an integral part of Ayurvedic treatment of psychopathologies. "Sattvavajaya is because medicine alone will not work in a mental problem. We also have to stimulate the patient with different aspects, morally, psychologically," said Dr Mangalam, a teacher of Ayurvedic psychiatry at the college.[209] Sattvavajaya is described only once in a verse of the Caraka Samhita Suthrastana (11:54) that lists yuktivyapasraya, daivavyapasraya and sattvavajaya as the three types of therapy. This verse describes sattvavajaya as restraining the mind from unwholesome or harmful objects (cf. Langford 2002). When I asked students and practitioners for an explanation of sattvavajaya, the most frequent answer I received translated it as "defeating the mind", "controlling the mind" or "disciplining the mind". Other common translations included "winning the mind" and "attaining a sattvika [pure] state". Monier-Williams translates sattvavajaya as "self-command, strength of mind or character" (1899: 1135.3, in Smith 2011, 23). Smith (2006, 538) speculates that sattvavajaya was regarded as part of daivavyapasraya. Several Ayurvedic psychiatrists, college teachers and students instead speculated that sattvavajaya should be considered part of yukti treatment. Dr Shankaran elaborated his understanding of sattvavajaya as mind control:[210]

> Whenever we get immersed with some bad things, that will affect us. So we have to draw our mind away from bad things. The person has to have control over harmful activities. Our mind is like a monkey. It is going here and there, without any concept of what is good and what is bad. But we have to realize what is good, what is bad, and we have to get some control over these things. To bring back the mind from things that are not good and only allow the mind to immerse with good things, that is sattvavajaya.

Sattvavajaya is a bio-moral concept because thought and behavioural changes in accordance with local moralities transform the physiology of the body, and reciprocally, diet and daily regimes are transformative to the gunas. It aims at restoring social harmony and social reintegration by means of controlling mental upheaval that arises within oneself as a result of passions and strong emotions (which are understood as causative of depression). Moral advice, dietary changes and suggested daily regimes such as early awakening, exercises, bathing, good dietary habits as forms of self-development are the most important techniques of sattvavajaya. Additionally, supportive techniques like reassurance and encouragement as well as social intervention are also common practices.

Since sattvavajaya, conceptualized as helping the mind to refrain from unwholesome objects, is open to multiple interpretations, it is deployed in many ways. Several Ayurvedic psychiatrists and general physicians told me that reassurance of the patient by the return of a lost object or person and the inducement of emotions opposite to those associated with the patient's distress, as described in another verse of the Caraka Samhita,[211] are integral parts of Ayurvedic psychotherapy or *adravya* [drugless] treatment. Dr Mangalam explained:[212]

> Those who have a lot of worries should be made happy. Those who are highly aggressive should be given peace. Those who have a lot of anger and hatred should be controlled with *kama* [sensual attachment or desire]. Those who feel dejected in the society should get attached to something.

As an illustration of the displacement of strong emotions by invoking their opposites, he recounted an example:

> An old father and mother had a son. This son married a girl who was not from their caste or community. The parents were totally against the marriage. This caused the son to separate from his family and to move somewhere else. Years later, when the son had a child and brought it to his parents, naturally their anger came down. They felt attachment and affection towards the child. So anger was replaced by affection. In a similar way we should impart a kama [sensual attachment] attitude to a person feeling *krodha* [anger].

When talking to his patients, Dr Mangalam often referred to Hindu mythology to explain this principle:

> When Lord Siva was doing *tapas* [literally heat, also meditation, austerity, discipline], Kama Deva [the god of erotic love, desire] shot an arrow at him. After being struck by this arrow, his tapas broke and he got up from tapas and simply looked at Kama Deva with his third eye. Through the regard of Lord Siva's third eye, Kama Deva got burnt. That means that kama can be controlled with the anger only. If you have a lot of attachment to something, how can we get detached? We should feel aversion towards it. All the psychological features are opposite in character. If somebody is too much afflicted with sadness we should try to make him happy.

The replacement of emotions by their opposite mirrors dramaturgic ideas in classic Sanskrit theatre of replacing the emotions of the audience by more refined *rasas* [emotions, tastes] represented by the divine characters on the stage. Likewise the aim of sattvavaja is not to evoke and lay open hidden emotional conflicts but rather to replace emotions by more refined and sattvik ones.

When I discussed sattvavajaya with Dr Kumar at GAMH, he began by defining sattvavajaya as "living according to the rules of the society, according to moral and religious rules.[213] These rules", he maintained, "are made aiming at good health." He enumerated examples including going to temples, lighting a religious lamp [*nilavilakku*] and associating with elders and wise persons. He further mentioned general advice such as controlling your emotions, telling the truth and having compassion for every living being. In other words, "All these advices we give are according to scriptures. Our patients should learn to live according to scriptures," Dr Kumar concluded. This is what several other Ayurvedic psychiatrists also meant when they told me that traditional Kerala culture with its norms and religious rules has contributed to the mental health of the people and that this mental health is eroding now in tandem with the erosion of traditional culture and its values. In a similar mode Dr Joshua explained sattvavajaya at a press conference on Ayurvedic psychiatry[214]:

> Sattvavajaya is very different from modern psychotherapy. Why it is different is that it promotes or develops the goodness in you. It restricts the person from seeing what is not good to see, and hear what is not good to hear, and so on. It grows the good attributes in the patient. It encourages good thoughts and action.

Sattvavajaya, beyond psychotherapy, is about wellness through living in accordance with social, religious and gender norms. This is what Dr Sundaran writes:

> There are many treatments which help to inculcate healthy thoughts in the mind by bringing in an improved awareness of social norms, cultural values and ethos, manners, good demeanour principles, and principles of societal accuracies. The sattvavajaya is powerful to bring back the patient's mind from fraying into undesired thoughts.
>
> (Sundaran 1993, 68)

Sundaran does not stop here but goes further and includes several other treatments that contribute to "streamlining the mind-sense complex" such as snehapana, dhupanam, vamanam and religious treatments that are "helpful in bringing the patient's mind into this proper state" also under sattvavajaya. For Sundaran, "sattvavajaya is a comprehensive treatment of mental diseases" (Sundaran 1993, 68). Although this inclusive notion of sattvavajaya is somewhat exceptional and practitioners usually distinguish purifying and pacifying medical treatments from sattvavajaya and spiritual treatment, it was not unusual that the demarcation between these three kinds of treatments became blurred.

Dr Mangalam told me how he taught sattvavajaya to his students:

> A person with a psychiatric abnormality has a psyche which is not under his control. We try to help him to gain control over his sattva. And *jnana* [general knowledge], *vijnana* [specific knowledge], *dhairya*, [courage], *smrti* [memory], and *samadhi* [higher consciousness] are the five tools to win over the sattva. Jnana is general knowledge or awareness. In clinical practice I ask students to impart certain general rules and regulations to the patients. How they perform, what is lacking, what is the ideal in our society to behave, certain activities should be advised. They should advise them to behave according to the requirements and norms of their family, the society, their occupational field, and other areas. Vijnana is specific knowledge. Students should try to educate them about their actual clinical problem, their disease. Dhairya is imparting courage to the patient. In Ayurveda, vishada can be overcome with courage, courage to live according to *dharma* [duty, norm]. If an individual is not capable of using his logic, brain, intellectual activities, to do what is right and refrain from doing what is wrong, then we should impart it. And smrti is memory. I tell students they should impart memory in the patient. The patient should remember that some years ago he was full of energy and active. From this memory

> comes self-realization and knowledge that what I am now is not right. These are the steps we will teach the students. In Ayurveda, a physician should have a perfect moral, psyche and balance. Otherwise when you counsel others it will not work properly.

Sattvavajaya is not only a psychological or moral process, but also a physiological one. Zimmermann (2014) is right when he states that sattva, which he translates as "will-power" or "human agency", though designating the ethical dimension of health and disease, is materialized as a fluid in the body channels. Morals are closely interconnected with physiology in the Indian context, as Marriott (1976) demonstrates with the example of dharma as a bio-moral notion. Many Ayurvedic psychiatrists see diet as an integral part of sattvavajaya. "How we tame our mind, that is sattvavajaya basically. We are telling them to use their mind correctly and decide which food to take and which not to take," the manasika student Dr Pritha reflected.[215] Another Ayurvedic physician, with whom I talked about sattvabalam, easily combined cognitive, emotional, and behavioural changes with the consumption of ghee and milk. Talking about different psychological measures to improve mental strength as prevention of depression at another Ayurveda College, Dr Girish switched from a psychological to a physiological notion of depression when he suggested, "We have to improve the sattvabalam. We have to apply daily ghrta and milk."[216]

Sattvavajaya is a specific kind of introspection in an effort to monitor the mind and to use the mind properly. Rather than the self-explorative introspection of Western biodynamic psychotherapy with its aims of emancipation and autonomy of the self, in sattvavajaya the mind is brought into accordance with the social and cosmological order and streamlined according to moral norms and ideas of the good life. As such, sattvavajaya is closely related to prajnaparadha that I have described in "Depression as a problem of perception" (this chapter, subchapter 3) in that the aim is to avoid faulty behaviour and re-establish the right connections between sense objects, senses and mind. The aim of the Ayurvedic psychiatric treatment of bringing the patient back to reality and normality so they can again experience conjugal, familial and social harmony and live well and in accordance with social norms resonates with local notions of recovery that can also be found in the context of ritual healing in Kerala. What Tarabout writes of the treatment at Poonkudil Mana is equally true for the Ayurvedic sattvavajaya:

> The cure does not aim at becoming conscious of inner conflicts and tensions so as to elucidate them, but at providing the patient serenity through his reintegration in his milieu, preserving all his previous beliefs. This can be seen as a logical outcome of an explanation of illness in terms of disharmony and disorder in the patient's relation to his environment.
>
> (Tarabout 1999, 139)

Rather than making inner conflicts conscious, the aim of sattvavajaya is to suppress and replace unhealthy thoughts and emotions and to prevent them from moving into the conscious mind, keeping the mind and senses away from unwholesome objects, thinking the right things, feeling at the right intensity, or in other words controlling thoughts and emotions as opposed to venting and expressing them. The aim of Ayurvedic psychotherapy then is not to make conscious the processes of the unconscious mind or to solve hidden conflicts. Whenever I heard Ayurvedic psychiatrists mentioning the unconscious mind they talked about it in terms of "purifying the subconscious mind", "eliminating bad thoughts and emotions" or "removing the subconscious mind" while others asked their patients to pray to God in order to heal their subconscious mind. In these cases, the unconscious was not merely "a name, a mere sign, empty of any vaster terrain of reference", as Langford (2002, 252) argues. Rather, it was something different in that it was not granted the epistemological power of being the source of or revealing one's true authentic inner self. The unconscious of Ayurvedic psychiatry as I observed it in Kerala is something to be overcome, something epiphenomenal; its content to be replaced by more refined and morally superior contents in line with the socio-moral norms of the society.

For Foucault, psychotherapy is one of the modes of pastoral power which "cannot be exercised without knowing the inside of people's minds, without exploring their souls, without making them reveal their innermost secrets" (Foucault 1982). Through the process of revelation, psychotherapy is an institution in which authentic interior selves are produced as much as they are healed. Through the different kind of judgmental introspection that takes place in sattvavajaya, it is selves as rooted in the moral and social realms rather than authentic interior selves that are produced. The revealed emotions and thoughts, then, do not become signs of an inner authentic self as they are in Western psychotherapy. Rather they become symptoms of a distance from an ideal sattvik state and are targeted for replacement by inner processes that are both productive and expressive of sattva and mental strength.

Most doctors did not see these differences between the aims of Western psychotherapy and sattvavajaya. For them, sattvavajaya is equivalent to psychotherapy. "Both increase mental strength," Dr Kumar explained, "and both aim to modify thought and behavioural patterns."[217] When they related sattvavajaya to cognitive behavioural therapy, Ayurvedic psychiatrists not only made both approaches commensurable but also reframed the latter as creating mental strength through adjustment to moral values. Some Ayurvedic psychiatrists such as Dr Joseph John described differences between what he called "modern" and "Indian psychotherapy".[218] The modern approach was, he said, "to let everything out even if it leads to divorce," whereas the Indian approach (sattvavajaya) aimed to control the senses and emotions and to adjust to often difficult familial circumstances.

> This is why I teach my patients to forgive, forgive your mother-in-law even if she is mean to you, forgive your husband even if he drinks and harasses you. Pray for them, change your state of mind. Do not oppress your feelings but change them.

Once I asked him why he did not advise a specific patient to separate from a destructive husband and in-laws. "Then the problems will only aggravate," he replied.

> In this culture it is not possible. She has to adjust to her husband and her in-laws. I can try to give her strength for that. But she has to cope with this situation. Husband and wife, this is meant by God. God had this plan with them, we cannot know why.

Although Ayurvedic psychiatrists stressed that the word "sattva" in sattvavajaya refers to the mind and not to the sattva guna, sattvavajaya is closely related to the promotion of sattva guna and sattvabalam as a predisposition and equivalent to mental health and protection against depression. This is linked to the decrease of rajas and tamas in order to reduce vulnerability to mental illness (cf. "Gunas, sattvabalam and mental health", this chapter, subchapter 3). The deterioration of mental health expressed in terms of sattvabalam is also linked to a modernization critique when doctors stressed that in former times people had better manobalam. The advice Ayurvedic doctors give to their depressive patients to improve their mental strength is likewise conducive to sattvabalam. Medical management mainly targets the doshas but sattvavajaya directly affects the gunas, and both the doshas and the gunas have physiological *and* psychological components. Sattvavajaya aims at increasing the proportion of sattva that is again related to local ideas of a good life and at decreasing rajas and tamas that are seen as responsible for passions, ignorance and immoral behaviour. This is why sattavajaya as mental discipline to promote the development of sattva can also be used as preventive treatment and ideally should start in early childhood. "If we find that someone has some weakness in the mind or sattva is reduced then we can use sattvavajaya," explained Dr Kumar.[219] "We don't have to wait for this person to develop mental illness. Because there is a chance that any bad incident in her life may precipitate a psychiatric illness. Better we don't wait."

Sattvavajaya as psychotherapy is often linked to psychological and philosophical ideas in the Bhagavad Gita and to what is described as "counselling" following the form of the archetypal Indian counsellor, Sree Krishna.[220] The Gita is used in Ayurvedic pedagogics to teach what is seen as the quintessence of Indian psychology and psychotherapy: Krishna advised Arjuna, who was suffering from vishada in the face of having to fight his relatives, to gain clarity of mind and of his dharma by freeing himself from attachment to the consequences or fruits of his actions. This is especially interesting since Arjuna's condition (vishadam) is often translated as "depression" and Krishna's advice is therefore interpreted as psychotherapy for depression. Dr Mangalam made this quite clear:[221]

> In Mahabharata, when the battle was about to begin, Arjuna was going to lead the battle. Initially he fell into vishada rogam [depressive disorder], he felt terrified, trembling, his mouth got dried up, he got totally exhausted,

> fainting, and felt like not being able to do anything. At that time Krishna advised him, this is your duty, you are supposed to do this duty. Don't think about the result; perform your duty. He maximum tried to encourage Arjuna. By that methodology he got courage.

For women, Dr Varghese linked mental health and prevention of depression to conservative and self-sacrificing gender norms.

> By performing without any attachment, the mother is doing her duties. That is what Lord Krishna told. The woman in the kitchen, she is not concerned about the credit, the praises, or the drinking husband's torture. She never minds. She just keeps on her duties. Indian families are good. Indian family life and bonds are so strong. Why? Because of the mothers. The husband may be a drunkard; he may be a useless fellow. She is not running after men, she is content though unhappy. She makes herself content, she is in the house, she is doing her duties, she is securing her family, protecting the family. That womanpower is saving India, that is my opinion.

Other doctors also linked sattvavajaya to elements of the Qu'ran and the Bible. However, these connections arose only out of their private engagement with these texts while the Bhagavad Gita is part of the syllabus of the Manasika postgraduate course.

Is sattvavajaya a technology of the self or a mode of treatment? Is it practised by the patient or by the physician? Is it the doctor or the patient who is "winning the mind"? Does it refer to a mental discipline or a relationship between the doctor and the patient? The way this term is used and taught by Ayurvedic psychiatrists suggests that sattvavajaya may refer to both: It can be both an inner transformative process and refer to the guidance of the doctor in this process.[222]

Smith (2011) argues that in its original meaning, sattvavajaya was neither a technology of the self nor a kind of ancient psychotherapy because the idea of self-care is a modern one that is not anchored in the classic texts. According to Smith, the word "sattva" in sattvavajaya as it appears the classical texts does not denote "mind" but rather refers to spirits. He argues that the term sattvavajaya lacks "the explicit descriptive sense of most early medical terms" and denotes "conquest or submission by sattva, by a sattva, or of a sattva" (Smith 2011, 23). For Smith, sattvavajaya is "a form of ancient Indian therapeutic practice in which ritual possession was a probable component" (Smith 2011, 23). According to this interpretation, sattvavajaya in the classical scriptures refers to non-Brahmanical healing forms involving the removal of spirit possession "whose traces can still be seen in ritual healing centers such as Balaji temple and many others throughout India". Smith speculates that sattvavajaya was "a therapeutic practice in which a disease was subdued (*avajaya*) by a sattva, an existent being." Sattvavajaya would then not have been akin to psychotherapy but to practices that involved possession. It may have been so. However, my focus is the way sattvavajaya is understood and practised by Ayurvedic psychiatrists today, and none of the Ayurvedic psychiatrists with whom I spoke related sattvavajaya to forms of possession. If Smith is correct and sattvavajaya was in previous times a form of exorcism, this meaning has been completely extruded from present-day understandings of sattvavajaya. This would, then, resemble the purification processes that gave rise to the discursive extrusion of bhutas as spirits from contemporary academic Ayurvedic discourse.

Several Ayurvedic authors merge sattvavajaya with other *upayangals* [drugless remedial practices] and translate this package of therapeutic techniques as Ayurvedic psychotherapy. The aim seems to be not only to make these ancient techniques commensurable with and anticipatory to modern psychological techniques but also to boost this (re)invented field with concrete techniques mentioned in several *slokas* [verses] throughout different texts beyond the single vague reference to sattvavajaya in the Caraka Samhita. This merging of sattvavajaya and upayangal as Ayurvedic psychotherapy resembles the complex translation processes through which bhutavidya is reconfigured as Ayurvedic psychiatry. In the case of the latter, diverse sections and slokas scattered through the texts are summarized under "bhutavidya" to invent psychiatry as a branch of Ayurveda. In the merger of sattvavajaya and upayangal as Ayurvedic psychotherapy, various techniques described in the texts as treatments for different forms of unmada are clustered together to form this new field of Ayurvedic psychotherapy. Some of the upayangal that Sundaran (1993) suggests and that doctors at GAMH occasionally use are scaring, shocking, ridiculing, insulting, beating or shouting at the patient, threatening to kill the patient, and tying the patient with a cloth.[223] Smith calls these practices "psychodrama" (Smith 2006, 135) and they are sometimes used by contemporary Ayurvedic psychiatrists. Other less dramatic measures that are sometimes applied at GAMH include exposing a patient to opposite emotions, friendly talk, reassurance and consolation, chaining and confining patients who try to harm themselves or others, causing fear in patients if they refuse to take food or medicine, or, to subdue a violent patient, telling them that a loved one is dead.

Since the content of the upayangal is not rigidly prescribed in the texts, Dr Kumar opined, it can also include techniques of modern psychotherapy.[224] To date, no clinical psychologist has been employed at GAMH. This is due in part to financial constraints, but also because Ayurveda is seen as already comprising the mind *and* the body, psychiatry and psychology[225] and therefore a clinical psychologist is seen as being unnecessary. Another cause is that the proponents of shuddha (pure) Ayurveda want to keep Ayurvedic and allopathic psychiatry – to which they count psychology – separate. Dr Kumar, however, confirmed the limits of the Ayurvedic approach when he suggested that a clinical psychologist should be employed at GAMH:

> In the Ayurveda system itself the use of upayangal[226] for mental illness is recommended. Modern clinical psychology and psychotherapy are a

> developed form. So we can adopt that. We hope that a psychologist assistant will be here in the future. That is needed. There is a limit for medicines; there is a need for some kind of psychotherapy also. It is said in Ayurveda itself. It is said, these upayangal methods you should use according to time. Now the time has changed, so we can adopt the new methods. The basic principles are the same.

The reconfiguration of sattvavajaya as Ayurvedic psychotherapy, as one part of (re)invented Ayurvedic psychiatry next to yuktivyapasraya chikitsa (rational treatment), aims to correspond to the bifurcation of treatment in pharmacological therapy and psychotherapy in mainstream psychiatry. Through complex processes of translation in the Latourian sense sattvavajaya is established as a field of specialization to correspond and anticipate psychotherapy. As it is understood by Ayurvedic psychiatrists in Kerala, sattvavajaya is a specific kind of introspection in an effort to monitor the mind and to use the mind properly. Rather than the self-explorative introspection of Western psychotherapy with its aims of emancipation and autonomy of the self, in sattvavajaya the mind is brought into accordance with the social and cosmological order and streamlined according to moral norms and ideas of the good life. Rather than venting and expressing thoughts and emotions, the aim of sattvavajaya is to suppress and replace unhealthy thoughts and emotions. Moreover, sattvavajaya is a biomoral technique because thought and behavioural changes in accordance with local moralities transform the physiology of the body, and reciprocally, diet and daily regimes are transformative to the gunas. In the latter sense, sattvavajaya is closely associated with a framing of mental health in terms of sattvabalam and vulnerability to mental illness in terms of rajas and tamas.

The psychologization and ontological epoché of daivavyapasraya treatment

Daivavyapasraya chikitsa or spiritual therapy is the third part of what Ayurvedic psychiatrists postulate as the treatment triad of Ayurvedic psychiatry, next to rational treatment and sattvavajaya. The poster that I mentioned at the beginning of this subchapter exemplifies this tripartite model of Ayurvedic treatment that students of the manasika course are taught and that practitioners conveyed to me. To explain daivavyapasraya treatment, clinicians explicitly or implicitly referred to one verse in the Caraka Samhita[227] that specifically mentions this treatment triad. This verse lists, for example, reciting mantras, wearing gemstones, and Hindu practices such as fire offerings [*homam*], the chanting of names of God [*japam*], sacrifices [*bali*] or pilgrimage as elements of daivavyapasraya treatment. Through these ritual practices, the consequences of a moral transgression effected in this or a previous life may be overcome. Zimmermann (2014, 93) translates daivavyapasraya as "placed in [the hands of] gods (daiva)" or "based on fate".[228]

In spite of occasional textual evidence of daivavyapasraya treatment in the canonical texts, so far there is no historical or ethnographic evidence that this treatment has ever been practised by vaidyas. Although students study the treatment triad and doctors refer to it in college teaching, in health magazine reports and in TV broadcasts, daivavyapasraya treatment is not part of the clinical practice in institutionalized Ayurvedic psychiatry. "Professional Ayurvedic practitioners have limited their realm to rational treatment",[229] Dr Sundaran emphasizes and adds, "Perhaps these ways of treatment don't have the backing of reason, which may be the reason why they are not dealt with in detail in the classical texts" (Sundaran 1993, 72). Although Sundaran excludes daivavyapasraya from rational treatments, he writes: "Some of the daivavyapasraya treatments are also indicated in the conditions of mental illness" (Sundaran 1993, 68). Doctors do not explicitly encourage their patients but they nevertheless do not dissuade them from seeking the help of Hindu, Muslim or Christian religious healers. I also found a tolerance for religious healing among mainstream psychiatrists "as long as they do not interfere with our treatment," as doctors often expressed it. There was greater sympathy towards religious healing amongst Ayurvedic psychiatrists: "We don't say, 'don't go', because basically we want to help them to get well", a student on the manasika course told me, repeating what students are taught at the college and by GAMH doctors.[230] "If they believe in that, if they believe it will help them, why not? So we don't say, don't go." Another student added,

> We direct some patients to religious healers if they have faith in that; according to their beliefs and their wishes. They ask us, "Can we go to a temple or do puja?" They come to us for treatment, and along with that they will go for religious treatment. If they continue the medication, we allow this. This is daivavyapasraya treatment that we can't do, so let them [religious practitioners] do it.[231]

Dr Rasheed told me that on those occasional cases in which astrologers or priests refer patients to GAMH, he asked them to continue with the treatment the ritual practitioner had recommended.[232] In line with a pragmatic approach that characterizes much of the help seeking behaviour of South Asians (Nichter 2010; Quack 2013), most Ayurvedic psychiatrists are convinced that *vishvasam chikitsa* [faith treatment] may aid patient recovery. I suggest that this tolerant stance – though also an adaption to the local help seeking behaviour of their patients – is a consequence of the fact that daivavyapasraya treatment is an integral part of the texts that form the corpus of what is regarded as Ayurveda today even though it is considered to be superstition and not in accordance with reason, modernity and science.

There are three ways Ayurvedic psychiatrists deal with the challenge arising as a result of the clear textual evidence of daivavyapasraya treatment and the conflict that arises between appreciating the authority of the texts on the one hand and adhering to a scientific model on the other. In the first, doctors engage a narrative of Ayurvedic decline and postulate that these passages are not original but later additions to the texts; in the second, doctors reinterpret the effects of daivavyapasraya treatment in psychological terms and thus psychologize and interiorize their effect and importance for recovery; and in the third, doctors engage in a kind of epistemological and ontological epoché or suspension from judgement and hold that the effects of daivavyapasraya treatment is unknown. Several doctors told me that the exclusive emphasis on medical or rational treatment is the result of patients' expectations of GAMH as a medical institution. Just as patients tend to emphasize their somatic symptoms in a doctor's consultation room because they expect doctors to treat physical problems, patients also expect medical treatment from their doctors. "If I tell them to tie a *elassu* [protective amulet] on their arm, they will not believe us," explained Dr Sarasvati.[233] "But if a priest in a temple gives it they will believe. That's why we cannot do daivavyapasraya chikitsa here. And they come for medical treatment. Otherwise they will go to some temples, churches, or mosques."

Although daivavyapasraya treatment is not an integral part of the treatment in institutionalized Ayurvedic psychiatry and doctors regard it as unscientific and irrational, most clinicians highlight the psychological benefits and positive effects of ritual healing practices as bringing peace of mind and thus contributing to recovery. Religious and spiritual activities such as visiting temples, worship and meditation produce mental peace, doctors stressed. In this sense, daivavyapasraya treatment practices may be included under sattvavajaya. According to Dr Sundaran (1993), "Prayers, homams, japas and so on are also helpful in bringing the patient's mind into its proper state. The mind-senses-complex is streamlined through these. So all these treatment modalities can be said to be sattvavavajaya." Likewise, Dr Mary, a Christian Ayurvedic psychiatrist practising in her own private clinic, expressed religious treatment in terms of sattva:[234]

> For me, previously if I had a depressed mood and I went to Potta Ashram [a famous Christian religious healing centre, see Jansen and Lang 2012], all my problems would be solved. The problems themselves did not leave me, but I could cope with them. That capacity I gained at Potta. Going to Potta increases my sattvik parts in me, sattvabalam increases. Earlier I was not *pravara sattva* [a high level of sattva]. *Rajo tamo avarana* [obstruction through rajas and tamas guna] was there. For small, small things I got into a depressed mood.

Similar to the transformation of daivavyapasraya into sattvavajaya or upayanal, which are then both reconfigured as Ayurvedic psychotherapy, Dr Sundaran speculated that some of the techniques employed by religious healers are comparable to the Ayurvedic techniques of upayangal.[235] Ritual healers may transform emotions – for example, fear into anger or revenge when resorting to sorcery and other techniques of occult violence – thus re-establishing the patient's agency. Others transfer hatred from husband or in-laws to a third party thus guaranteeing conjugal or family harmony (Lang 2014). Still others reassure their clients that occult violence cannot harm them due to protective actions or devices. This is, Dr Sundaran opined, closely related to the Ayurvedic technique of replacing emotions with their opposites.

Other Ayurvedic psychiatrists stressed the effect of religious healing as instilling hope or as a placebo that can make a significant contribution to recovery. "It is the belief of the patient," a student said in a classroom presentation, "that plays a key role in the process of recovery."[236] Generally doctors stressed the importance of engagement in religious activities to the healing process in cases of depression. They may also, as Dr Sundaran remarked, be seen as a kind of behavioural therapy for depression in that a pilgrimage draws patients out of a pathogenic environment, and regular visits to temples, mosques or churches, and prayers establish a positive daily routine and prevent a patient from falling into a lethargic state.[237] "We can interpret some of the modes of action of daivavyapasraya chikitsa through yuktivyapasraya chikitsa", Dr Ganapati (a general Ayurvedic physician) noted, then continued:

> For example pilgrimage can cause a change of atmosphere. The atmosphere can lead to a change of the disease of the mind. So pilgrimage is yuktivyapasraya, the causative factor is removed, by the change of environment or change of atmosphere. The disease-causing factor will be the father or the mother, so the causative factor is removed, so it is yuktivyapasraya.[238]

This is why many doctors not only tolerate but also encourage prayers and spiritual exercises. When doctors emphasize the psychological effects of daivavyapasraya treatment or interiorize agency and efficacy into an inner psychological space within the patient, this is another aspect of the general process of eliminating external [agantu] influence and shifting the agency for healing into inner or psychological processes in the treatment of mental suffering that some authors have described as "psychologization" of ritual healing (Tarabout 1999; Lang 2014).

Some doctors emphasized the physiological effects of daivavyapasraya treatment. Dr A. Raghunadhan (2001) describes what he calls the "pharmacodynamics of adravya [drugless] treatment" by which he mainly understands daivavyapasraya treatment as including elements such as rituals, pilgrimages, wearing gems, chanting mantras and prayers. He maintains that,

> wearing jewels and divine material as well as chanting mantras are the matters of intense research today and these can be emphasized elaborately with the parapsychology and newer biological branches. The principle in these methods is that by these, the nervous system of the patient is stimulated, vigil is recovered, and the bodily channels are cleansed well. Automatically then the mind does function in proper way.
>
> (Raghunadhan 2001, 168)

This kind of evidence-based research on religious practices is also emphasized by other Ayurvedic doctors and others I spoke with who use evidence-based research to study the effects of mantras, tantric practices and other treatments on neurotransmitters, physiological processes and in certain allopathically defined disease conditions such as depression.

Several times I heard doctors saying that recovery is easier for those with faith or belief [*vishvasam*]. This is true in terms of belief in Ayurveda but also belief in religious treatment. Interestingly, I have never heard mainstream psychiatrists say that a patient should have "belief" in psychopharmaceuticals. Dr Ganapati framed daivavyapasraya as that part of the treatment in which doctors utilize their patients' "beliefs":[239]

> Daivavyapasraya means that we make use of the beliefs of the patient, that's all. It is very easy to treat those who are having astikhyam, faith in the god. Actually this is a manipulation or some therapeutic usage of their beliefs. If they don't have some belief, then we cannot do deiva viapasraya chikitsa.

The majority of Ayurvedic psychiatrists discarded the ontology of spirits and occult violence and psychologized ritual healing, but others showed an agnostic stance or a kind of epistemological and ontological epoché [bracketing] by stressing that the effects cannot (yet) be explained in terms of logic and rationality [*yukti*], deliberately leaving questions of ontology and agency open and unresolved. "Wherever we cannot understand the mode of action, then it is daivavyapasraya chikitsa," was Dr Ganapati's short definition. And, Dr Sundaran (1993) writes: "Daivavyapasraya chikitsa is something which benefits the patient in a way which cannot be explained in terms of fact-reason logic." Psychologization and bracketing ontologies while simultaneously discarding or distancing from what they perceive as superstitious assumptions characterize how most Ayurvedic psychiatrists negotiate daivavyapasraya chikitsa today.[240]

6 Ayurvedic psychiatrists beyond the clinic: the politics of recognition

In March 2014, the recently founded Association of Ayurveda Psychiatrists (AAP) held a half-day meeting with a subsequent two-hour press conference for local newspapers at a hotel in Thrissur. Dr Praveen, then president of the Thrissur unit of the Ayurveda Medical Association of India (AMAI), Dr Joshua, the president of the recently founded AAP, Dr Joseph John, Dr Mary and two other young Ayurvedic psychiatrists were present. At the opening of the press conference, around twenty journalists from the local sections of the major Malayalam newspapers and channels were in attendance. During the event, Dr Praveen made the following demands. In Kerala, he started, stress and depression are prominent mental health problems. After introducing Ayurveda as a holistic and indigenous system well suited to treating mental health problems, he demanded that Ayurveda be included in India's new Mental Health Care Act and in national and state mental health policies and programmes. Moreover, all Ayurveda colleges, he insisted, should have a psychiatry department and all district hospitals at least five beds for psychiatric patients and one psychiatrist on staff. Additionally, mental health care should be included in public Ayurvedic primary health care in state dispensaries in Kerala. The Government Ayurveda Mental Hospital in Kottakkal should be made a centre of excellence and all five posts for medical officers should be filled. With these measures, all Ayurvedic postgraduates who complete their MD (Ay) with a manasika specialization could work in psychiatry and on the front lines addressing this prominent problem, and would not be forced to work in other areas. Moreover, all medical officers should be trained in diagnosis and treatment of mental diseases. Similar to demands made by the Indian Psychiatric Society, he suggested more teaching hours in mental health for undergraduate BAMS students. Finally he recommended that Ayurvedic psychiatry be included in the syllabus of the 11th and 12th class in Kerala. These demands directly target the recognition of Ayurvedic psychiatry as an important actor in the mental health care network, the urgent need to address depression and the risk of losing trained Ayurvedic psychiatrists due to a lack of posts in Kerala. Then, Dr Joshua reported on the AAP and he, Dr John and Dr Mary reported from their clinical practice in Ayurvedic psychiatry. This was the second time I attended a press conference of this type. The first took place one year before in February 2013, when Dr John organized an event in Kottayam with a similar goal of promoting Ayurvedic psychiatry. At both press conferences, doctors pushed me speak about my research and my interest in Ayurvedic psychiatry. Indeed, it seemed a selling point of the events was the presence of a German scientist who had come all the way to India to research Ayurvedic psychiatry. Although I would have preferred to remain as an observer, my participation as small-scale action anthropology was the least I could do in return for the generous assistance of the Ayurvedic psychiatrists with my research.

Shortly before the first press conference, the doctors met to discuss the way they intended to present Ayurvedic psychiatry. Dr Joseph John wanted to introduce me as a foreign scholar conducting research on "Ayurvedic solutions for depression". Dr Joshua suggested that I – a foreign researcher – should underscore the efficacy of Ayurvedic psychiatry: "You should tell them that with Ayurveda we can effectively treat depression. This type of answer they are expecting. If an outsider tells that Ayurveda is effective we [Ayurvedic psychiatrists] will get more attention." I replied:

> I am not here to judge the efficacy of the treatment. This would be another approach. My approach is to try to understand how the topic of depression is negotiated within Ayurveda psychiatry and all the political issues related to it. Actually, the press conference is very much a part of the study. I aim to describe these processes, what is happening in Ayurvedic psychiatry, how it is established as a science, how it is located within the mental health care market in Kerala, how it goes public. So my work is a descriptive and analytic work. This is social science. It is not a question of how much patients with depression may benefit from Ayurveda or

> modern medicines, or from religious treatments. These are not the kinds of questions that I ask.

In a typical manner of ethnographic refraining from judgement, I explained that all I was able to do was to emphasize that Ayurvedic psychiatry is more culturally sensitive and that it creates another option or alternative for patients. As such, it should be included in BAMS and postgraduate training programmes and mental health policies should include Ayurveda, especially since policy makers and health planners postulate a treatment gap for depression and other mental health problems in India. It was against my deepest convictions as an anthropologist to do this because, after all, my intent was to study these processes not to influence or intervene in them. Thankfully, Dr Joshua was satisfied. "This answer is needed at the press conference. These things you have to say. If a foreign research scholar tells like that, this itself is effective." I did so but in the end, however, things took an unintended and disappointing turn. Instead of reporting on Ayurvedic psychiatry or engaging with the political and health care demands made by the four doctors, the articles that appeared in several local newspapers wrote only about my research and nothing about integrating Ayurveda into mental health policies.

At the beginning of the first conference in Kottayam in 2013, Dr Joseph made the aims of the conference clear right from the start:

> This conference has been convened, firstly, to explain the stand that Ayurveda be included in the Mental Healthcare Policy in Kerala. Secondly, it aims to bring to public notice that there is treatment in Ayurveda for mental diseases. Sincerity of the doctor and cooperation of the patient and relatives play a vital role in the cure of the patient. Modern medicines have undesirable side effects that can make the patient physically weak. Ayurvedic treatment helps to control the overuse of medicines and also wards off the side effects of modern medicine. The possibility of recurrence of diseases is very much lower. Along with the treatment, personality improvement and promotion of moral values in the patient is also possible through Ayurvedic mental healthcare. Ayurvedic treatment is also relatively inexpensive. Thirdly, we will talk about education opportunities in Ayurveda Mental Healthcare. Fourth, mental health treatment in Ayurveda has been divided into three sections. The first is the treatment with medicines. Second is sattvavajaya therapy, which is Ayurvedic psychotherapy. The third is daivavyapasraya chikitsa, a treatment based on spiritual methods.

This was a press conference on Ayurvedic psychiatry from the point of view of two Ayurvedic psychiatrists with a strong focus on Christian spirituality. Dr Joshua criticized "common misconceptions about the Ayurvedic treatment of mental diseases":

> We know about the role of Ayurveda in the treatment of mental disorders. This is an Indian system of medical treatment that has developed over

> several hundred years. Unfortunately few patients come for Ayurvedic treatment due to lack of awareness. Even in movies the Ayurvedic treatment for mental disorders has been discredited with scenes showing patients with *abhyanga* [oil baths/massages], *dhara* [warm oil pouring over the forehead] and so on. In other countries they try to promote their own systems of treatment while here it is discriminatory. Each new legislation effectively curbs the scope for ayurvedic medical practice.

Further, he complained that even if the media try to propagate Ayurvedic treatment for mental diseases they do not feature Ayurvedic practitioners who specialize in psychiatry. "They go to a general BAMS practitioner rather than to an Ayurvedic psychiatrist and the answer given is always about some dhara or *kizhi* [massage with warm herbal poultices]" which are too general in nature and send the wrong signals to readers. Dr Joshua then demanded the establishment of psychiatric treatment facilities in all district Ayurveda hospitals and the creation of specialty Ayurveda mental hospitals in all the major cities of Kerala. Additionally, he suggested a dedicated department for psychiatry at the Ayurveda College in Kottakkal and at other colleges. Moreover, "there are eighteen doctors studying for MD and there is only one guide. How can one doctor guide eighteen students? More guides should be appointed." In conclusion, Dr Joshua argued that there should be more money allocated for research: "We do not have the benefit of a research base to validate our work. Everything must be proved through research. Adequate funding must be provided."

Two months later, in April 2013, the Ministry of Health & Family Welfare of the Government of Kerala launched the "Health Policy Kerala 2013" (Ministry of Health & Family Welfare 2013). One important difference to previous policies is the integration of non-communicable diseases, mental health issues and geriatric care within the primary care system. It further includes the shift of mental health care from specialty hospitals to primary health in primary health centres, community health centres and other general hospitals. According to the Policy, the state aims "to incorporate the mental health services with the general health care services up to the primary health center level". However, one of the major handicaps, it continues, is the "shortage of mental health professionals". Although the draft lists different professional and lay mental health care providers in the prevention and treatment of mental disorders, Ayurvedic practitioners are not mentioned in the sections on mental health care. Ayurveda is only mentioned later in the Policy as a separate category (before Homeopathy and Oral Health) but not as part of the mental health service system of the state. The Policy provides for improving the Ayurveda sector through the promotion of research and documentation, quality assurance, support of manufacturing and support for the availability of raw materials, and awareness regarding the benefits of Ayurveda. The sections on Ayurveda are a shortened version of an earlier draft titled "Kerala State Comprehensive Health Policy – Draft for Ayurveda" by the Ayurveda doctor M.R. Vasudeven Nampoothiri.[241] In it, Nampoothiri argues for mainstreaming Ayurveda, a vision already formulated in the

National Health Policy of 2002 that, he states, still needs to be implemented through state policy and regulation. Although he does not explicitly mention mental health, he stresses that Ayurveda education should included "basic elements of primary health care and public health" which may implicitly also mean depression and mental health as important elements of public health. He further suggests the revitalization and protection of certain Ayurvedic fields (again without explicitly mentioning psychiatry) and that "all specialties of Ayurveda must be available to the public in the district level, and selected specialties to the *thaluk* [sub district] level hospitals". Moreover, his draft provides for interdisciplinary research according to international standards, the incorporation of Ayurveda into national and state insurance schemes, and the integration of Ayurveda into the health system of the state on all levels through co-allocation and the establishment of an AYUSH department in Kerala. As a reply to the Health Policy Kerala 2013 draft, AMAI published "Suggestions for Additions in Health Policy" (Ayurveda Medical Association of India 2013) in May 2013. The letter to the state health minister starts by relating positive health indexes in Kerala to the wide availability of Ayurvedic specialities – psychiatry explicitly among them – long before the spread of allopathic medicine in Kerala. The letter continues:

> The national health policy of 1983 clearly envisages incorporating traditional systems to strengthen the health care delivery system in the country. The draft [Health Policy 2013] does not give a comprehensive approach in the utilization of total health infrastructure available in the state as directed by our national Health Policy and central government policy on AYUSH. The policy only deals with the modern medicine and does not give any idea about the role of other recognized medical systems including Ayurveda, which is considered as the indigenous medical system of Kerala.

Like Nampoothiri's draft, Ayurveda Medical Association of India suggests the establishment of an AYUSH department in Kerala, the co-location of AYUSH disciplines in primary and community health centres, and the inclusion of AYUSH practitioners into public health schemes. Moreover, the Association insists on restructuring the Ayurveda education system so as to develop a "specialty cadre" and demands that MD and postgraduate diploma courses in all specialties should be started in all Ayurveda colleges. Apart from one exception, mental health does not explicitly appear in the AMAI's draft or in Nampoothiri's draft, even though mental health is one of the major health concerns formulated in the Kerala Health Policy. The policy papers stress that all Ayurvedic specialties need to be given more emphasis in public health in Kerala.

Concerning public mental health, it was as early as 2000 that the Kerala State Mental Health Authority (KSMHA) proposed the integration of mental health into Ayurvedic training and "to start full fledged psychiatric departments in all Ayurveda Colleges and psychiatric units in all Ayurvedic District Hospitals with minimum five beds".[242] However, the KSMHA has made no efforts to integrate Ayurvedic mental health care into mental health programmes. Likewise, a WHO (2008) report in the chapter "India: Integrated Primary Care for Mental Health in the Thiruvananthapuram District, Kerala State", although otherwise fairly inclusive, excluded Ayurvedic clinicians from contributing to mental health care in the state. On the national level, the first National Mental Health Policy "New Pathways, New Hope", launched by the Government of India in 2014, does indeed mention Ayurveda in two paragraphs: "Practitioners of Ayurveda and Yoga systems are a resource who need to be included as activists for promotion of mental health", it notes, and under the rubric "research" it suggests conducting "research to evaluate the potential of traditional knowledge, practices and alternative therapies to address mental health problems."

In August 2015, the Government of Kerala fulfilled one of the most urgent demands of Ayurveda interest groups in Kerala: to launch a state AYUSH department. In its preamble the Kerala AYUSH Health Policy (Department of AYUSH 2016) formulates the goals as follows.

> As part of its efforts to promote AYUSH by way of improving production, sale, quality of education, acceptability and employment opportunities the Kerala Government has decided to frame a dedicated AYUSH Health Policy for the state. This is the first concrete step being taken by the Kerala Government to strengthen the basis of the traditional treatment systems after the formation of AYUSH department in the state.

Under the point Mental Health, the Policy states: "The existing Govt. Ayurveda Research Institute for Mental Diseases in Kottakkal, the only one of its kind in India, would be upgraded as the Centre of Excellence in the field of Ayurveda Mental Health Care". With this recommendation the policy picks up on the advice of Shailaja Chandra who in a 2011 report suggested, "There is a need to strengthen this hospital [GAMH] and to modernize it. It should become a center for Ayurvedic treatment of mental disorders and should provide information on doctors/treatment and private board and lodging for families of patients" (Chandra 2011). Moreover she writes that, "regional mental health centers for AYUSH would be started. The feasibility of treatment of mental diseases through other systems of AYUSH would be assessed and explored" and "techniques in yoga for emotional control and life style modifications would be propagated across the state."

These examples demonstrate that most mental health policies and projects including the National Mental Health Programme and the different District Mental Health Programmes ignore the Ayurvedic discourse on mental health and depression that I describe in this chapter. While Ayurveda has been integrated into general public health schemes in India (Wujastyk 2008) and in other South Asian countries such as Nepal (Cameron 2008) and Sri Lanka, Ayurveda has, apart from some rare exceptions, not played a significant role in the public mental health care either in Kerala or elsewhere in India (Weiss 2015).

But this is changing. The AAP and individual doctors lobbying for Ayurvedic psychiatry – along with the AYUSH department – not only aspire to the integration of Ayurveda into public and private mental health care of Kerala on the level of policies and schemes, they are also working to make Ayurvedic psychiatry a taken-for-granted part of public knowledge about mental health. As active contributors to health magazines and TV programmes on depression and other mental health issues, doctors are taking their message directly to wide public audiences. *Arogya Masika*, a prominent Malayam health magazine, released a special issue on manasika rogam [mental disease] on 1 June 2009 with contributions from psychiatry, psychology, Ayurveda and other fields. In one article, "Ayurveda for curing mental diseases", Dr Sundaran (the former superintendent of GAMH) describes the Ayurvedic etiology of mental diseases including "unsatisfied desires, unexpected tragedies, guilt or bad food" and the Ayurvedic theory of vulnerable personality types expressed in terms of the level of sattva guna. This is followed by a description of the two kinds of mental diseases, dosha and bhuta unmada. It is noteworthy to quote the paragraph on bhuta unmada at length to demonstrate how Ayurvedic psychiatrists sell bhutavidya to the public. Sundaran writes:

> The treatment of mental disease is known as bhutavidya. This is, however, a misnomer. The term "bhutavidya" has created a lot of confusion. The word bhuta in Malayalam means ghost or evil spirit. This has lead many people into believing that mental diseases are caused by the possession of ghosts or evil spirits. In Ayurveda the word "bhuta" means having physical existence or living organism. The word "panchabhuta" means the five elements [...]. Bhuta is not used to mean ghost or evil spirit in Ayurveda. Guidelines of Ayurveda instruct to name a mental disease based on the way the patient behaves or acts. A patient may imitate a creature (bhuta) by appearance, behavior, movement or language. The disease should be named after that bhuta. If a patient is like a *deva* [god] in appearance or behavior the disease is called *devonmadam* [god madness].[243] If the patient's eyes are red, walks in a zigzag manner, be angry, breath noisily or put tongue out the disease is called *sarponmadam* [snake madness]. As the patient behaves and appears like a snake the unmada is named after snake. If a patient is like *rakshasa* [demon] the disease is called *rakshasonmadam*. As the naming of mental diseases is on the basis of creatures (bhutas) imitated by patients the general term for this treatment is called bhutavidya. Ayurveda does not endorse the view that mental diseases are caused by gods or spirits. Ayurveda says that the view that mental diseases are caused by gods and spirits are silly.

Then follows a list of different Ayurvedic treatments including purifying and pacifying treatments for dosha unmada, fumigation, application of medicines to the eye, and other procedures for bhuta unmada. The article also includes dietary advice, recommends specific medicines and suggests upayangal including "beating the patient, shocking the patient, locking up in a room, giving training to forget, consoling, and so on". Helping the patient to plan future projects, creating awareness and sympathy are also important. Sundaran also includes a list of key points and behavioural advice for preventing mental diseases and possible symptoms of mental diseases.

Some months later in April 2010, *Arogya Masika* published a special issue on vishadam [depression] that again included different perspectives. The Ayurveda contribution was written by Dr K Ravishankar, Head of the Panchakarma Department of the Ayurveda College Hospital, Thripunithura who does not specialize in psychiatry but sees many patients with depression. The teaser text points to passions such as "intense desire to possess something, intensified anger or aversion, fear of depossession or apprehensions about losing something and irresistible longing" as the most important factors for despair. Controlling these passions, Dr Ravishankar continues, means "controlling depression and other diseases that affect the mind". The basic cause of all pains, he states, is the mind or rather the "mind-body-complex". Somatic problems affect the mind and problems of the mind aggravate physical maladies. Like Dr Sundaran, Dr Ravishankar then elaborates on three kinds of dosha unmada (vata unmada, pitta unmada and kapha unmada) and the three kinds of personality types in terms of the gunas sattva, rajas and tamas. Then he comes to passions as an important triggering factor.

> A mind which has a craving to be loved will be pained when love is denied. The phenomenon of despair arisen out of the non-accomplishment of a desire can turn into turbulent anger. When deprived of desired objects or the aspired is not achieved, a person will often fall into a depression state. If this condition continues and a person becomes possessed by it, she is said to be conquered by a mental disease called depression.

Although, he goes on, "there is not much mention in the books of Ayurveda about a disease referred to as depressive disorder", common symptoms such as lethargy, fatigue, morbid thoughts and so on are mentioned and treatments discussed in detail. For treatments, first and foremost he describes yoga and pranayama as "natural remedies" for depression, treatments that are not practised at GAMH but which are offered to inpatients at the Ayurveda College hospital, Kottakkal and in some private clinics of Ayurvedic psychiatrists. He then lists dosha purifying treatments that "affect primarily the body to provide relief from the mental problems". In the last paragraph, titled "*Rasayana chikitsa*" [rejuvenation treatment] Ravishankar describes this as "useful in many types of mental diseases including depression". He concludes by stressing the importance of medhya rasayana, which he translates into "neuron tonics" in the treatment of depression.

While *Arogya Masika* and other Malayalam health magazines address a middle class Malayalam readership, the Kochi-based English magazine *Ayurveda & Health Tourism* mainly targets foreigners and members of India's upper-middle and upper classes interested in Ayurveda. The March 2011 issue featured a special section called "Open Your Mind: Ayurvedic treatment for mental diseases". The issue contains (heavily edited) contributions from Ayurvedic general physicians and Ayurvedic psychiatrists. Two articles deal with the notion and etiology of mental diseases in Ayurveda and a description of the usual treatments, medicines and diet regimes that mostly aim at purifying the body and cooling the head. The other two contributions by Dr M.P. Parvathi and Dr Tom P. Paul who specialize in Ayurvedic psychiatry are case studies. Although these last two articles describe the medical management of severe depression [kaphonmada] in one case, and reactive depression [adhijonmada] in the other, they both underscore the importance of the doctor-patient relationship. "With my experience as a doctor", writes Dr Parvathi, "I will say that a touch or a word with compassion helps more than any medicine."

As contributors to health magazines and TV programmes on depression and other mental health issues, Ayurvedic psychiatrists are lobbying to make Ayurvedic psychiatry a taken-for-granted part of public knowledge about mental health. Doctors describe Ayurvedic etiologies and vulnerabilities to mental health problems in terms of gunas, doshas, passions and diet and delineate the purifying and pacifying treatments to wide public audiences. Many contributions make clear the distinction in dosha and bhuta unmada and distance from the interpretation of the latter as related to possession or spirits. In "From Expert to Popular Knowledge" (Chapter 3) I traced how mainstream allopathic mental health professionals represent and disseminate depression in the media and stabilize psychiatrists and psychologists as authoritative experts, expand depression diagnosis to encompass ever-wider dimensions of everyday life and ever-wider segments of society. While mainstream psychiatry and psychology have become part of popular knowledge, Ayurvedic psychiatry has not (yet) entered popular psy discourse. In organizing press conferences and contributing to media reporting about the Ayurvedic contribution to depression and other mental health problems, Ayurvedic psychiatrists stabilize mainstream psychiatric disease categories, but first and foremost aim to secure their discipline's place as alternative and complement to mainstream psychiatric treatment. More than mainstream psychiatry, Ayurvedic psychiatrists are confronted not only with public reservations against psychiatry as not scientific, but doubly so since Ayurveda is also often presumed as not scientific. The politics of recognition of Ayurvedic psychiatrists then aims to establish this (re)invented discipline as an alternative scientific *and* genuine Indian actor in mental health care of Kerala.

The general argument of *Depression in Kerala* is that the transformation of depression from a rare severe disorder into a widely diagnosed and treated, common mental disorder is closely related to the intertwined processes of drug development and marketing, institutional shifts, and ideological and ontological transformations of emotional suffering. Public education and awareness campaigns as technologies of psychiatric governmentality (Orr 2010) disseminate the psychiatrization, individualization and pharmaceuticalization of emotional suffering and despair and degrade local socio-centric and cosmological etiologies and moral worlds as superstitious and incompatible with modernity. Emotional suffering, once dealt with primarily by family elders, religious experts and *vaidyas* [traditional Ayurveda practitioners], is now increasingly handled by biomedical experts, thereby transforming an existential, moral, religious or humoral problem into a biomedical condition that can and should be treated with pharmaceuticals. As a result, popular psychological idioms such as depression or tension have either marginalized local concepts of possession or occult violence (Halliburton 2005) or become linked with them in a hybrid or syncretic manner. The global circulating psychiatric disorder depression is described as resulting from the impacts of modern lifestyles, often in conjunction with stress. Whether diagnosed by allopathic physicians or psychiatrists, by Ayurvedic doctors or religious healers, or in magazine self-tests and online questionnaires, patients demand a quick cure. In this chapter I followed depression into the context of an indigenous medical system. I described the translation and reframing of depression in Ayurveda in conjunction with the (re)invention of institutionalized Ayurvedic psychiatry as an emergent field of specialization.

I have described the Ayurvedic physio-moral notion of depression that is deeply intertwined with the Ayurvedic concept of mental health humoral balance, involving mental strength, self-control, equanimity and clarity which is, I argued, closely related to South Asian notions of the self that can be described, following Marriott's (1976) anthropological research, as bio-moral or physio-moral selves. It is fluent bodies in addition to embodied substantial minds and morals that make up depressive patients in Kerala, which makes it more compatible with notions of neurochemical imbalance than with the biodynamic model. I have then analysed the reconfiguration of *bhutavidya* into Ayurvedic psychiatry, and the engagement between Ayurvedic and allopathic psychiatric nosologies and mental health policies in terms of translation and autonomy. These processes of engagement serve to enrol Ayurveda into the network of global and local mental health care while at the same time maintaining its basic incompatibility. At the same time, Ayurvedic psychiatrists are engaged in the double process of demarcating their field from the vernacular sector while also engaging in translation processes to make their practice legible to patients and wider discourses of mental health. By the rhetorical manoeuvre of translating their field into psychiatry, Ayurvedic psychiatrists lay claim to the modern science of psychiatry as one of the classic fields of Ayurveda. By a second rhetorical manoeuvre, they include the treatment of dosha unmada and apasmara along with graha unmada under this (re)invented Ayurvedic field of bhutavidya or psychiatry. I described parallel processes of translations and purifications, and while the "work of purification" (Latour 1991) is an effort to maintain separation and distinction between mainstream psychiatry, Ayurvedic psychiatry and occult violence, the "work of translation" (Latour 1991) creates hybrids of allopathic and Ayurvedic psychiatry on the one hand and of Ayurvedic psychiatry and spirits and sorcery on the other.

In accordance with a physio-moral notion of depression, Ayurvedic psychiatrists treat the mind through the body by use of purifying, cooling and pacifying procedures and medicines. Apart from various treatment procedures, patients get a host of classical and patent and proprietary Ayurvedic medicines. It is noteworthy that these latter branded "Ayurvedic antidepressants" fit well with the allopathically informed preferences of India's modern urban middle class, and also the international market for alternative and complementary medicines. Ayurvedic branded medicines for depression promise natural, holistic, gentle and genuine Indian healing and wellness and the enhancement of mental capacities thanks to the help of traditional Indian wisdom. The commodification and pharmaceuticalization of Ayurveda in this form assures the patient of the ability to maintain a modern lifestyle with the support of ancient authentic Ayurvedic knowledge of holistic wellness, free of side effects. It is mainly (though not exclusively) through patent and proprietary drugs that Ayurvedic pharmaceutical companies enter the market of mental health care. Through a focus on problems related to a lack of mental well-being, stress and tension rather than mental disease they cover a wide range of minor problems, everyday distress and stress, especially in relation to what are perceived to be the exigencies of modern life.

The reconfiguration of sattvavajaya as Ayurvedic psychotherapy as one part of (re)invented Ayurvedic psychiatry next to yuktivyapasraya chikitsa (rational treatment) aims to correspond to the bifurcation of treatment in pharmacological therapy and psychotherapy in mainstream psychiatry. Through complex processes of translation in the Latourian sense, sattvavajaya is established as a field of specialization to correspond and anticipate psychotherapy. Rather than Western psychotherapy with its aims of emancipation and autonomy of the self,[244] however, sattvavajaya aims to bring the mind into accordance with the social and cosmological order and to streamline it according to moral norms and ideas of the good life. Psychologization and bracketing ontologies, while simultaneously discarding or distancing from what they perceive as superstitious assumptions, characterize how most Ayurvedic psychiatrists negotiate daivavyapasraya chikitsa today.

The reconfiguration of bhutavidya into Ayurvedic psychiatry, the translation of depression into Ayurvedic categories in training, research and treatment, and the development and marketing of specific Ayurveda products that address depression not only contribute to legitimize and stabilize this (re)invented branch of Ayurveda as an actor in public and private mental health care of Kerala but also as an emergent actor in the glocal network of depression. In their effort to mainstream Ayurvedic psychiatry in training, treatment and in state mental health policies, Ayurvedic psychiatrists maintain they are providing a "traditional" treatment – holistic, scientific, reliable and free of side effects – for depression and thus helping to close the postulated treatment gap. The reconfiguration of sattvavajaya as Ayurvedic psychotherapy and the marginalization of daivyavyapasraya treatment are important elements of teaching and clinical practice of institutional Ayurvedic psychiatry. But how is Ayurvedic psychiatry practised outside institutionalized Ayurvedic psychiatry? How is daivavyapasraya treatment dealt with in private clinical practice? The next chapter provides an analysis from the margin of institutionalized Ayurvedic psychiatric health professionalism of the practice of an Ayurvedic psychiatrist with his own idiosyncratic approach.

Notes

1 I would like to thank David Mosse for his comments on an earlier iteration of this idea.
2 *Mathrubhumi*, 12 February 2014. This report was one of five articles in the series "Kerala Seeks Mental Peace".
3 cf. "We are damn sure about it": research and evidence in Ayurvedic psychiatry" (this chapter, subchapter 3).
4 Dr Kumar, Kottakkal, 25 January 2013.
5 Dr Chandra, Kottakkal, 1 March 2013.
6 "General medicine" or "internal medicine" is only a rough translation of *kaya chikitsa*, although practitioners, students and teachers of Ayurveda commonly translate it in this way.
7 The other two postgraduate courses at the Ayurveda College, Kottakkal are in the more prestigious fields of *agada tantra* [toxicology] and *panchakarma* [literally the five treatments, consisting classically of the purifying procedures vomiting, enema, purgation, nasal purification, and blood letting and certain associated procedures]. Beyond the Ayurveda College in Kottakkal, two other colleges offer a psychiatric postgraduate qualification: SDM College of Ayurveda & Hospital, Hassan, Karnataka, and the Faculty of Ayurveda Institute Of Medical Science Banaras Hindu University Varanasi, Uttar Pradesh.
8 This is the degree title for the qualification "Doctor of Ayurveda".
9 The *Regulations, Curriculum and Syllabus of Postgraduate Course (MD/MS) in Ayurveda*, edited by the Kerala University of Health Sciences, prescribes: "Only a department defined as an independent academic entity of a teaching institution having the minimum facilities as per norms of the CCIM shall be permitted to commence a post graduate training programme to qualify for the award of the MD/MS Degree" (Kerala University of Health Sciences 2012).
10 Students at the Ayurveda College, Kottakkal, 16 March 2011. The council argued, they told me, that in the Ayurveda classical texts, the treatment of mental disorders comes under *kaya chikitsa* [general medicine] and therefore there is no need for a separate *manasika* department. According to senior staff at the college, the problem is more a question of profitability. Psychiatry is simply not an attractive subject for most students. However the Arya Vaidya Sala, to which the college belongs, supports the development of a department of psychiatry, according to P.K. Varier, the managing trustee and chief physician of the Arya Vaidya Sala.
11 Dr Kapur, Kottakkal, 7 February 2014.
12 Pritha, Kottakkal, 10 February 2014.
13 This is not to imply that "depression" existed as a concept in Ayurveda, which is not the case. Rather, depression occurs in response to the "glocal" priority of the term and the pressure on Ayurveda to acknowledge it.
14 cf. "The politics and pragmatics of nosologies and their translations" (this chapter, subchapter 3).
15 I refrain from giving translations here. Translations are multi-layered and messy and each of these will be treated separately and at greater length below. Readers may also refer the glossary.
16 Dr Rasheed, Kottakkal, 7 March 2010.
17 Alter (1999) criticizes what he calls the "remedial bias" in medical anthropology. Halliburton criticizes the "limitation of the ideology of curing" as "the return-to-balance metaphor may involve importing biomedical assumptions about curing as ridding of symptoms and restoring functionality" (Halliburton 2009: 47). But it

was the restoration of functionality that was emphasized to me as the main goal of treatment by the Ayurvedic practitioners I spoke with in institutional Ayurvedic psychiatry and at Poonkudil Mana who combined Ayurveda and religious treatment. When I mentioned Alter's argument that the aim of Ayurveda was to make the patient "better than well", most Ayurvedic psychiatrists said that they would be content enough to see a patient return to normal functioning. The same was true of practitioners at Poonkudil Mana. Only Dr Joseph John (cf. Chapter 5) regarded a spiritual transformation as the aim of the treatment.

18 The seven dhatus are *rasa* [lymph or plasma], *rakta* [blood or hemoglobin], *mamsa* [muscles], *medas* [fat], *asthti* [bone or cartilage], *majja* [marrow], and *shukra* [semen and reproductive tissues]. The vital essence of this transformative process is *ojas* [vital essence].

19 Dr Nayar, Kottakkal, 23 July 2009.

20 cf. "The reconfiguration of bhutavidya into Ayurvedic psychiatry" (this chapter, subchapter 2).

21 Dr Mangalam, Kottakkal, 11 March 2011.

22 Dr Rasheed, Kottakkal, 19 February 2010.

23 Dr Hari Namboodiri, Aluva, 4 February 2013.

24 Dr Manikandan, Kottakkal, 6 August 2009.

25 Although vishadam also denotes a mental state similar to melancholia, this translation was rarely used by my Ayurvedic psychiatric interlocutors.

26 Dr Krishnan, Kottakkal, 2 March 2010.

27 Dr Krishnan, one of the teachers at the college, told me, "We [Ayurveda people] correlate the stage of a disease, not the disease entity." As far as mild depression [vishada] and severe depression [kaphonmada] are concerned, mild depression is an earlier stage of the *samprapti* [the course of the disease], followed by moderate and then severe depression" (Dr Krishnan, Kottakkal, 15 August 2009).

28 Dr Krishnan, Kottakkal, 2 March 2010.

29 cf. "Manovahashrotas" (this chapter, subchapter 4).

30 Dr Nayar, Kottakkal, 27 July 2009.

31 This is an example where Ayurvedic knowledge is seen to both anticipate "modern" discoveries and to be confirmed by modern neuroscientific research.

32 If the mental illness does not follow the path of any of the doshas, graha unmada [madness of graha kind] is – theoretically – suspected.

33 Anwar (2004) identifies the symptoms of kaphonmada as they are described in Caraka Samhita: tastelessness, loss of interest, vomiting, reduced activities, little desire for food, reduced talk, increased libido, desire for solitude, increased salivation and discharges from mouth and nose, disgusting appearance, aversion to cleanliness, increased sleep, swelling of the face, aggravation in the night and after taking food, remaining on one place, white and timid eyes, paleness of nails and skin, indigestion, cough, decrease in intellectual capacities, fondness for warm things, increased fatigue (Anwar 2004).

34 Dr Sarasvati, Kottakkala, 12 March 2010.

35 Dr Shaila, Kottakkal, 1 March 2013.

36 Dr Kumar, Kottakkal, 11 March 2011.

37 Dr Rasheed, Kottakkal, 7 March 2010.

38 Dr Rasheed, Kottakkal, 7 March 2010.

39 Dr Krishnan, Kottakkal, 15 August 2009.

40 I also encountered a few Ayurvedic practitioners (both general and specialized in psychiatry) who differentiated between vata, pitta and kapha kinds of depression. Dr Joshua, trained in Ayurvedic psychiatry but working in his own clinic, elaborated: "Those who are daily not able to sleep, they will get the vata type of depression. Those who are taking greater amounts of meat or alcohol or spicy food, they will get the pitta type of depression. Those who take more sleep and kapha food

items, they will get the kapha type of depression. If a person has been psychologically weak from the childhood onwards, then according to their lifestyle and diet she will get the kapha, vata, pitta type of depression." (Dr Joshua, Thrissur, 1 February 2013).

41 cf. Chapter 5.

42 This might be a vernacularization of Sanskrit terms since *adhi* in Malayalam means stress, tension, severe worries or emotional breakdown.

43 Keraleeya Ayurveda Samajam Hospital in Shoranur.

44 Dr Ganapati, Trippunithura, 21 September 2010.

45 Mark Nichter, "Hybrid Medicine for Hybrid People", lecture delivered in Heidelberg, Germany (12 June 2009).

46 Dr Praveen, Thrissur, 5 August 2009.

47 Dr Sundaran, Kottakkal, 23 July 2009.

48 Dr Devan, Kottakkal, 13 February 2014.

49 Dr Krishnan, Kottakkal 15 August 2009.

50 Pranayama are breathing exercises that are part of Asthanga Yoga. Dr Praveen described the effect of pranayama from an Ayurvedic point of view: Pranayama promotes *prana* [breath, life force] that is equivalent to *vayu* [wind], the element that is the basis of vata, which is responsible for transporting the thoughts. Pranayama is thus for "streamlining vayu in the body".

51 Dr Hari Namboodiri, Aluva, 4 February 2013.

52 Dr Nayar Kottakkal, 15 August 2009.

53 Dr Ganapati, Trippunithura, 21 September 2010.

54 Dr Nayar, Kottakkal, 15 August 2009.

55 Dr Nayar, Kottakkal, 15 August 2009.

56 Osella and Osella (2008) describe the gunas of Samkyha philosophy as they are understood by upper caste Hindus in Kerala in relation to the classification and hierarchy of food: "sattvik is associated with ideas of whiteness, brightness, purity, coolness, and so on; rajasik is associated with heat, vitality, energy, and the colour red; tamasik is associated with the colour black and with darkness, sluggishness, stupidity and impurity" (p. 177). These food classifications also play an important role in Ayurvedic diet recommendations (*pathya*). In Ayurvedic psychiatry, sattvik food is recommended while rajasik and tamasik food should be avoided.

57 Dr Sundaran, Kottakkal, 27 July 2009.

58 Dr Praveen, Thrissur, 5 August 2009.

59 Dr Rasheed, Kottakkal, 7 March 2010.

60 Dr Nayar, Kottakkal, 25 July 2009.

61 This last detour into psychoanalysis gives an indication of how the psychoanalytic notion of subconsciousness is locally appropriated. In the context of Ayurvedic psychiatry, I occasionally heard the subconscious or subconscious mind constructed not as something deep and essential but as an impediment to mental health, an obstacle to be overcome. Religious healers and self-titled counsellors made similar statements.

62 Dr Devdas, Kottakkal, 10 August 2009.

63 Dr Shankaran, Trippunithura, 21 September 2010.

64 Dr Rasheed, Kottakkal, 22 July 2009.

65 Dr Kutty, Guruvayur, 9 March 2010.

66 Dr John, Kottayam, 20 March 2011.

67 Dr Mary, Thrissur, 4 March 2014.

68 Dr Deepak, Kottakkal, 8 March 2010.

69 Vegetarianism is one of the major strategies for social mobility in India and in Global Hinduism (cf. Osella and Osella 2008).

70 Dr Sundaran, Thiruvananthapuram, 9 October 2012.

71 Dr Chandra, Kottakkal, 1 March 2013.

72 *Vikara* (literally disturbance, abnormality, pathology or transformation) is the opposite of *prakrti* (in this case normal, healthy state or physiological condition). Vikara is generally translated as "disease" and used synonymous with *rogam* [disease]. In several Ayurvedic textbooks and websites, *manovikara* is translated as "mental illness".

73 As discussed in this chapter, Ayurvedic theory and practice does not differentiate between mind and emotion or the cognitive and the emotional realm – manas denotes both mind and emotion. Similarly, South Indian dramaturgic, aesthetic, and poetic traditions do not differentiate reason and emotion (Lynch 1990). Clinical psychologists practicing cognitive behavioural therapy in Kerala often complained that their patients often had enormous difficulties clearly discerning their thoughts and their emotions, which is an important prerequisite of the treatment.

74 Frustration or passion as the cause of mental illness is a trope that also pervades popular psychological discourses of depression. A disappointing marriage or conjugal life, a failed love affair, poor educational results, or unfulfilled desires for high-status consumer goods such as mobile phones, motorbikes, or cars are often noted as causes for depression and suicide. In these situations, the satisfaction or replacement of these desires would have the power to prevent suicide, and head off or cure depression. Unsatisfied passions or frustrated desire are also related to local discourses of occult violence that arise in a social climate of envy, jealousy and competition. Moreover, individuals who die with unsatisfied desires and attachments might become spirits and have to be released from their attachments to the world of the living to become ancestor spirits instead of restless spirits.

75 Dr Nayar, Kottakkal, 13 August 2009.

76 cf. "Purifying the body, controlling the mind, and excising the spirits" (this chapter, subchapter 3).

77 Dr John, Kottayam, 19 September 2010.

78 This is also how depression was framed on the television programme, *Eternal Health*: "Most people when they suffer from these heavy depressive states, they are in the state of ignorance". "The essence of Ayurveda, jiva, Ayurveda and depression", 17 March 2008, *Eternal Health* (television series), www.youtube.com/watch?v=ITX0R_akcCw [accessed on 23 June 2016]. Episodes of *Eternal Health* target an Indian audience and can also be watched on Sadhna TV, Shraddha Channel and Care World Channel.

79 In the Asthangahrdaya, prajnaparadha is described both in the context of dosha-related illnesses and bhutavidya. In the bhutavidya chapter that describes possession, prajnaparadha is listed as one of the main causes.

80 Dr Devdas, Kottakkal, 12 August 2009.

81 It resembles a similar conceptual shift in the causation of *dhat* [semen loss] from masturbation and excessive sexual activity to the guilt resulting from it.

82 I do not agree with Alter (1999) on his critique of a remedial bias in Ayurveda especially with regard to his sources and also his argument that "better than well" is the aim of Ayurvedic treatment. However, his concept of the "physiology of self-improvement" is helpful for understanding depression and its treatment as a moral-physiological process. Alter speaks of the treatment as a "form of metabolic, humoral body-building" (Alter (1999, 45). This "body-building" includes body, mind and self.

83 Removing inappropriate passions from the mind is a concept of purification that closely resembles the notion of removing contents from the subconscious mind or purifying the mind from the subconsciousness.

84 AYUSH is an acronym for Ayurveda, Yoga and Naturopathy, Unani, Siddha, Homeopathy, and, since 2012, Sowa Rigpa (Tibetan Medicine). These are the medical systems promoted by the Ministry of AYUSH that replaced the former Department of AYUSH of the Ministry of Health and Family Welfare that again

replaced the former Department of Indian Medical Systems and Homeopathy created in 1995.

85 Chopra (n.d.) differentiates three outcomes of the translation process: (1) A classical Ayurvedic disease entity continues to exist in its own right unaffected by allopathic notions; (2) an allopathic disease entity is translated with an Ayurvedic term whose meaning is narrowed down compared to the traditional usage, and (3) a new Sanskrit term is coined for a disease which is purely based on biomedical physiology. The first and latter cases are rare, Chopra argues, but the second is the most common one in contemporary Ayurveda.

86 "Unmada" is the Sanskrit spelling while "unmadam" is the Malayalam version. Both forms are used in teaching and diagnosis. The Old English term "unmod" to denote an illness that arises from the stomach is etymologically related to the Sanskrit unmada (Jadhav 2000).

87 Weiss (1977) and Meulenbeld (1987) offer different answers to the question of whether or not there is historical development from the early to the later authoritative texts away from spirits and towards a more rational (i.e., physiological) understanding of unmada (Meulenbeld 1997) or, using the narrative of the decline, vice versa towards a greater elaboration of the number of bhutas described under the heading of bhutavidya and to place less emphasis on endogenous (nija) forms of mental illness (Weiss 1977; cf. Trawick 1987; Langford 2002).

88 Dr Sundaran, Kottakkal, 23 July 2009.

89 Dr Sundaran, Kottakkal, 23 July 2009.

90 Dr Devdas and his students, Kottakkal, 25 August 2009.

91 Dr Sarasvati, Kottakkal, 10 February 2014.

92 Dhupana is used for doshic disorders but is also described in the texts and practised in the context of Hindu religious healing as treatment for possession.

93 Ayurvedic psychiatrists used the terms "bhuta" and "graha" as well as "bhuta unmada" and "graha unmada" interchangeably.

94 Dr Joshua, Kottakkal, 2 March 2014.

95 Dr Sarasvati, Kottakkal, 10 February 2014.

96 It is difficult to know the authentic, original meaning of bhuta and graha. It can be speculated that there have always been multiple readings of these terms at the times of origin of the classical texts and over the centuries. An understanding of bhuta as "living being", a metaphorical understanding of grahas and an understanding of bhutas and grahas as referring to inner rather than to external processes might have existed along with a reading of these terms as spirits. As Smith (2006) and Langford (2002) have argued, however, the texts that form the textual corpus of institutional Ayurvedic clinical practice do refer to spirits and deities in their bhutavidya or graha chikitsa sections. For example, the Caraka Samhita (6.9.16) writes, "Externally induced [āgantu] [madness, unmada] has as its [direct] cause attacks by gods, seers, celestial musicians, flesh-eating demons, semidivine protector demons, dangerous demons, and deceased ancestors; [indirectly] it is the result of incorrectly performed internal and external vows, etc., and actions from a previous existence" (translated in Smith 2006, 488). Moreover, the notions used in the texts that Smith translates as "inhabited", "overwhelmed", "tormented" or "possessed" (Smith 2006, 488–497) suggest spirit possession.

97 Dr Rasheed, Kottakkal, 7 March 2010.

98 http://ccimindia.org/draft_syllabus_pg_mana.html, accessed 17 May 2016.

99 A more full discussion of the terms suddha and mishra Ayurveda is taken up in the conclusion of this subchapter.

100 Ayurvedic practitioners often used the term "modern" to denote biomedicine.

101 Draft syllabus PG course *Manovigyan avum Manas Roga* [Knowledge of the mind and of mental diseases or, for that matter, Psychology and Psychiatry], (www.ccimindia.org/syllabus/first_year_syllabus.html#ab13) accessed on 14 April 2016. For

more on Ayurvedic modes of treatment, cf. "Purifying the body, controlling the mind and excising the spirits" (this chapter, subchapter 3).

102 In the section "Depression of two kinds" (this chapter, subchapter 3) I showed the complex pathogenesis for kaphonmada, vishadam, and adhijonmada which are often translated into depression.

103 Dr Krishnan, Kottakkal, 15 August 2009.

104 Dr Nayar, Kottakkal, 15 August 2009.

105 Dr Varghese, Kottayam, 17 February 2010.

106 Dr Nayar, Kottakkal, 15 August 2009.

107 Pitta is made up of the elements fire and water. In clinical practice, pitta is often related to fire, activity, change and metabolism.

108 Kapha is made up of earth and water.

109 Patients and families do not have much knowledge of these Ayuvredic diagnostics. But they do share an understanding of the treatment practices as cooling and purifying body and the mind.

110 Dr John, Kottayam, 13 September 2012.

111 Dr Rasheed, Ernakulam, 25 January 2013.

112 This quote shows one of the problems of psychiatric epidemiology. The "cultural epidemiology" developed by Weiss (2001) challenges epidemiology including psychiatric epidemiology which is based on professional concepts as inadequate to the cultural patterns of distress, perceived causes and help seeking of patients and focuses instead on local representations of illness.

113 Dr Sarasvati, Kottakkal, 10 February 2014.

114 Dr Mangalam, Kottakkal, 11 March 2011.

115 Dr Lakshmi Nair, Ernakulam, 29 January 2012.

116 There still exists among allopathic doctors a rhetoric about the absence of scientific studies in Ayurveda. In fact, there are studies of the effectiveness of Ayurvedic treatments using controlled clinical trials well outside of the world of student theses and some of these have appeared in mainstream medical journals. A search of the Medline database produces several such studies including publications in mainstream biomedical journals of successful clinical trials of Ayurvedic treatments for cirrhosis, arthritis and other problems. Moreover, there are American psychiatrist Nathan Kline's classic studies of Rauwolfia serpentina for psychopathology in the 1950s (Kline, 1954) which are well known in Ayurvedic circles in India.

117 Dr Shaila, Kottakkal, 1 March 2013.

118 Dr Krishnan, Kottakkal, 15 August 2009.

119 For a detailed description of the five phases in clinical trials, see Friedman et al. (1998).

120 The NIMHANS has had an Ayurvedic clinical and research unit. Since 2002 it also has a yoga treatment centre, which has been promoted and managed by the current director B.N. Gangadhar.

121 The ingredients are *sankhapushipi* (Clitoria ternatea), *sarpagandha* (Rauwolfia serpentine) and *gokshura* (Tribulis terrestris).

122 In Ayurveda, medicinal substances are characterized by five properties: *rasa* [taste], *guna* [properties], *vieerya* [potency], *vipak* [post-metabolic effect] and *prabhava* [specific effect].

123 In order to evaluate patients according to assumed authentic Ayurvedic criteria of mental health for research as well as for diagnostic ends, students of Ayurvedic psychiatry in Kottakkal use two Ayurvedic rating scales: The Rajas Rating Scale and the Tamas Rating Scale. Both were developed by former students of the college and are based on the descriptions of the three gunas [basic qualities] collected from Caraka Samhita, Sushruta Samhita, and Asthagahrdaya.

124 See the discussion on prajnaparadha in the subchapter "Depression as a problem of perception".

125 Abraham writes: "When the *manasika bhavas* [mental states] become excessive or inappropriate that is termed as *vikaras*" (Abraham 2009: 41). According to Anwar (2004), the term *vikara* means abnormal conditions in opposition to *prakrti* [natural or healthy state]. Excessive emotions or passions are caused by rajas and tamas.
126 cf. "Gunas, sattvabalam and mental health" (this chapter).
127 "Scientific" is understood here as exact (i.e., quantitative) exegesis of the classical texts.
128 Anwar concludes an elaborate discussion of different forms of endogenous and exogenous unmada in the classic texts with a short note that indicates the openness of graha unmada for social change resulting in new forms of graha unmada such as computer graha or internet graha (for those who are highly obsessed with computer or internet) and IAS unmada for officers of the Indian Administrative Service (in India, this is highly prestigious position).
129 For preta graha, 47 per cent; for pitre graha, 69 per cent (Anwar 2004: 95–97).
130 Dr Kumar, Kottakkal, 18 February 2014.
131 On Ayurveda in general, cf. Langford (2002).
132 Ayurveda College Kottakkal, 24 February 2010.
133 Dr Kumar, Kottakkal, 20 February 2014.
134 Some vaidyas and a few BAMS trained Ayurveda practitioners took the horoscope into consideration and asked for the *nakshatra* [birth star] and other planetary constellations, none of these questionnaires enquire about the horoscope.
135 Dr Kumar, Kottakkal, 11 March 2011.
136 Jayanthi, Kottakkal, 4 February 2014.
137 Dr Rasheed, Kottakkal, 7 March 2010.
138 Dr Vidya, Kottakkal, 7 February 2014.
139 This was exceptional, and I was not able to verify that a graha diagnosis had been recorded in this case. In all the GAMH case records I consulted I never saw a graha diagnosis.
140 For an ethnography of pisachu see Shukla (1980); for textual sources see Smith (2006).
141 Dr Sundaran, Kottakkal, 31 July 2009.
142 Dr Rasheed, Kottakkal, 22 July 2009.
143 Jayanthi, Kottakkal, 4 February 2014.
144 This corresponds to the stance most allopathic psychiatrists took with regard to religious healing. When patients employed other (and multiple) types of treatments, Ayurvedic and allopathic psychiatrists were both tolerant so long as these did not interfere with the treatment they were pursing.
145 Dr Sarasvati, Kottakkal, 1 March 2013.
146 Dr Shankaran, Trippunithura, 21 March 2010.
147 Dr Sarasvati, Kottakkal, 10 February 2014.
148 Dr Vidya, Kottakkal, 7 February 2014.
149 Dr Sarasvati, Kottakkal, 12 March 2010.
150 Babu Panikkar, Kuttipala, 2 October 2010.
151 Dr Paul Thomas, Kottakkal, 8 March 2011.
152 Dr Sarasvati, Kottakkal, 12 February 2014.
153 Dr Rasheed, Kottakkal, 24 February 2010.
154 Dr Sarasvati, Kottakkal, 6 February 2014.
155 Dr Ganapati, Ernakulam, 21 September 2010.
156 Dr Paul Thomas, Kottakkal, 8 March 2011.
157 Xavier Francis, Kottayam, 18 March 2011.
158 Dr Joshua, Kottayam, 14 February 2013.
159 Though pathyam includes both diet and daily activities, it is often used synonymously with diet.
160 The physiology of digestion plays a vital role in Ayurveda (Zimmermann 1987; Alter 1999; Ecks 2004).

161 In general Ayurvedic practice, virechanam is the treatment of choice for an imbalance of pitta, vamanam for kapha and vasti for vata. However, this rule is often modified in Ayurvedic psychiatry due to pragmatic and medical considerations.

162 *Rasayana* or rejuvenation aiming at nourishing the tissues [*dhatus*] is one of the eight branches of Ayurveda. Indian gooseberry is one of the main ingredients Ayurveda's best selling rasayana medicine *cyavanaprash* (Bode 2015).

163 Dr Sundaran, Kottakkal, 12 August 2009.

164 Neena, Kottakkal, 14 February 2014.

165 Dr Kumar, Kottakkal, 18 February 2014.

166 Dr Vidya, Kottakkal, 7 February 2014.

167 The duration depends upon the reaction of the patient.

168 Dr Sarasvati, Kottakkal, 12 February 2014.

169 Panchagavya are the five [*pancha*] products of the cow [*gavya*]: milk, sour yogurt, ghee, urine, and liquid squeezed from the dung. Smith speculates: "Animal products were deemed more antithetical to the possessing spirits, thus indirectly influencing, and even rectifying, humoral imbalances" (Smith 2006: 540).

170 These two yogams [compounds] are discussed in the Caraka Samhita, one of the canonical texts, in the context of *apasmara* [convulsion, epilepsy], demonic incursion, and other kinds of unmade.

171 Asthangahrdayam 3.5.1–53.

172 Asthangahrdayam 3.5.13a.

173 Krishnakumar, Kattumadam Mana, 15 March 2010.

174 Insulin shock (or insulin coma therapy) was introduced into psychiatry in the 1930s in Germany and became a standard procedure in the treatment of schizophrenia in the middle of the twentieth century. Critiques of this therapy as potentially brain damaging resemble later critiques of electro-convulsive therapy. According to psychiatrist Moncrieff (2008), insulin coma therapy was the first treatment that was claimed as specific treatment for schizophrenia. In contrast to insulin shock therapy, snehapana produces neither hypoglycemia nor coma.

175 Dr Joshua, Thrissur, 1 February 2013.

176 Dr Mary, Thrissur, 4 March 2014.

177 Dr Narayanan, Thrissur, 3 September 2009.

178 Dr Sarasvati, Kottakkal, 6 September 2010.

179 cf. "Translations undercover" (this chapter, subchapter 4).

180 In cases of kaphonmada, the oil used is *Dhanvandharam thailam*, a *yogam* [compound] of twenty-eight ingredients including cow's milk, *ashvagandha* (Withania somnifera), *amla* (Indian gooseberry), and others usually used for vata-related diseases and applied both internally and externally.

181 If patients were able to consume enough ghee during snehapanam, thailavasti was given with ghee instead of oil. Also disorientated or chronic patients usually receive thailavasti with ghee.

182 Dr Shaila, Kottakkal, 1 March 2013.

183 For their head purifying effects, some Ayurvedic psychiatrists also call these measures *shiroshodanam* [head purification].

184 Dr Sundaran, Kottakkal, 14 August 2009.

185 Dr Sarasvati, Kottakkal, 18 February 2014.

186 Dr Sundaran, Kottakkal, 14 August 2009.

187 Some religious practitioners also give extremely irritating medicines for the nose or the eyes to clients affected by spirit possession, occult violence, or behavioural disorders (Lang 2014).

188 Vital spots [*marma*] play an important role in Ayurveda and Siddha medicine (Sieler 2015).

189 Apart from dhupanam, inpatients are also given dhumapanam – a treatment that involves smoking medicine in cloth rolled like a cigar. Here, a paste made of the

ground ingredients mixed with cow's urine is applied to a light cloth [*jaganadhan tunni*], dried in the sun, rolled, tied, dipped into grtham and burnt. As in dhupanam, the very strong smoke stimulates the nerves and sense organs in the brain and aids recovery from depression, one student explained.

190 For a more detailed description of dhupanam and its ontological ambiguities cf. "Translations undercover" (this chapter, subchapter 4).

191 The Sanskrit term "medhya" denotes mental strength, intelligence and purity, terms that are often seen as equivalents in Ayurveda.

192 The oils [thailam] that used include, for example, *chandanadi thailam, shangupushpa thailam, ksheerabalam thailam* – all of which are classic yogam preparations with dozens of ingredients.

193 Dr Joshua, Thrissur, 1 February 2013.

194 Dr Sundaran, Kottakkal, 23 July 2009.

195 Dr Vidya, Kottakkal, 7 February 2014.

196 Dr Sarasvati, Kottakkal, 6 February 2014.

197 For the problematic epistemological and ontological translations involved in Ayurvedic drugs and yogams addressing a biomedical disease entity, see Naraindas (2014b).

198 Pradeep and his father Manikandan, Kottakkal, 4 September 2010.

199 A lakh denotes 100 000. 12 Lakhs (1.2 million Rupees) is worth about $18,000 USD

200 Madhavan and Punam, Kottakkal, 10 February 2014.

201 A para is a unit of measurement. One para is approximately 10 kg.

202 The difference is that Western polyherbals can draw from a worldwide pharmacopoeia whereas Ayurvedic polyherbals are circumscribed by the Ayurvedic canon (Naraindas, 2014b, 16–17).

203 Exotic India, 2016, Stresscom Ashvagandha Capsules, www.exoticindiaart.com/product/ayurveda/stresscom-ashvagandha-capsules-for-stress-strain-fatigue-combats-price-per-strip-of-10-capsules-AMH06/ (accessed 23 June 2016).

204 Classic Ayurvedic yogams must quote the textual source but do not have to list ingredients on the packages.

205 Hebbar, J.V., Ayurvedic Medicine Information, http://ayurmedinfo.com/2015/12/03/alert-capsule-uses-dose-ingredients (accessed 24 June 2016); Vasu Pharma Herbals, http://mall.coimbatore.com/bnh/vasupharmaherbals/alert-capsule.htm (accessed 24 June 2016).

206 "Brain fag" was identified by the Canadian psychiatrist Raymond Prince in the mid-twentieth century as a disorder found among male students in Nigeria who complained of having lost the capacity to retain information that they read in books or heard in lectures. In a most cases, patients also experienced physical ailments including crawling and burning sensations in the head. Prince published two articles (Prince 1960) on the discovery of "brain fag syndrome" and it soon became a common diagnosis for Nigerian psychiatric patients. The cause of the disorder, Prince argued was the stress associated with earning a European degree (this was very important, particularly for young men, because it had become the avenue to wealth and prestige in Nigeria). The learning style and institutional setting of British-style education conflicted with communal Nigerian lifestyles. For Prince, brain fag represented a subconscious rebellion of the Nigerian personality, a rejection of European education by the "traditional African mind". As Heaton identifies, Prince's work built direct links to colonial ethnopsychiatry and theories regarding negative psychological consequences of "psychologization" (Heaton 2013). The concept of brain fag that emerged in the 1950s was widely criticized as a racializing concept, but migrated from Nigeria to India where it fell on fertile ground due to the educational demands put on children. Further research is needed to explore this hypothesis. Although I have never heard this term mentioned by allopathic or Ayurvedic psychiatrists, it nonetheless appears here on the promotional material for Ayurvedic medicine for depression.

207 A further association might be the "Mentats" in the English-language science fiction book and movie Dune by Frank Herbert. In this fiction, Mentats are a type of human whose brains are adapted to function like computers.
208 In this case, they are part of what are called "ethical products", which are sold on prescription in contrast to "over-the-counter" products that clients can purchase without a doctor's prescription.
209 Dr Mangalam, Kottakkal, 11 March 2011.
210 Dr Shankaran, Ernakulam, 21 September 2010.
211 Caraka Samhita, Chikitsasthanam, 9, verses 85–86
212 Dr Mangalam, Kottakkal, 11 March 2011.
213 Dr Kumar, Kottakkal, 1 March 2013.
214 Dr Joshua, Kottayam, 14 February 2013
215 Dr Pritha, Kottakkal, 17 February 2014.
216 Dr Girish, Thrissur, 5 March 2014.
217 Dr Kumar, Kottakkal, 18 February 2014
218 Dr Joseph John, 20 March 2011.
219 Dr Kumar, Kottakkal, 18 February 2014.
220 See also the work by Indian psychiatrists such as A. Venkoba Rao (1978), Reddy (2012) or Bhatia et al. (2013) on the Bhagavad Gita.
221 Dr Mangalam, Kottakkal, 11 March 2011.
222 From numerous talks with practitioners and students of Ayurvedic psychiatry I got the impression that the difference between yukti, daiva, and sattvavajaya treatment was located in agency. In yukti treatment agency rests with the physician, therapeutic procedures, and medicines while in sattvavajaya agency may lie with the patient or with the doctor, and in daiva treatment agency is distributed (Sax, 2009: 133) between gods, spirits, healers, therapeutic substances, or (in the context of efforts to psychologize religious healing) the crucial role of what is called "belief" for recovery, and for the patient.
223 These points are made in Caraka Samhita 6.9.80–84. These lines are found just prior to the passage on sattvavajaya.
224 Dr Kumar, Kottakkal, 18 February 2014.
225 The postgraduate course at the P.S. Varier Ayurveda College, Kottakkal is called Manovigyan avum manorogam [knowledge of the mind and mental diseases], which students also translate as "psychology and psychiatry".
226 It is interesting to note that Dr Kumar mentions upayangal but not sattvavajaya when in relation to psychology or psychotherapy.
227 Caraka Samhita, Sutrasthana 11.54.
228 The Sanskrit term "daiva", literally "divine", derives from *deva* [deity]. Daiva has been extended and usually denotes "fate", often though not always related to actions performed in this or in previous lives (Zimmermann 2014).
229 As demonstrated above, Dr Sundaran includes sattvavajaya under rational treatment.
230 Dr Shafik, Kottakkal, 5 February 2014.
231 Jyanthi, Kottakkal, 5 February 2014.
232 Dr Rasheed, Kottakkal, 24 February 2010.
233 Dr Sarasvati, Kottakkal, 1 March 2013.
234 Dr Mary, Thrissur, 4 March 2014.
235 Dr Sundaran, Kottakkal, 3 August 2009.
236 Student of Ayurvedic psychiatry, Kottakkal, 24 February 2010.
237 Dr Sundaran, Kottakkal, 3 August 2009.
238 Dr Ganapati, Ernakulam, 21 September 2010.
239 Dr Ganapati, Ernakulam, 21 September 2010.
240 For an exception see Chapter 5.

241 Nampoothiri, Vasudevan M.R., n.d. "Kerala State Comprehensive Health Policy – Draft for Ayurveda", last accessed 3 March 2015. This document is no longer available on the Internet.

242 Kerala State Mental Health Authority, 2000, Mental Health Policy for Kerala State, www.ksmha.org, last accessed 15 August 2011. This document is no longer available on the KSMHA website.

243 Devonmadam is the Malayalam term for the Sanskrit "deva unmada". Likewise the following Malayalam terms for different forms of bhuta unmada in the other elements of the list in this quote.

244 Langford (2002) makes a distinction between Western psychotherapy as self-explorative introspection uncovering an authentic interior self and Ayurvedic psychotherapy. This distinction does not, however, account for the fact that exploratory psychotherapy has been systematically de-emphasized over the past several decades when supportive therapy and cognitive behaviour therapy orientations have supplanted exploratory psychodynamic psychotherapy.

5 Possession to depression and back: Ayurvedic psychiatry from the margins

This is an account of how one Christian Ayurvedic psychiatrist in Kerala, Dr Joseph John, reinterpreted and reclaimed spiritual therapy as an important component of Ayurvedic psychiatry. This analysis of one figure "from the margins" of institutionalized Ayurvedic psychiatry highlights negotiations in everyday healing practice that are obfuscated by homogenizing narratives of the "scientization" of institutionalized Ayurveda. Dr John's relatively peripheral location vis-à-vis institutionalized Ayurveda allowed him greater freedom from the kinds of gate keeping that would be more substantial in an institutional setting. This is not a story of borrowing scientific authority from biomedicine alone, but also the reconfiguration of Christian healing into a scientific endeavour. Using the case of Anita, I analyse how Dr John understands, translates and treats depression and how depression becomes multiple in his treatment regime. I argue that it is these multiple authorities and the multiple or distributed healing agency that allows depression to become multiple in Dr John's diagnostic and therapeutic practice.

A private Ayurvedic psychiatric clinic

My research assistant Dr Nayar, who had completed his BAMS at the Ayurveda College in Kottakkal, recommended Dr John to me. I had asked him about Ayurvedic psychiatrists with private clinics, outside the institutional frame of GAMH or the Ayurveda College. Dr Nayar made an appointment and I visited Dr John on my way to Kollam where I had intended to stay with my family and my colleague Eva Jansen. My first visit was to one of his two private clinics, located in an old building in a town near Ernakulam. The practice board proclaimed in English, "Dr John, BAMS, PGDCP, Consultant physician in Ayurveda, P.G. diploma in counselling and psychotherapy|" and was transliterated into Malayalam. Later, we became good friends and he told me that our first meeting was a bit overwhelming for him. The big car arriving in front of his building, the presence not just of me but also my colleague and my research assistant Sanat: all this did not make Dr John feel very comfortable that first visit. He said he felt very unprepared. However, he invited us to come back a few days later to visit his second clinic, situated in a rural area about fifteen kilometres away from the first, surrounded by rather wealthy houses in a Christian neighbourhood where many of the homes belonged to his extended family. This clinic was part of his residence where he stayed with his wife and his three daughters. His house was surrounded by trees and green lands and was, apart from the buses and cars that passed the building, so calm and quiet that the loudest sound I usually heard there was the cry of a crow. This clinic had four simple and very basic rooms with two beds and a small shelf in each, connected by a large balcony where the patients, their family members and therapists would sit and chat, read the Christian spiritual books that Dr John used to give them as part of the therapy, or watch TV. Patients also prayed the rosary here along with the therapists and Dr John's family, and the balcony was additionally where Dr John's counselling took place. Two huge boards read "A centre for ayurvedic treatment, counselling & psychotherapy, especially for psychosomatic diseases" in English, and "Dr John arogya & manovikan kendra" [health and psychology centre] in Malayalam. Dr John's patients were mostly middle class, though not exclusively and he sometimes also had upper middle class patients.

Dr John was prepared for our second visit. He had invited three of his former patients who had been diagnosed with depression to come and speak with us. Also invited was the yoga practitioner he had appointed, who not only showed us the yoga postures he offered to patients but was also supposed to take photos of us for the local section of the newspaper *Malayalam Manorama*. Later in the course of my research, when I was in the habit of residing at Dr John's clinics for several weeks each year, I came to understand that Dr John organized his patients for me quite carefully: he would invite selected patients who had undergone successful treatment with him to come and be interviewed. He also allowed me to speak to all his inpatients, to attend outpatient consultations, counselling sessions, and to shadow him wherever he went, including to meetings of the Association of Ayurveda Psychiatrists (AAP) or the Anthropologists of Ayurveda Medical Association of India (AMAI), to press conferences, to visits to his relatives, and to church and retreats. He had a large network of mainstream psychiatrists, psychologists, members of mental health NGOs and priests and it was through him that I built much of my network in the area around Ernakulam. What he told me about his approach towards mental health, about his patients, Ayurveda and Ayurvedic psychiatry, religion and many other things, did not happen only in formal interviews. We talked and chatted in and between consultations, in the evening when he was free, during the daily car rides from his house to his clinic in the town and on many other occasions. As we were sitting together as we did during many consultations, he told me how he came to a decision regarding his diagnosis and treatment and explained his treatment rationale. He tried to increase his credibility and status vis-à-vis his patients by having a foreigner sitting with him as a student. He never introduced me as an anthropologist but as a doctor from Germany. So I was often asked (despite my protests) to use the stethoscope or sometimes even to do counselling in which he expected me to give guidance to his patients to get them on the right track. I was on the horns of a dilemma: to do this was contrary to my convictions and against my research training, but not to do so risked offending the doctor and breaching culturally appropriate norms of behaviour. So in practice my "counselling" consisted mostly of ethnographic narrative interviews, asking questions instead of giving advice. I wanted to learn about his approach and treatment and he wanted to teach me and to initiate me into his Christian practice of Ayurvedic psychiatry. When talking to his patients I often had different interests than he did, and he sometimes admonished me for not formulating my questions according to what he perceived to be medical or Ayurvedic history-taking.

Dr John often contended that he was "a man of faith, not of theory". And in fact, his ideas, especially with regard to Ayurvedic psychiatry, often differed from those as taught and propagated in institutional Ayurveda and training in Kottakkal. However, there were also many similarities, due in no small part to the fact that Dr John maintained regular exchange with Ayurvedic psychiatrists trained or working at the college or GAMH in Kottakkal, and that he had studied Dr Sundaran's Malayalam book *Treatment of Mental Diseases in Ayurveda* (Sundaran 1993). In order to keep pace with the scientific progress of academic Ayurvedic psychiatry, he continuously kept himself up-to-date with the latest developments in the Ayurveda College in Kottakkal by attending their seminars or adopting new Ayurvedic measuring tools emphasizing that "this is more scientific". When I spoke with Ayurvedic doctors in Kottakkal, however, it turned out that apart from a few Christian postgraduate students of psychiatry in Kottakkal, Dr John was not known to most of the practitioners of Ayurvedic psychiatry there.

When I first met him, Dr John presented himself to me as holder of a BAMS degree and a postgraduate diploma in counselling and psychotherapy who had worked for ten years with an allopathic psychiatrist. Thus, he had experience with both Ayurvedic and biopsychiatric diagnostics and treatment. He explained:[1]

> I took my BAMS degree from Trivandrum Ayurveda College in 1989. After my degree I took a postgraduate diploma in counselling and psychotherapy. I was practising after the course with a modern psychiatrist, Dr Shankadevan. He was my guide. He was an Ayurvedic doctor as well as a modern psychiatrist. He had taken his postgraduate degree from NIMHANS, Bangalore. But he is no more. He was situated as a famous treatment centre in Middle Kerala. The whole centre integrated Ayurveda and modern medicine. In this hospital I was with Dr Shankadevan ten years as medical resident. Through him I got much experience. He was very interested in Ayurveda and in Indian psychology, Yoga, acupuncture and Christian disciplines such as desensitization of enmity, jealousy and aggression, the cardinal principles of Christian ideology. This he did by counselling.[2] This attracted me more than the medicines.

This was his short introduction when we were sitting in his small office where he usually saw his outpatients in the morning and evening. Behind him, there was a board saying, "God heals we help". A bit later he added, borrowing authority from mainstream psychiatry and psychology, "I took a PG diploma in modern psychology. So I treat the patient in the modern view. No other Ayurvedic (psychiatric) doctor is doing it in the modern way. They only go through the Ayurvedic only." Dr John diagnosed in mainstream psychiatric terms first and then mapped these diagnoses on to Ayurvedic ones for determining the appropriate treatment. The way he described his diagnostic process indicates his politics of translation:

> I follow the way of the ICD-10 and use the diagnostic criteria of the ICD-10 and connect them with the Ayurvedic treatment. I make a diagnosis in modern terms first, correlate them with Ayurvedic principles and give the Ayurvedic medical management. Diagnosing in modern terms is important nowadays because all the patients want to be convinced. In Kerala, they don't know what is Ayurveda but they know what is modern medicine. So we have to convince them.[3]

Dr John's most frequent diagnosis was "reactive depression" or "agitated depression" which he translated into *adhijonmada*. "Reactive", he explained to me, designates that it is a reaction to some external cause, while "agitated" describes the kind of symptoms that involve anger, irritation and crying. In Ayurvedic classics, physiological mental diseases are divided into six types: *vatonmada* [a state characterized by unsteadiness of thought and emotions and psychotic features]; *pittonmada* [a state characterized by excessive emotions or passions]; *kaphonmada* [a phlegmatic, despondent state], *samnipadunmada* [mental disorder involving all the three doshas]; *visha unmada* [mental disorder due to poison] – and *adhijonmada*.[4] The Caraka Samhita and Asthangahrdayam describe adhijonmada as *unmada* [madness, mental illness] due to or following a loss, often the death of a family member. At the Ayurveda College and GAMH in Kottakkal, adjijonmada was very rarely diagnosed and I never saw this diagnosis in patient charts. Dr Mangalam at the Ayurveda College told me that adhijonmada is similar to bereavement or grief.[5] A Malayali friend told me that in former times people used to express distress using the Malayalam term *adhi* [mental pain, grief, anguish, anxiety, agony] and that this term is now increasingly being replaced by the English term "tension" to indicate distress.[6] Adhijonmada would then denote mental disease [*unmada*] related to tension [*adhi*]. This would come close to how Dr John conceptualized adhijonmada as depression due to stress and strain. It is exogenous depression in the sense that it is a reaction to external circumstances and relates individual suffering to difficult social or economic circumstances.

As I demonstrated in Chapter 2, the rise of depression in Kerala is often related to deep socio-economic changes in recent decades. I suggest that depression due to "stress and strain" is probably more socially accepted and less stigmatized than endogenous depression. Once, Dr John also equated adhijonmada to post-traumatic stress disorder (PTSD), which for him was nearly the same as reactive depression. As reactive depression, he understood adhijonmada as neurotic depression other than kaphonmada that he framed as endogenous depression. According to Dr John, adhijonmada as a condition primarily related to *vata dosha* [vata humour] often presents with somatic symptoms including gastric problems, low appetite, tiredness, weakness and palpitations in addition to the more psychological and behavioural symptoms such as anxiety, tension, anger, irritability, crying, shouting and violent behaviour. In his conceptualization, there was no sense of somatic symptoms acting to mask psychological ones.[7] Depression with purely psychological symptoms such as self-doubt, guilt and despondency is different, Dr John explained: "This is kaphonmada or severe depression." I rarely saw him diagnose kaphonmada.

Dr John used another diagnostic technique which I suggest be called "reverse diagnosing" ("Marketing depression, marketing a 'cure'", Chapter 3). He inferred allopathic diagnoses from the pharmaceutical prescriptions his patients brought with them from prior visits to mainstream psychiatrists. Then, he translated these diagnoses into Ayurvedic ones – if this step was necessary at all. Sometimes my sense was more that he (as did other Ayurvedic psychiatrists) made these translations more for the sake of demonstrating Ayurvedic mental health literacy and giving credibility to Ayurvedic classifications as an independent and parallel classificatory system than for reasons relating to effective treatment of the patient. Dr John – and others – often skipped the step of translating allopathy into Ayurveda and skipped immediately to assigning an Ayurvedic treatment protocol to an allopathic diagnosis. Reverse diagnosing presupposes "floating prescriptions" (Ecks and Basu 2009) through which knowledge about pharmaceuticals and, I argue, psychiatric diagnoses, travel from psychiatrists to non-specialists but also to Ayurvedic psychiatrists. Floating prescriptions help Ayurvedic psychiatrists diagnose patients in line with mainstream psychiatry. This is only possible since mainstream psychopharmaceuticals are clearly assigned to ICD or DSM diagnoses – "the pill matches the ill", as one Ayurvedic general physician critically put it[8] but can be complicated by the practice of mainstream psychiatrists to prescribe several psychopharmaceuticals at the same time (Chapter 3). Of particular significance is how well known and prestigious is the doctor or the institution where this prescription came from. A prescription (and implicit diagnosis) from an experienced and renowned psychiatrist or institution carries much greater weight than from unknown individuals or minor institutions.

One of the first things that Dr John told me at my initial visit to his clinic was his specific treatment approach to Ayurvedic psychiatry.[9] Although idiosyncratic, he traced his approach back to the Ayurvedic classical scriptures themselves. "Ayurveda has three parts," he started. "First is *yuktivyapasraya chikitsa* [rational treatment] which is the medical management. It has two parts, *shodana* [purifying] and *samana* [dosha pacifying] treatment. Second is *sattvavajaya* or Ayurvedic psychotherapy. Third is *daivavyapasraya* treatment, spiritual therapy." I was familiar with all three terms. I also knew from the Ayurveda College and GAMH at Kottakkal that sattvavajaya was translated into "Ayurvedic psychotherapy" by Ayurvedic psychiatrists. Yet, what Dr John told me about daivavyapasraya treatment contradicted what I heard in Kottakkal, namely that daivavyapasraya treatment as it is described in the classical texts and which includes Hindu practices such as fire offerings, the chanting of the name of God, sacrifices or pilgrimage is not practised by Ayurvedic psychiatrists. But here was an Ayurvedic physician who said that daivavyapasraya chikitsa was an important – if not the most important – part of his treatment. And this was a Christian doctor! I was curious. It soon turned out that Dr John understood the "spiritual treatment" or "spiritual management" as he called it, quite differently than it is described in the codified texts and in Kottakkal. He reframed it within a Christian framework, more specifically, within a Catholic Charismatic framework and included practices of Charismatic healing, deliverance and exorcism into the treatment of depression and other mental health problems. Later it turned out that the integration of Christian religious practice into Ayurvedic treatment, although not frequent, was nevertheless not that unusual. Dr Varghese, an older Catholic Ayurvedic physician from a lineage [*parampara*] of Ayurvedic doctors who specialized in the treatment of mental illness and had treated inpatients living in small huts on the family's compound until some years ago, told me similar stories.[10] If it was needed, he told me, they had referred patients to a Catholic priest for exorcism.

According to Dr John, Ayurvedic psychiatric clinical practice would not be complete without daivavyapasraya chikitsa. With all three forms of treatment, the patient gets "a total cure, not a partial cure."[11] In fact, he argued, Ayurveda is closely related to religion and the Ayurvedic knowledge written in the classical texts was given by the God, and there was no problem whatsoever with correlating this to the Hindu and the Christian gods. This did not mean, however, that in his practice religion trumped science. For Dr John, religious treatment was in fact equal to science. He often emphasized the scientific nature of his practice in front of patients and to me. He used biomedical devices such as the stethoscope or the sphygmomanometer, or ICD categories and explanations to testify to his scientific approach. But he also understood the retreats, deliverance prayers and exorcisms, to which he used to refer his patients, as scientific treatments. Like many Christian priests I met, and resonating Charismatic notions of healing, Dr John had no problem marrying Freud to God or, in other words, connecting ideas of the subconscious to prayer. "All experiences will be stored in the subconscious mind and control our behaviour in the future," he stated.

> If our past experience was bitter, our subconscious mind is not able to give a good stimulus for good health and good thought. These persons will always be angry, feel depression or fear, sadness and selfishness. So we have to pray to God to heal our subconscious mind, to heal us from these wounds.[12]

Moreover, Dr John had an idiosyncratic interpretation of sattvavajaya. In theory, he followed institutional Ayurvedic psychiatry and described sattvavajaya as "refraining the mind from unwholesome objects or winning the mind", and translated it into Ayurvedic psychotherapy or counselling. The "personality development programme" that his patients underwent included "personal and social discipline", "self-control", or "control of the thoughts and senses" and "proper judgement". Moreover, patients were instructed to refrain from "passions, strong affects and violent thoughts and actions".[13] It was a means to control and coordinate mind and behaviour to correspond with social and religious norms. In practice, however, sattvavajaya or counselling for Dr John meant strengthening the religious faith of the patient of any denomination that rendered his personality development equal to spiritual development, as he often stressed. His counselling was therefore oriented towards bringing the patient on the right path, both socially and spiritually. For this aim, he offered his patients an assortment of Malayalam and English "spiritual books" and DVDs. In one of his many efforts to explain his concept of sattvavajaya to me, as he saw me struggling to understand it, he explained:

> We should purify ourselves from unwanted impulses. We should just look at the right things, not the wrong ones. We have to control all urges. I try to connect Christian, Muslim and Hindu philosophy. God gave us Ten Commandments. If we obey them, we will get peace. Or if we give alms without looking at the benefits as Bhagavad Gita asks us to do, we will be happy in our mind. This is sattvavajaya. If people do service for their own benefit and not for the grace of God, it will make them *ahamkara* [selfish].[14]

Reassurance of the patient was another important aspect of Dr John's counselling. "I tell them, 'I will help you to get rid of the disease.' I reassure them. Then there will be some changes in them and the medication will act more positively." What doctors often refer to as "supportive therapy" is not specific to Dr John or to Ayurvedic physicians alone. Indeed, reassuring the patient of the benefit of the treatment was part of almost every consultation I witnessed. Sattvavajaya also means strengthening or developing *sattva* [purity] *guna* [quality] and reducing *rajas* [activity] and *tamas* [ignorance] gunas, as I have shown in "The physiology and morals of depression" (Chapter 5). The solution to stressful or harmful social constellations or circumstances was not to change them but to enhance mental strength or willpower [*manobalam*] to better endure or deal with them since, as Dr John stressed, mental health can only be achieved if a person lives in harmony with their society. With regard to marriage, this often meant that he counselled women to adjust to their husbands and in-laws, or not to engage in a culturally unsanctioned "love marriage" (a marriage that stands in opposition to culturally appropriate "arranged marriage"[15]). If the patient is young enough, such as in the case of Anita (see below), Dr John's counselling also addressed the parents and called on them to act and to behave in accordance with social and religious norms, to lead a morally good life, and to support and be at peace with one another. More than once he underlined his strong connection between mental health and conformity to social norms and religiosity with his interpretation of how the World Health Organization defines mental health. "WHO says clearly that mental health is psychological, physical, social, and spiritual well-being and not only the absence of disease".[16] Interestingly this was a local interpretation of the WHO's definition of health as "complete physical, mental and social well-being and not merely the absence of disease or infirmity" (World Health Organization 1946) that I often heard referenced by Ayurvedic and mainstream psychiatrists, clinical psychologists and psychiatric social workers in Kerala to emphasize the pioneering role of what is framed as Indian psychology in a comprehensive understanding of health.

Like practitioners at GAMH and the college hospital in Kottakkal, Dr John treated patients with depression with purifying [shodana] and pacifying [samana] treatments. The usual shodana treatment for a patient with depression lasted fourteen days. It started with two days of *takrapanam*, the drinking of large quantities of buttermilk to make the body dry and rough. If *pitta* [bile, transforming principle] is involved which manifests as anger, irritation or as a feeling of heat in the body, this procedure is replaced by purgation with *avipathi churnam* [a powder used as a purgative to induce a bowel cleaning motion] which pacifies pitta and kapha. This is followed by about five days of *snehapanam*, the drinking of large quantities (from 80 to 150 mL in increasing dose) of ghee in order to lubricate and prepare the body. For snehapanam in depression he used *panchagava ghrtam*, a ghee made of "the five products of the cow" with vata and kapha pacifying qualities. This is followed by one day of therapeutic vomiting [*vamana*]. Like at GAMH and the college hospital, vamana has two effects. It balances vitiated kapha and detoxifies patients who are taking host of psychopharmaceuticals. It is often only after vamana that the Ayurvedic samana drugs are said to be effective. Vamana is regarded as the essential purifying treatment for kapha-related disorders including depression. During my early visits, Dr John always emphasized that he did not like to apply vamana treatment in depression for several reasons. During later visits, however, he proudly announced: "You will be happy to hear that I changed my treatment regime. I now include vamana in the treatment". In a kind of "samyogic experimentation" (Obeyesekere 1992), he had tried vamana in treating a patient with severe depression on the suggestion of and in collaboration with the patient's brother, who was an Ayurvedic general doctor and a college mate of his and, in his words, got "wonderful results".[17] From then on, Dr John integrated vamana into his treatment line of moderate and severe depression.

I add an excerpt from my field notes to provide a clearer idea about this procedure, and also to indicate how unpleasant and challenging therapeutic vomiting can be for patients. This extract also shows how Dr John demarcated vamana from the vomiting that is part of kaivisham treatment ("Translations undercover", Chapter 4):

> In the morning, 5:30 a.m. I was woken up by Aisha, the Ayurvedic therapist in one of Dr John's clinics, who knocked on my door and said "vamana" and I was allowed to watch a patient doing vamana. Today Rose, a female patient in her early twenties with mild depression receives vamana. Doctor takes BP and pulse and prepares some vomit-inducing paste and mixes it with milk. Rosa sits on a chair, Aisha next to her. Rosa is given a glass of milk, after that the milk with the paste, after that milk again several times, then *kashayam* [cooked decoctions], then milk alternating with kashayam. Rosa has a dislike for milk, also for kashayam. In the beginning she is very cooperative, later she has to develop new will power in order to drink. After almost every glass she vomits. Doctor explains to me that 50% of the patients believe that their problem is because of something bad in the stomach; some substance that was given by somebody else. "We do it the scientific way," he says. "Mantravadis and priests in Cherthala [a kaivisham treatment centre], they look for some substances to come out".[18] Rosa vomits at least 15 times after she was given 15 glasses of either milk or kashayam. I think of Western patients in resorts speaking about "gentle Ayurvedic treatments". Rosa really has problems drinking the fluids. The end is marked by some pitta [bile] coming up. Half a bucket full of vomit. It smells in the room. Aisha massages her back in the upward direction to stimulate further vomiting. The procedure takes one hour and after it is done, the doctor smears some ghee [*neyyu*] on a piece of liquorice, lights a candle and burns it and it is held under the face of the patient in order for her to smell the smoke. This is to stop the feeling of vomiting, Dr John explains. After that, BP and pulse is measured and she is asked to rest. The whole day, she gets first rice water, then *kanji* [a soup of broken rice], then some rice with green leaves (?) to eat. Rest is indicated.

After vamana follows a day of *abhyanga* [oil baths/massages] and *svedana* [steam therapy]. The last part of the purifying procedures is *nasyam* [nasal drops] with a dose of five to nine drops in increasing quantity to purify and to eliminate the kapha in the head. Along with this, the patients must follow a diet [*pathiya*] that contains kanji in the beginning and the same light vegetarian food in the further course of the treatment for every patient. It is only after the patient's body and embodied mind are purified that the pacifying part of the medical treatment, counselling and daivavyapasraya chikitsa, can be started. Patients diagnosed with depression usually get *thakradhara* [pouring medicated buttermilk on the forehead], a treatment that Dr John described as cooling and clarifying. Additionally, he prescribed both yogams and branded drugs for depression. Though Dr John has a franchise contract with a local Ayurvedic company, he also prescribed products made by other companies. The kashayams and *aristhams* [fermented decoctions] that he prescribes are basically the same *yogams* [unions, compounds] prescribed by GAMH doctors. Additionally, his patients receive powders and pills. For depression, Dr John gave *Manasamitram vataka*, a yogam made out of several dozen ingredients used for mental health problems and restlessness which mainly induces sound sleep, to be crushed and mixed with an *arishtam* [fermented decoction]. But he also prescribed branded pills that he regarded as more powerful than yogams. Typical branded pills used by Dr John to treat depression are Mentat by Himalaya, Stresscom by Dabur or Jessica by Imis.

Many patients who come to Dr John were on psychopharmaceuticals, most of who took more than one of these medicines. For example, a patient with bipolar disorder had been on the mood stabilizers lithium and sodium valproate, the antidepressant escitalopram and the anxiolytic and tranquilizer lorazepam (a benzodiazepine). Usually Dr John cut dosage in half, quartered it or cut some drugs out completely, continuing only with one or two. In severe depression, he regarded it necessary for the patient to continue allopathic antidepressant(s) "because of the risk factor for suicide".[19] Although legal restrictions prohibit Ayurvedic doctors from prescribing allopathic drugs, Dr John sometimes encourages his patients to re-use older prescription leaflets for psychopharmaceuticals.

The god of small things

Anita hailed from a middle class Syrian Catholic family. She was twenty-three years old, and had just finished the B.Sc. nursing course at a college in Bangalore when I met her and spent about two weeks with her in March 2011. She was about to be married and her parents had decided that her mental problems needed to be addressed before the wedding. She had already received several diagnoses and treatments. Anita had been diagnosed with bipolar disorder and major depressive disorder, respectively, by two mainstream psychiatrists and with dual personality disorder by a Brahmin priest. She had taken the mood stabilizer lithium carbonate, the antidepressant fluoxetine, the neuroleptic olanzapine and different anxiolytics, which all seriously affected her studies. She had already made several suicide attempts and suffered greatly while at the college. Anita was intelligent and eloquent, interested in reading books on philosophy, psychology and poetry, and controversial Kerala feminist writers such as Kamala Das or Arundhati Roy, and watching films dealing with spirits, ghosts and other occult themes. She was very curious about different kinds of spiritual practices and experimented with them. She liked to write poems and to draw. Once she told me that most people would probably call her mad when they got to know that she was creative and read all these things. Her mother who accompanied her was indeed afraid that her daughter's reading and art would influence her negatively and enhance her mental distress.

It was already dark when I first met Anita and her mother on the rooftop of Dr John's clinic. I was surprised to run into somebody there. Usually the patients stayed down on the storey below sitting, chatting or watching TV. The two women stood there talking and watching the stars, Anita holding her mother's arm tightly. Together we watched the full moon, so close that night, when Anita slowly started to speak about her life in Bangalore. We were talking in English, which became our habit because Anita had studied at an English language school and spoke it fluently. When studying she used to get harassed by some senior girls, she began, which made her suffer a lot. She became depressed and tried to commit suicide by cutting her veins several times. Moreover, she had developed breathing problems that showed up again recently after her father had shouted at her. "Not asthmatic," Dr John explained to me later, "but somehow hysteric".[20] Her mother, Anita continued, came from her home in Kottayam district to stay with her in her college lodgings in Bangalore for the remaining four years of her nursing course. "My Mummy is my only friend", she told me that night while hugging her mother. "But at the same time she is over-protective. She is afraid when I cross the road alone that some accident might happen." Living back in rural Kerala where she grew up (a several-hour car journey from Dr John's clinic), she tried to hide the fact that she studied in Bangalore from neighbours and friends "because everyone will think bad things about girls having studied in Bangalore". When we went down to our rooms Anita invited me to sit with her and we chatted about her other interests. She was fascinated by the teachings of the famous charismatic spiritual teacher Osho Sri Rajneesh who drew many young followers from Europe and North America in the 1970s. She told me she especially liked his preaching on inner emptiness and bliss. She also spoke about Arundhati Roy and Kamala Das, two highly controversial writers from Kerala. When we talked about marriage, she commented, "After marriage all women become slaves." She could not imagine getting married since, she said, she had difficulties "adjusting" to new situations. She also told me that sometimes she went on a hunger or sleeping strike to manipulate her parents. Recently she had not slept for three days to blackmail her mother into sleeping in Anita's bed through the whole night. Anita's mother used to get up every morning at three o'clock to do the household chores, and as Anita used to sleep on her mother's shoulder, this disturbed her own sleep.

On the following days we often sat on the balcony and chatted. Or we would take walks through the neighbourhood, and Anita would talk about different birds and plants that we saw or eagerly tell me about different recipes that she was fond of experimenting with. She would instruct me on so many small details, such as expounding upon a small bird that we watched stick his bill into a flower and suck the nectar out. Other times she would sit gloomy and depressed in her room or on the balcony, not at all interested in talking, not wanting to be disturbed. At other times, she talked like a waterfall, stories tumbling out of her without pause. She seemed very inspired when she talked about films she liked, books she had read, little stories she had overheard in her childhood of spirits and ghosts, and the interest of some of her Syrian Christian family members in Hindu ritual practice.

When we talked about how she felt in depressive states, Anita told me that for her depression meant first and foremost that she cried for no reason.

> If somebody tells me a simple thing, actually there is nothing in that word to get sad but I start weeping like crazy. For example, last time I collected

> the pistachios on the ground and my grandmother swept them away. Actually that was a simple thing but I wept like anything.

Then she talked about emptiness. Conditioned by my reading of the feeling of emptiness and of being cut-off from the world as characteristic for the phenomenology of depression in "the West," I was interested and probed Anita further about this feeling of emptiness. To my surprise emptiness turned out to be a positive feeling for her, something she was striving for rather than she suffered from, a state she regarded as the opposite of depression.

> Emptiness means, if we are in a good environment, a calm and quiet atmosphere. Sometimes I used to feel like that, empty. I felt like an ocean, like the Pacific. It means forgetting everything, not being bothered about anything or not remembering anything ... simple ... we are free.

Using the generalizing "we" she continued narrating how depression felt for her.

> But in depression, we feel that we are alone. Then we feel hopelessness, we don't want to live, sometimes there is a tendency toward suicide, for a simple, simple reason. We want to end our life. Nothing will enter our mind. If somebody says, "I have a problem," nothing will enter our mind. When severe depression came, at that time only. We feel that we are nothing in this world. All are teasing us.

Later she added, "I lost all my interest even in daily activities, eating, cooking, sleeping. Then I refused to bathe twice. Usually I bathe twice a day but at that time I felt difficulty even brushing my teeth." "Could you tell me a bit more?" I asked.

> It might start with a headache. Or else, I was so talkative at that time, before that, then became silent, depressed, would go and sit alone in my bedroom, and cry. And I felt that everyone was criticizing me. Then I didn't have any hope to live for. When the depression was severe, I felt that my heart was going to break; something was inside here [pointing to her heart-mind]. If you want to cry but the tears won't come, that time we have some pressure inside, no? Even though we cry, it means our emotions will break us and what can I say. During the time of slight depression, I became so irritated, talkative. In the other [mania] state, sometimes I was hyperactive. I felt so excited, so much excitement, I felt like I was just floating. But I liked that mood, when I had this hyperactivity. But sometimes when I had only slight depression, I was so irritated. And so, I lost my temper. Sometimes I threw all the things in my room, whatever I got in my hand. Actually, I was sad inside. But I showed it as irritation, as loss of temper. Because I wanted to be alone at that time and if somebody came and disturbed me, for example my father, I got irritated. Sometimes I would say something but they didn't understand my mood and didn't accept it.

> And again I got irritated and threw things. And sometimes I tried to kill them also, their neck, throat. Then I felt I was cruel.

Depression feels, she continued, like an inner turmoil, like the huge waves on the surface of the ocean. This resonates with other narrations I heard in Kerala, from patients and their family members, from doctors, psychologists and counsellors as well as from ritual healers, for many of whom anger featured as one of the main characteristics of depression (Chapter 4). For Anita, depression was the opposite of emptiness and calmness. This idea of emptiness, bliss and an enhanced state of wellbeing resonates with Buddhist ideas of emptiness and especially with Osho's teachings on inner emptiness that she had read and was fascinated by. She showed me a book by Osho in which it was written that there is nothing else other than emptiness or nothingness after the different layers of one's being are peeled away, a state that he called enlightenment. This emptiness or tranquillity is what Anita experienced as the calm eye of the cyclone (depression). "When I was depressed", she remembered, "my mind was just like an ocean, full of waves, like that. And I would long to calm down, like a river. Because then there are no waves."

The following narrative of Anita's childhood is an amalgam of the stories she told me over several days and nights of chatting and of what Dr John told me about her. She had a difficult childhood. "The parenting of her parents was not good," said the doctor. She told me that very often she was alone in the house. When she was six years old, nobody cared for her. Her mother was often away in her natal home for months, her father worked and she was taken care of by her father's parents. Anita's uncle and aunt did not really care for her and often spoke badly of her mother. "That was the real cause for Anita's personality disorder," Dr John explained, engaging a psychodynamic model. Once she had an accident and was badly burned and nobody really cared about her. "At other times my grandmother didn't allow me to take enough curries [side dishes]," Anita recounted, using a local idiom of complaint to signify the lack of care and love. She had also been sexually abused by an older male family member. Anita's father was an alcoholic and when drunk he often used to shout at her and her mother and verbally abuse them. When her father's sister married a Hindu man, a love marriage lacking the family's consent, "it was a big tragedy for this aristocratic family", said the doctor. "The father was stunned by his sister's disobedience. He was very strict with Anita and never allowed her to meet with friends or neighbours." "So many restrictions," Anita remembered,

> I should not make my clothes dirty, should wear *chappels* [sandals] always, should not climb trees. One day I did and fell down. I had a fracture in my arm. This was a wonderful time. I couldn't write my homework so my Mummy would sit next to me, she wrote and we did the homework together.

When her mother was pregnant, five-year-old Anita was very jealous. She would beat her mother's belly and force her to carry her. "My relatives used to make fun of me saying, ‘You are not our child, the coming one is our child. We don’t want you’, things like that. At that age, it wounded me a lot.” Her anger was mainly directed toward her father, and she sympathized with her mother who had to suffer at the hands of her husband and his relatives. “My mother often went to her natal house,” Anita told me,

> because she was afraid of my grandfather and grandmother. They used to make fun of her. My grandmother made her do all the work in the house. Often, they used to accuse her of not finishing the work on time. My grandmother also didn’t allow my mother to be with my father at some times. The property belonged to my grandfather. My father had no voice. My mother got so weak when she was pregnant with me. Once my father wanted to take her to the hospital because she was so weak because of the vomiting in her pregnancy but his parents didn’t allow him to spend money on this. My mother was not able to tolerate all this. So she prayed to God and tried to abort me.

On the evening after her first deliverance session at a nearby Catholic retreat centre (see below), Anita told me about the abortion attempt and how she went through her own experience as a foetus during the priest’s prayers:

> I was able to see a womb with a foetus. The foetus was in a disturbed mood. It was rejected. That was me. I was rejected by my mother. I can’t believe that my mother had done this to me. Maybe because of all the rejections she got from others. Maybe all her feelings that she felt. My mother was very depressed during my pregnancy. She felt that she couldn’t have me at that time. She was only nineteen.

According to Dr John, it was the fact that Anita’s father was a liquor distributor that made the family vulnerable to the influence of evil spirits. From the doctor’s point of view, engaging in this kind of business made the father responsible for many tragedies and sufferings of other people. It is not only that distributing liquor was morally questionable. This type of business also attracted evil spirits into his family, Dr John opined. This was further exacerbated through the father’s interest in Hindu temples to which he used to take Anita. Anita’s problem, Dr John stated, was thus in fact a spiritual problem relating to the larger family.

Dr John diagnosed Anita with *adhijonmada* [reactive depression] that was growing into *kaphonmada* [endogenous, severe depression] and with “personality disorder”. One feature of what Dr John called “psychosis” was suicidal tendencies. That is what he told me. To her, he explained it differently in one of their first encounters, sitting on the balcony, “counselling” her:[21]

> Daughter, I don’t want to see you as a patient. The doctors have named your disease. But you don’t show its typical symptoms. There is a

> personality disorder. But personality disorder is there in everyone. [...] Personality disorder should not be treated as a disease. But at present, this has changed from neurosis to psychosis. Good counselling and spiritual management would have prevented you from reaching this state. It requires treatment. Ayurveda treatment will not adversely affect your health.

He started his usual treatment for depression. As preparatory procedures he prescribed drinking of large quantities of buttermilk [*thakrapanam*] for two days to dry the body, drinking of large quantities of ghee [*snhepapanam*] for six days, external application of oil [*abhyanga*] and steam therapy [*svedana*]. These were followed by purgation [*vamana*] and seven days of nasal applications of medicated oil [*nasya*]. She also received pacifying treatments [*samana*] like thakradhara in which medicated buttermilk was poured over her forehead. To induce sleep, she was given a large dosage of Ashvagandharistham and two pills of Manomitra at night. Allopathic medications were cut. Dr John talked to her about her family problems, especially her alcoholic father, and counselled her how to help him and how to love him. According to the doctor, Anita could not be successfully treated before the family problems were solved, which mainly meant that hatred within the family had to be dissolved. This is part of his etiology of "personality disorder" which can go back as far as several previous generations and thus becomes an intergenerational fault [*parampara dosha*] – that is, the sins of the forefathers which, if not addressed by spiritual (Christian) treatment, might affect all generations to come. According to Dr John, the causality of Anita's "personality disorder" included both problems in her upbringing and family conflicts on the one hand, and evil spirits on the other. In the following pages, I focus on this "personality disorder" aspect of her disease.

After a two-week treatment, Dr John usually referred many of his Christian and some of his Hindu and Muslim patients to Father Kurien in a nearby Roman Catholic Charismatic *ashrama* [religious centre] for deliverance or exorcism. Dr John told me that, in recent years, "I became more and more aware that mental problems are often caused by evil spirits". As Anita was acutely suicidal, Dr John sent her immediately to Father Kurien for help after he had told her that the depressive mood was part of her disease, also that evil spirits might be involved, but that the power of God was stronger and she did not need to be afraid. As this was an urgent case, he could not wait for the parents to arrive from their home (several hours away by car) and so Anita first saw Father Kurien without them present. At a second visit, on which I also accompanied them, both Anita and her parents participated in the religious treatment.

I accompanied Anita to her treatments in the ashrama. I had been there several times before to chat with Dr Kurien and the other priests or to attend the masses or shorter retreats. The ashrama included a church where most of the activities took place, a small chapel for silent prayers, a building where the priests lived with a kitchen and other rooms, and a new building for retreat attendants. Before they established the monthly retreats, priests at the ashrama had been engaged in ministry with prisoners.[22] Sometimes they housed ten or more male prisoners who lived, worked and prayed with the priests. Although this ministry had come to an end since they started the retreat centre, there were still a few men who remained. Of one, Father Kurien told me that he had lived a good life, was hardworking, had three jobs and lived together with his mother, his wife and his daughter whom he loved very much. One day, all of a sudden, he was, in the words of Father Kurien, taken over by an evil spirit.[23] He killed the three of them and wanted to commit suicide but was prevented from doing so.

Father Kurien was a modest and "simple" man, as Malayalis would say, in his sixties. People who had been treated by him often described his penetrating gaze from his warm and compassionate eyes. Others described his powerful voice. Those seeking help often came to see him for healing on Fridays, when he offered deliverance prayers and people waited in the church for their turn, or they made an appointment to come on any other day and he treated them either in the church or in a visitor's room.

Father Kurien had been in Tanzania for nine years where, he told me, he had seen and treated many people being afflicted by or possessed by evil spirits.[24] Before that he had served as a volunteer at the Divine Retreat Centre in Chalakkudy (Jansen and Lang 2012) where one of the officiating priests had already sent certain people to him to have spirits removed. But his main experience with deliverance and exorcism came from Tanzania where, as he recounted, he had seen many people healed of diseases that he called "spirituo-somatic" such as asthma, arthritis and cancer. "Doctors say it is psychosomatic, but it is spirituo-somatic more than psychosomatic," he explained.[25]

In Kerala, Father Kurien was a figure at the margin, marginal even among Christian priests who all receive a psychological training in their years at seminary and many of whom work as clinical psychologists. I use Father Kurien as an example of a counter discourse to hegemonic psychiatric-psychological discourse. As an analysis from the margins, it is not a discourse unaffected by psychiatry and psychology, but rather one that engages the psy-ences, criticizes them and offers an alternative. Father Kurien had mental health literacy, knew the basic diagnostic terms and criteria, and could attribute symptoms to diagnoses. Yet he situated psychiatry within a larger framework of spiritual attack and discarded psychology as insufficient in treating what he regarded as spiritual problems. As it later turned out, he was very familiar with psychology. In fact he also used what he called "psychological tricks" in his treatments. But what he criticized was the way psychology replaced the knowledge and belief of spiritual attacks in priests (and in the wider population), something he found deeply problematic.

> Here in Kerala, the priests are not aware of spirits, most of the priests don't believe in such things. I say, "unfortunately," it is not a very good thing. Many people think, education goes up, people become more and more aware of these psychological things, but I don't call it as a good thing, I think it is an unfortunate thing.[26]

Psychological or mental health literacy, Father Kurien opined, in which spiritual problems are reframed as psychological problems leads to a decline of other forms of knowledge that are then lost. As the priests "don't believe in such things" any more, they also lack the knowledge of how to deal with these problems appropriately. They offer psychological treatment while deliverance and exorcism might be indicated and thus only scratch on the surface of the problem and do not reach its deeper layer that is spirit affliction. "I have seen many people with depression or psychotic problems, really violent people getting healed by deliverance prayer. And people who had been undergoing treatment for several years, after two or three retreats completely they have become quite normal." And spirits manifest only to those priests who "believe in evil spirits", that is who stabilize the ontology of spirits by means of their therapeutic practice.

> Suppose a person has an evil spirit and the priest goes there and prays for that person but does not believe in evil spirits. He may pray for long and long hours but he will not see any change or the evil spirits will not manifest. But if the priest believes that it can be a result of an attack by an evil spirit and starts talking to it, then it can manifest and come out.[27]

"Do psychologists or psychiatrists refer patients to you for deliverance?" I asked. There were not many, he replied. Apart from Dr John, there was only one homeopathic doctor who referred patients for physical problems and there was a priest-cum-clinical-psychologist who used to refer but he had moved to another place. "Most of the priests do not have this kind of faith, especially those people who are practising psychology. They will always say it is a psychological problem. This latter priest believed because he himself came across some of these problems." Father Kurien was well aware of the modernist discourse that denies contemporaneity to priests like him who cast out spirits: "It is not well accepted because those people who pray for casting out demons, they are considered to be kind of superstitious, maybe to live in the last century, not modern people. So they are looked down upon."[28] What many Christians diagnosed with depression do is to seek "spiritual counselling" either from a priest, a nun or a layperson who are said to "get visions" of a person's problem in the wider context of their life or what they describe as hindrances of their spiritual growth, such as "living in sin" or hatred that they regard as impurity and as blockage for spiritual growth. In spiritual counselling, the counsellors "see" the larger trajectory of the afflicted person's life, locating their problems in a larger spiritual framework and receiving visions of appropriate passages from the bible and offering prayers. Spirits are usually not involved in spiritual counselling, which is different from the deliverance prayers and exorcism that Father Kurien practised.

Attacks or possession by spirits can happen either because the individual, their parents or forefathers have "invited" the spirits by a moral transgression that attracted evil spirits. Or spirit attacks happen because an individual deliberately invited a spirit by engaging in certain forms of occult worship. A spirit can also be sent by a jealous or malevolent person who seeks the help of a specialist to do so. Or it can reside in a haunted house and can catch the people who live or visit there. This is why "house deliverances" were part of the routine tasks of Father Kurien. Anxiety or depression can also provide an opening for as well as being symptom of attack by evil spirits. Father Kurien explained to me:

> If I hate myself and the world and am desperate and lose my faith, this can be an opening as well as an effect of a spirit attack. It's a vicious circle. But once you just start thanking God for your whole life the whole perspective changes and then the evil spirit cannot enter or remain in you. If there are people who are not able to receive the power of God when I pray or the evil spirit is not ready to go away it is because that person still is very depressed and full of hatred [...] Because of hatred, many people become unclean, that is why evil spirits use them. Some people might think that only because of sexual immorality people become unclean. The Bible says, if there is hatred, you can become unclean. It says, the root of hatred grows and makes the person unclean. I have seen when people become possessed by evil power; if they are not able to forgive it is very hard to completely deliver them. I don't say it is impossible but it is hard. If they can forgive that will be easier to get rid of the evil powers.

The spirits of the vernacular Christian Charismatic universe fall into several categories. According to Father Kurien there are specialized spirits for different diseases, such as the Spirit of Depression or the Spirit of Asthma. Other spirits are Hindu deities reinterpreted as evil spirits. Indeed in the deliverance of Anita I demonstrate that Bhadrakali, one of the many manifestations of Devi [a Hindu goddess], is reinterpreted and exorcised by Father Kurien as an evil spirit. Others are the spirits of people who have died without repenting, a type that the father called *preta*. In Father Kurien's cosmology, spirits and deities are reframed as aspects of demonic evil. At the top of the cosmological hierarchy stands Satan. "Satan is the commander or chief of them. It is a well-trained army. And there are ordinary soldiers and captains, commanders, commanding officers and others, and finally the captain. It is a well-trained, organized army," he explained.[29]

Anita was taken twice to Father Kurien, once alone and once with her parents. I accompanied Anita to both of these sessions and participated as an observer. The deliverances took place in the room where the priests also used to welcome guests and meet in the evening to talk and read the newspaper. It was a casual room with a sofa, a wooden table and some rattan and plastic chairs to the right and left against the wall. Anita took a seat on one, opposite the priest. I sat on the sofa between them. The deliverance comprised five parts. In the first visit, the father waited for the spirit to manifest while he struck up a conversation and in fact a battle with it. The second visit some days later comprised another deliverance session of further spirits, which was followed by a session where Father Kurien counselled Anita's parents separately from their daughter. This was followed by a part where the priest healed Anita's wounds (Csordas 1997) and culminated in the healing of the family in which each member was asked to beg each other's pardon and to forgive them. Father Kurien had no issues with me recording the healing with a voice recorder and a small camera. He also made an audio recording of Anita's first deliverance session with his mobile phone.

After the completion of the deliverance, I asked Father Kurien if he could explain it to me, and he began to tell me what had happened.

> At the first moment she saw me [at the door of the house where the deliverance took place, after we had rung the bell] she was not able to come in. Because that thing in her would not allow her to come in.[30] Some people who come to me say that even though they are trying to give their very best to come inside it is as if someone is pulling from behind, they cannot enter the gates.

Anita had told the priest that she had seen a huge snake when she reached the gate and that she had never seen such a big one. "After some time I saw it going away and then I entered the gate," she said. "That is why," Father Kurien explained, "it was not comfortable to talk to me in the beginning. Although I was trying to smile at her, she was not at all feeling at home. When I was talking to her, this convulsion of her hands was the manifestation of the spirit." When Anita had taken a seat, Father Kurien asked about her problem. "Do you have some terrible dreams in the night?" She did, and told him that she saw snakes and similar things and that she was attracted to the Hindu goddess Bhadrakali and often felt like going to the temple of Bhadrakali to worship her. Anita was sitting on a chair and light fell on her face. She said that she could not bear light. "If someone likes sitting in the darkness, that is also a spiritual problem, not a psychological problem," Father Kurien explained to me.

> These people want to be in the dark and to join with the powers of darkness. Physical light sometimes even hurts them. So that is why I asked her to sit there in the darker part of the room. This is also why I asked her if she has dreams of snakes. Because when there is Satan in them, they often dream of snakes.

Anita acknowledged that sometimes snakes appeared in her dreams and also that she sometimes dreamed of temples and participating in worship there. When the priest asked her, she told him that her father sometimes went to church but not for mass. Her mother did not go to church. She herself used to go to church, but now she was more interested in going to temple and in the Hindu gods and goddesses, she recounted. She had taken an interest in temples as she had sometimes accompanied her father to them and made offerings and worshipped there. When Father Kurien asked her if she was of a violent nature, she said that she had tried to destroy herself with a knife and attempted to strangle herself. He further probed her whether she liked to see blood. "Yes," she replied. Father Kurien later explained to me,

> she likes to see blood and sometimes scratches herself. Though it is always painful, she likes to see blood. This is not necessarily a suicidal tendency, but because of rage and of that persistent destruction mentality. It is painful but she cannot control herself and she is so happy to see it and compelled to see the blood.

Anita added that she often felt herself getting angry and so violent that she was not able to control her anger and that she felt like she wanted to cut everyone's head off. Moreover, she sometimes quarrelled with her father and he tried to beat and abuse her. Once, she told the priest, when she realized that her father was a heavy drinker and that he was destroying their family, she had a desire that everything should be destroyed. Her father had abused her with very bad words, had cursed her and her mother, and called them prostitutes, which caused her extreme hurt. Several times she repeated that she was not able to control her anger. Sometimes, she said, the anger became so strong that she suffered feelings of suffocation like an asthma patient. Following further questions by Father Kurien, she later told him that she had become interested in knowing about the black mass. She searched online and wrote down what she found. Although she did not practise such things, she was very much attracted to them, she said. Father Kurien asked whether she could pray, whether she knew God, whether she could pray to Jesus. She said that she felt so far away from God that she could not pray, that she could not come closer to God. Anita had been in a convent school till tenth standard and she was able to pray there. After that, she moved away from God. Then she spoke about the treatment she had been undergoing. She had seen many doctors, taken herbal medicines and other medicines. And she then went to "people who are praying for others, one was a Muslim, the other a Brahmin priest." The Brahmin priest told her that what she had was bipolar disorder, and he also mentioned dual personality.

Then Father Kurien started to pray and Anita fell to the floor. This was the moment when Father Kurien went to the door and locked it. "Because it might make her run away from this place," he told me later. It was around half an hour after Anita had entered the room that the spirit started speaking and Father Kurien engaged it in conversation. As he later told me, it was Bhadrakali who manifested in her. It was also Bhadrakali that Anita remembered most when the priest asked her later if she remembered anything. Bhadrakali plays an important role for Hindus in Kerala. She is a manifestation of the Goddess Devi and is also one of the goddess' manifestation at the Chottanikkara temple where she plays an important role in possession rituals. But during the conversation and the deliverance, although repeatedly requested to do so by the priest, this spirit refused to reveal her identity. The conversation between Father Kurien and Bhadrakali (in Anita) mainly dealt with power and mutual humiliation in which Bhadrakali, first so proud, grew increasingly weak. The subsequent deliverance ended with a final victory of God/Jesus/Mary/the priest against Bhadrakali and symbolically, of Christianity against Hinduism.

BHADRAKALI: I will not go.
FATHER KURIEN: Jesus is the lord of the lord, the saviour of the saviours.
BHADRAKALI: I pity him. [laughing]
FATHER KURIEN: How long?
BHADRAKALI: As long as I like. Until I finish my projects, I will not leave her body.
FATHER KURIEN: Have you heard about Holy Mary, mother of God?
BHADRAKALI: She is such a poor lady. She can do nothing to me [laughs]
FATHER KURIEN: Only she can crush your head.
BHADRAKALI: Oh, that is not going to happen.
FATHER KURIEN: Let me call her?
BHADRAKALI: No. Everybody will run away from me in the war against me. I am so powerful. It is better for you to go away from me or you will be defeated. It is of no use. You also will be defeated. I will not go away. I am so powerful now. I am a fire. You don't need to threaten me. You want to destroy me? I am fire itself. How can you burn the fire? You are just a fool. The whole world is depending on me and you also depend on me. How can you fight against me? You don't need to attempt. It's of no use, I will not leave her, this is my body, this is my body!
FATHER KURIEN: How?
BHADRAKALI: I have established my domain over her. She likes me, then why should I go away?
FATHER KURIEN: You trapped her.
BHADRAKALI: I am smart.
FATHER KURIEN: Now she wants to get rid of you.
BHADRAKALI: She wants to get rid of me? If you are smart enough, send me away. No, I am not going to go away. I will destroy her family. I will completely destroy her family. All her people will have a disastrous death. I want their souls to wander and never be redeemed.
FATHER KURIEN: How long?
BHADRAKALI: I am able, I am able. You don't try to chase me away from this body. I will not leave until my job is finished. I will not go.
FATHER KURIEN: What is your duty?
BHADRAKALI: To destroy her family and her life and destroy everything. I am assigned to do.
FATHER KURIEN: Assigned by whom?
BHADRAKALI: A relative. I can't tell. I do not know. I cannot see everything. If I go without finishing my job there is a very cruel punishment waiting for me. Don't send me away. Don't send me away.
FATHER KURIEN: You are afraid of your superior? Because some harsh punishment is waiting for you?

BHADRAKALI: Yes. Yes. [Bhadrakali speaks in an imploring tone]. Please don't send me to Kodungalur, don't send me, the punishment is so cruel. Please let me do my work here. Don't send me away.

FATHER KURIEN: She [Anita] was born to the Grace of the living God.

BHADRAKALI: Please don't send me away.

[Father Kurien laughs contemptuously]

Don't be proud of that. If it is not her, I will destroy all her family. Then somebody else in her family will be destroyed.

FATHER KURIEN: I now call Holy Mary.

BHADRAKALI: Don't threaten me telling about her. I have to fear only my superior.

FATHER KURIEN: Your superior is afraid of Holy Mary.

BHADRAKALI: I don't know. I do not want to know. Did I tell you if I leave this body, I will get the other body, that is my purpose: to destroy everyone. If not her, then her sister. I will destroy everything. Even if you send me away from her, I will get into that person. Your prayer is of no use, you can do nothing to me. I challenge you. If you are able, compete with me.

FATHER KURIEN: You have already failed.

BHADRAKALI: That is only your feeling. So many people have felt like that and they were defeated.

FATHER KURIEN: Then I call Jesus.

BHADRAKALI: It is of no use calling him. We have the power now on earth, not him.

[Father Kurien laughs]

No, no.

FATHER KURIEN: Jesus is the Lord, he has power. His glory has filled the whole world.

BHADRAKALI: [sounding tired and very weak] No, no, no.

FATHER KURIEN: One drop of Jesus is enough to destroy you. Look at my hand.

BHADRAKALI: No, I will not look. I will not go unless you do puja [the rituals of reverence] for me.

FATHER KURIEN: Every ritual is over with the sacrifice of Jesus on the cross, and I am not going to do anything because everything is over on the cross of Jesus. You did not know, don't you read the newspaper? Jesus died on the cross!

BHADRAKALI: It is of no use. I am staying in the other world, not here.

[Father Kurien laughs]

FATHER KURIEN: Then you are such a fool.

BHADRAKALI: No, no, you are the fool.

FATHER KURIEN: [showing his hand] Look at me here.

BHADRAKALI: No, no, no.

FATHER KURIEN: Look at me here.

BHADRAKALI: No, no, I will not obey. You need to do all the rituals.

FATHER KURIEN: OK, I will do everything.

BHADRAKALI: Fool, fool! [very tired]

[Father Kurien blesses the water and pours it onto Anita's head]
It is so hard to go there. I am unable to go there. Don't punish me, don't punish me. Don't send me, don't send me away. Don't send me away. [crying]

She crawled along the floor groaning, trying to reach the door and to open it. Father Kurien went to the door and closed it. In a commanding voice he said, "I don't allow you [to go]." He positioned himself in front of the door and Anita was kneeling on the floor, her upper body moving to and fro, her eyes closed. "It's an order," Father Kurien commanded. "In the mighty name of Jesus." He whistled. "Say who you are." Anita shook her head vigorously. "Tell me." He whistled and blew upon Anita in a manner that closely resembled what I have seen in the treatment of *thangals* [Muslim healers] blowing Qu'ranic verses over a patient. Anita sat on the floor, her head slowly moved backwards until she looked up. Father Kurien stood in front of her, pointing his index finger towards her. The power disparity between him and the spirit became obvious. He whistled and blew again. Anita groaned and, still kneeling, moved her body as if in deep pain and cramped from inside, her arms now behind her. She moved back and forth. Her body movements closely resembling those of the women I have seen possessed in Hindu temples and Muslim shrines. "In the mighty name of Jesus. Holy Mary, mother of God." Anita got weaker and weaker. "I surrender this child of yours, calm, calm, I surrender this child to you. Holy Mary, mother of God." When Anita did not move any more, the priest approached her saying "Holy Mary, Holy Mary, in the mighty name of Jesus" several times, his voice getting louder and louder, becoming more and more demanding. Suddenly he clapped her lightly on the forefront. He stretched out his index and pinkie fingers. "I bind you, by the power of Jesus." Now bowing down and speaking close to her face, he continued, "Where do you want to go? Tell me, where do you want to go. It's an order, by the mighty name of Jesus, it's an order." Anita – or the spirit – still moved, groaned, laughed and sometimes shook her head "no". Then Father Kurien held his outstretched hand in front of her face. "Can you smell it? The blood of Jesus that melts every sin." Disgusted and angry she turned her face away, eyes still closed. Her groaning got louder, as if something choked her, as if a strong force within her resisted. The priest now sat down in front of her. "Precious blood of Jesus." She got very calm and stopped moving. Father Kurien came closer, took Anita's head into his hands, blew on her head, and slowly and carefully held and moved her head down with one hand and supported her arm with the other, moved her head backwards and lay her down on the floor. When she was finally on the floor, he said, "Thank you Jesus." He now sat on a chair next to her face and drew the cross with his thumb on her forefront two times, laid his right hand on her forehead again and bowed her head carefully back. Anita groaned, the last scraps of resistance surfacing. Father Kurien said, "I cast you out," and whistled again. He held his hand over her saying, "Look at this sword of St Michael," whistled and blew again. "Look here, if you can." Anita clenched her right fist, beat his hand and pushed it back. Father Kurien continued his whistling and blowing with his hand offering a soft resistance against hers. Still lying on the floor and making occasional spastic movements, Anita's eyes were still closed. "Thank you Jesus," Father Kurien repeated several times. She now lay calmly on the floor, only the last groans were audible. "You have proved that you are the Lord, thank you Jesus." Finally, he drew another cross on her forehead.

The deliverance proper was marked by a shift in Father Kurien's language. After Anita tried to crawl toward the door as if to escape, he began to speak in English, addressing and commanding the spirits, and he continued in English for the remainder of the deliverance. In this and in the next session, when addressing the spirits, Father Kurien spoke in English to Bhadrakali but spoke to Anita in Malayalam. With regard to the specific deployment of the two languages, he told me that English is the language that he used for most deliverances. Even the people who do not know English, he said, will respond when he speaks in English. The presence of Bhadrakali in Anita was also marked by a language shift. In Kerala there are many Malayalam dialects connected to different areas and as such it is usually easy to tell from someone's speech where they come from. Father Kurien recognized that the dialect Bhadrakali spoke was different from the one Anita spoke.

Father Kurien later told me that he stopped here although he had already sensed another spirit. But the fact that she was physically weak due to the Ayurvedic treatment she was undergoing led him to postpone the second part of the deliverance until another day. After, Anita and I took an autorickshaw and went back to Dr John's clinic.

Some days later, her parents arrived and the family went to see Father Kurien. It began with another deliverance session. Anita sat on one side of the room while Father Kurien sat opposite. Her eyes were closed, her arms on the armrest of the chair, her head bowed slightly downwards. Father Kurien started talking to the spirit, contemptuously, and whistled and blew upon her again. "You shall be afraid," he addressed the spirit, "of the king of kings, spirit of death, of the lord of life. He is the way, he is the life, he is the truth." All the time, Anita sat almost motionless, the only movement a slight and slow shaking of her head indicating a trace of resistance. Father Kurien constantly fixated closely on her eyes. "The powers of death have no chance in those people who believe in Jesus", he said. "Spirit of death," he whistled and blew, "right now, I bind you on the cross of Lord Jesus Christ. At the glorious and mighty name of Jesus." Then he suddenly got up, went to her, took her head with his two hands and drew a cross on her forehead, slowly bowing her head back a bit.

After the talking had gone on some time, Anita's left foot and left hand started to move, a ring on her finger beating against the armchair and producing a rhythm that her foot followed also. Her eyes were wide open, staring to the floor in front of her. She slowly moved her head to the rhythm. In insulting tones, Father Kurien started speaking. "Michael, Michael", he said, interrupted by whistling and blowing. The rhythm of Anita's hand and leg became faster. The priest then said, "Finally the Holy Spirit will burn you. You are afraid?"

Anita's body started to writhe as if she was dancing while still sitting on the chair, her eyes now closed. "You cannot stand before Jesus," Father Kurien addressed the spirit. "You are dancing?" Her movements resembled the movements of the women and men at Chottanikkara temple who were possessed by snake deities ("Experiencing Spirit Affliction and Occult Violence", Chapter 4). The sound made by her movements resembled that of a rattlesnake. Father Kurien continued to whistle and blow. Anita's movements and rhythm slowed. "Thank you Jesus," he repeated several times. "Where do you want to go? In the mighty name of Jesus. One angel is more than enough to bind you." The whistling and blowing transported his prayers through the air towards her. Her movements got slower and almost subsided, her eyes opened slowly. "Amen, amen, amen," concluded Father Kurien.

He went out of the room to get some holy water and returned a few minutes later. Meanwhile Anita was sitting quietly on her chair, eyes closed. When he came back, she opened her eyes, staring towards the floor in front of her. The priest approached her carrying a jar with holy water. Her left index finger moved slowly in the way people in Kerala do to say "no". Father Kurien prayed in Malayalam and poured some drops over her body. Her index finger stopped moving, her left hand closed into a fist. Father Kurien poured drops of the holy water over her head saying, "In the mighty name of Jesus." Anita kept staring on the floor, not moving, rigid. "Thank you Jesus." Anita's eyes were now closed, the drops of holy water dropped down from her face. She opened her eyes and closed them again. Father Kurien came to her, laid his hand on her forehead, drew the cross and gave her the jar to drink. Anita drank it. Father Kurien did not want to give me further details on this second spirit. He only revealed that this "thing", as he called it, was a far more powerful one than the first one.

After the second deliverance session, Father Kurien called Anita's parents and talked to them alone. He told them how important it is to forgive each other and to stand together as one family. They should be thankful for each other and regard the others as gifts from God. If you abuse other people, it is as if you abuse God, he explained. There should be peace in the family: "Where there is peace and love, that is the least basis where God can come and stay. If there is always fighting, that's a place for Satan." Then he asked them to go to the church and pray. "And then I told them to give up hatred. I didn't tell them that hatred attracts spirits. I just told the mother that as long as she keeps the hatred within her, it is hard for her husband to give up alcohol." Father Kurien told Anita's father that if he continued drinking, it would destroy the whole family. "I didn't say it attracts spirits. I didn't want to get deep into this", he explained to me later.

When Anita was called in, Father Kurien gave the family instructions on how to beg pardon from one another and to forgive each other. Anita's father began by begging pardon and her mother replied that she forgave him. Her mother was next. Father Kurien told me later that although Anita's father begged pardon of Anita, he did not really realize the hurt he had done. "Drinking and using abusing words. Psychologically, that is what hurt her," Father Kurien later explained to me. "And taking her to the temples. She did not hate him because of the latter, but it is because of the drinking and him hurting her that she developed hatred towards him." Further, he told me that it was not so important that people whole-heartedly beg pardon and forgive. Like in mantras, the merely pronouncing the words is enough. "Our words have spirit and life," Father Kurien told me. But in the end, it was Anita who could neither beg her father's pardon nor forgive him. The wounds were too deep.

After this, Father Kurien conducted a "healing of wounds" for Anita.[31] He started by praying for her. Different from the first part of the deliverance, the atmosphere was completely calm, quiet and relaxed. It was Anita who now spoke. She said that she felt she was floating like an embryo. She experienced herself as a foetus, a foetus that was rejected, rejected by her mother, a foetus in a disturbed mood. Father Kurien prayed for her, he prayed for these wounds to be healed, he prayed that she could forgive her father, and that her unconscious mind would be healed. "And he prayed to heal all my wounds that I got from others, from this rejection in the womb through different stages of my growing," Anita told me. And Father Kurien added, "If her mother could not accept her as a child or in the womb, and she did not get the love, there is only one remedy, divine remedy. I prayed to Holy Mary to come and fill her with the love of the Almighty." The remedy was not a psychoanalytical "working through" of pre- and postnatal experiences, a rational revisiting of the suffering to make it part of the conscious mind. Here, the remedy came from something else: that divine love would fill her. It was not the love of the mother or the father that Anita was granted retrospectively through this "healing of wounds", but rather the love of Mother Mary as a replacement for the love that was lost which was supposed to effect the healing of her psychological wounds.

Later, I asked Father Kurien how he thought that the family problem related to the sprit problem. "There is a direct relationship," he replied.

> Because if there is a good family, these spirits should not have been able to get into her. First of all, her mother is not going to church. Her father goes to church, but doesn't have any personal relationship with God [...]. If Jesus is a personal experience, that gives you protection for evil things. If Jesus and God stay in a person, then how can this small silly thing get into one person? [...] Once Mary came, then this demonic power lost all legal place. These demonic powers always look to legal matters. Legal in the sense, if somebody has invited them, they have to appear by themselves. If the parents invited these demonic powers to their families, they have a legal right, they say, we are invited. There is a legal block, it cannot leave, it has the legal right to be in her. Now Mary is with her as her mother and that will break that chain, break that block. No it has no legal right to be in her anymore.

So what happened in the end? After the healing of wounds, Anita was finally ready to beg pardon of her father and to forgive him. Then Father Kurien told her:

> Now there is no need of any medicine, because your problem is almost overcome. Maybe for some time, you have to continue some medicines to get rid of the side effects of the spirit, you take a few medicines. But in the due course, you can abandon, there will not be any problems. But you have to always forgive and thank God. Otherwise you will not be able to abandon drugs and you are going to lose your life. You have a good life. God created you for a good life. You have a good future, a good job, a good husband, a good family. So forgive them and love them. Otherwise you are not getting anywhere in this life.

Although the spirits as cause of the problems were removed and family relations successfully pacified, the changes that the spirits produced in Anita's body were still there and required treatment with medicines and therapeutic procedures. She completed her Ayurvedic treatment at Dr John's clinic. When I came back two years later, Dr John told me that Anita had married a Syrian Christian and had gone to the United Arab Emirates to live with him. Since her parents had been concerned that she overcome her mental problems before her wedding, the fact of Anita's marriage confirmed she had made a full recovery.

Anita's case clearly demonstrates how not only people but also the disease depression can traverse multiple epistemological and ontological spaces. If depression is the product of a stabilizing network of theories, professions, institutions and technologies, then depression becomes multiple and gradually changes shape when it flows and intersects with other local networks. The "diagnostic liquidity" (Lakoff 2005) of depression makes symptoms and experiences compatible and commensurable on the one hand while multiple therapeutic practices extend and change its ontology, which further shapes and transforms local phenomenologies of depression. If ontologies are created through therapeutic practices (Langwick 2011) and if depression is an "immutable mobile" (Latour 1986) that is combinable with other actors, then depression becomes multiple as it traverses various ontological spaces. In Anita's case, depression was first diagnosed and treated with psychopharmaceuticals as a psychiatric condition – both as unipolar and as bipolar depression – and experienced by her as deep despondency, anger and rage, as a feeling of suffocation and of waves overruling a feeling of emptiness as free floating and a subjective experience of freedom that she experienced in her manic states. In Dr John's clinic, depression became the Ayurvedic condition adhijonmada with a tendency to develop into kaphonmada, which required Ayurvedic dosha-purifying and pacifying treatments. There depression was further transformed into a personality problem understood in both psychological and spirit-related terms. As Anita was suicidal and an emergency case, spiritual treatment by Father Kurien was used to immediately target the root cause of the problem – the activity of destructive spirits in her – that Dr John usually prescribed after the completion of the medical management portion of treatment. In his practices of deliverance from spirits (another process of reconfiguring Hindu gods into Christian evil spirits) Dr Kurien not only removed the spirits in Anita and facilitated the healing of her psychological wounds, he also emphasized forgiveness and good familial relationships as a barrier to further spirit attacks or possession. He transformed depression and its physiological and psychological manifestations from a disease entity into a symptom, the sign of spirit attacks and possession. He stabilized the spirits through his therapeutic practice of negotiating and finally defeating them. In this way he stabilized both the ontology of depression and the ontology of the local Christian Charismatic cosmology. Depression became multiple also in Anita's experience. She not only experienced depression as neurochemical changes in her brain and feelings of despair and anger, she also experienced dejection in the womb of her mother, rage against her father and the presence of spirits in her. Physiology, psychology, and spirits formed an expanded network of depression.

Institutional gate keeping and an analysis from the margins

Towards the middle of my research and after spending several months at GAMH and the Ayurveda College in Kottakkal and several more several months with Dr John, I returned back to GAMH and had a discussion with Dr Rasheed.[32] When I told him that I had visited several Ayurvedic psychiatrists who were working in private practice he did not show much interest. "This is the only specialized mental hospital in Ayurveda," Dr Rasheed corrected me.

> This is the only place with an Ayurvedic approach to psychiatry. We don't know what they do in other institutions. But this is the only approved government institute for treating mental disease in Ayurveda. This is the only authorized institute. We don't know what is the authenticity of other clinics. Here we are following the Ayurvedic principles.

"Any other manasika treatment outside the GAMH is not real," he argued. "They don't offer inpatient treatment. Maybe they give some symptomatic relief, some medicines. What we are doing here, our shodana treatment, really purifies their bodies, cures their mind." Practitioners and teachers of institutionalized Ayurvedic psychiatry in Kottakkal were the gatekeepers of professional institutional Ayurvedic psychiatry. Although they acknowledged that some of what they called "faith healers" also used some Ayurvedic psychiatric medicine, they disparaged therapeutic practitioners who included religion as non-scientific and superstitious. In any case, they were *not* considered to be practising Ayurvedic psychiatry.

The separation of medicine and religion is part of institutional Ayurveda including institutionalized Ayurvedic psychiatry. Although in classical Ayurveda texts and in the local *vaidyam* [traditional Ayurvedic practitioner] tradition of Kerala there was no clear-cut separation between science and religion (Engler 2003) many scholars of Ayurveda (Meulenbeld 1987; Zimmermann 1987; Zysk 1991) as well as Ayurvedic clinicians (including psychiatrists) claimed that classical Ayurveda was scientific in a modern sense. Religious elements in the texts, they argue, were either Vedic remnants or later Brahmanic impositions and as such were marginal, non-essential, or inauthentic.[33] Yet, religious elements and astrology have been part of local vaidyam traditions in Kerala as much as Ayurvedic knowledge was part of astrological classical texts such as the *magnum opus* Prashnamargga which is still the basis of contemporary astrological practice in Kerala. For the modernization and professionalization of Ayurveda, however, institutionalized Ayurveda had to be purified from the religious and "magic" elements.

It had to be "cleansed of esoterica, cleared of contradictions, sanitized of ghosts" and marginalize healing mantras, supramental curing powers, and 'magical' rather than 'rational' uses of substances" (Langford 2002, 17). As described in Chapter 4, Ayurvedic psychiatrists struggle with the supernatural elements in the *bhutavidya* [knowledge of the bhutas] sections of the classic texts and with daivavyapasraya chikitsa as one part of Ayurvedic treatment (in addition to yukti vyapasraya chikitsa and sattvavajaya). For the project of reconfiguring bhutavidya as psychiatry, spirits had to be either excised or translated into mainstream psychiatric terms and thus internalized as aspects of the illness or personality of the patient. The result is an ontological gap that doctors struggle hard to fill with either translation or marginalization. The aim of purification of Ayurvedic psychiatry from spirits and religion and policing the boundaries with religion is to be recognized as scientific and an equally valid approach to mental health as mainstream psychiatry (or superior to it). This process requires translations and the "borrowing of authority" (Varma 2012) from both mainstream psychiatry and Ayurvedic classical texts. For mainstream psychiatrists and other mental health professionals outside Ayurveda, Ayurvedic psychiatry is quackery but Ayurvedic psychiatrists sustain a lively discourse on the genuineness or falseness of different Ayurvedic psychiatric practitioners (Pigg 1996; Langford 1999).

Institutional gate keeping motivates the efforts of Ayurvedic psychiatrists and their students in Kottakkal to control what they call "quacks" or false practitioners. In the context of institutional Ayurvedic psychiatry, "quacks" was a broad and not clearly defined term that might include non-institutionally trained Ayurvedic practitioners, religious healers of any kind, those religious healers without a heritage [parampara],[34] or sometimes practitioners who claimed to practise Ayurvedic psychiatry but had not completed the MD course in psychiatry. Practitioners at GAMH and teachers at the Ayurveda College in Kottakkal had the power of definition over Ayurvedic psychiatry. Institutional Ayurvedic psychiatry thus functions as a gatekeeper of authenticity, determining at once what is Ayurvedic psychiatry and what is quackery. Only those Ayurveda doctors who had completed the Manasika postgraduate course or who worked at GAMH should be regarded as professionals, only their voices counted, only they should be allowed to practise Ayurvedic psychiatry, or so Ayurvedic psychiatrists in Kottakkal argued. This stance made them not only intolerant vis-à-vis other forms of knowledge and training, but also "structurally blind" (Quack 2012; Sax 2014) to non-institutional Ayurvedic mental health care in the same way that mainstream psychiatrists are structurally blind to Ayurvedic psychiatry.

For Dr Rasheed and his colleagues, Dr John simply was not one of them although he was a qualified Ayurveda doctor and had additional qualifications and experience in counselling and mainstream psychiatry. And yet, several doctors who had posts at GAMH were not trained in Ayurvedic psychiatry but in another subfield and they were not judged like Dr John. The description of Dr John's approach and clinical practice demonstrated the uniqueness of his location in the wider world of Ayurvedic psychiatry, which allows for an analysis "from the margins". With this analysis I problematize (or at least add nuance to) homogenizing narratives of the "scientization" of institutional Ayurveda. The case of Dr John, who gently wove together science and religion, helps to make clear an integration of practices that analyses focusing exclusively on the push to institutionalize Ayurveda leave out. Dr John not only explicitly included daivavyapasraya treatment into his "management" of depression and other mental illness; he also reframed "spiritual treatment" in the context of Christian deliverance and exorcism.

Dr John borrowed authority from three sources: modern psychiatry, institutional Ayurvedic psychiatry as it is taught and practised in Kottakkal, and Christian healing. When he used mainstream psychiatric categories such as depressive disorder, conversion, somatization or somatoform disorder he not only displayed mental health literacy and mimicked (Bhabha, 1984; Langford, 1999) mainstream psychiatrists but also borrowed authority (Varma 2012) from them. Dr John not only used the stethoscope, the sphygmomanometer and mainstream psychiatric categories as to borrow biomedical authority and to bestow legitimacy onto his clinical practice: with these "mimetic acts" (Bhabha 1984; Pinto 2004) he also tried to make his clinical practice legible to patients more familiar with biomedical devices and popular psychiatric categories than with the Ayurvedic psychiatry. Moreover, Dr John highlighted his professional standing with regards to counselling and psychotherapy through a diploma, and in modern psychiatry through ten years practice with an allopathic psychiatrist. Furthermore, he not only emphasized his BAMS qualification but also referred to the authority of institutional Ayurvedic psychiatry in Kottakkal and his regular exchange with experts there by participating in their conferences, training programs, and Ayurvedic associations. The third source from which Dr John borrowed authority was Christian healing. He not only reframed daivavyapasraya treatment described as integral in the canonical texts as Christian healing including deliverance prayers or exorcism but also remade Christian healing into a scientific endeavour. With this approach he claimed to be doing more authentic Ayurveda than what was practised and taught in Kottakkal, where spiritual treatment was heavily marginalized.

It is worth noting that in Dr John's clinical practice, Christian healing was established as more "scientific" than Hindu or Muslim practices. Indeed, whereas Dr John legitimized Christian healing as modern and scientific, he denigrated Hindu and Muslim healing as "irrational" and unscientific. Often when talking to his patients, Dr John stressed, "I see the whole thing in a scientific way", or said "Father Kurien has a very scientific approach". How did he justify constructing Christian healing from spirit affliction as science and Hindu and Muslim practices as superstition and irrational? Although he never explicitly justified his position on this, Dr John did his best to convince me. He gave me books such as *An Exorcist Tells his Story* by Father Gabriele Amorth (Amorth 1999) who had been the exorcist in Rome until his death in 1992. He arranged meetings with several priests engaged in different forms of Christian healing and insisted I participate in several sessions of and masses for deliverance from spirits. After Anita's deliverance he told me, "Now you are forced to believe."

There are several other factors that, for Dr John, contribute to the scientific credibility of Christian deliverance prayers and exorcism. Father Kurien, as was the case with many other priests involved in deliverance and exorcism, had mental health literacy, knew the psychiatric and psychological discourse, and engaged psychiatric categories while also transcending them. Moreover Dr John regarded deliverance and exorcism as rational. He often stressed that even the pope had now acknowledged the urgency of professionalization of exorcism globally and introduced a course into Vatican university training. Moreover, while he regarded Hindu and Muslim healing from spirit attacks or spirit possession as locally bounded, for him Christian healing was Western and connected to global Christianity. Finally, for historical reasons Christianity in Kerala is related to modernity, education and development. Many of the private English-medium schools in Kerala and many private hospitals including big mental health centres are Christian. Dr John was engaged in the work of vernacularization (Goodale 2007; Varma 2012) of Ayurvedic psychiatry in a context in which mainstream psychiatry had already been vernacularized and acted as a "more culturally familiar buffer" (Varma 2012, 518) than was Ayurvedic mental health care. Dr John adhered to three paradigms – mainstream psychiatry, Ayurveda and spirit affliction – and smoothly moved between and also merged these three ontological universes. Through his practice and his collaboration with a Christian specialist in removing spirit affliction, Dr John simultaneously promulgated and stabilized depression as neurochemical imbalance, as a doshic imbalance, and as a spirit affliction.

Notes

1 Dr John, Kottayam, 28 August 2009.

2 At a later visit, Dr John told me that his teacher, Dr Shankadevan, also tried to develop a psychotherapeutic approach based on the nine emotions [*rasas*] of classical Sanskrit theatre [*kathakali*] in Kerala. Through rasa therapy he tried to induce opposite emotions such as joy or peace in his psychiatric patients who suffered despondency or anger by animating them to evoke and express these emotions in the way a Kathakali performer does.

3 Dr John, Kottayam, 28 August 2009.

4 The adhi form of unmada is not included in the Caraka Samhita, but it is in Asthangahrdaya Samhita (6.6.15) and Asthanga Samgraha (6.9.2) (Weiss 1977). Of the

three main texts (Caraka, Sushruta and Ashtanga), the Ashtangahrdaya and the second text attributed to the same author (Astanga Samgraha) are most important in Kerala.

5 Dr Mangalam, Kottakkal, 11 March 2011.

6 Bino, Tiruvizha, 11 February 2013.

7 Teachers and students at the Ayurveda College in Kottakkal also differentiated depression related to vata from kaphonmada or endogenous depression. Yet, they did not use an Ayurvedic term for the first but instead called it "mild depression", "neurotic depression", or "depression due to vata".

8 Dr Praveen, Thrissur, 5 August 2009.

9 Dr John, Kottayam, 28 August 2009.

10 Dr Varghese, Kottayam, 18 February 2010.

11 Dr John, Ernakulam, 2 March 2014.

12 This idea of praying to heal the unconscious mind is in stark contrast to psychodynamic ideas of healing as making the unconscious conscious by cognitively working through past experiences and subconscious conflicts that are, of course, no longer mainstream in psychiatry. In the Christian form of healing the subconscious in Kerala, it is not necessary to become aware of past experiences. On the contrary, it would be dangerous and detrimental to mental health to grapple with the traumas of the past. In the first, healing agency lies within oneself, in the second agency is with God. The aim is not to integrate the content of the subconscious into consciousness, as its content is regarded as exogenous and as trivial, as something to get rid of. In this respect, the idea and practice of healing the subconscious through praying resonates with other ideas of removing an exogenous agent perceived to be responsible for the suffering of the person in the context of spirit possession and sorcery. As also in Nura's case (Preface), this is one of many ways in which the Freudian notion of how the subconscious impacts our life is appropriated locally (Tarabout 1999; Halliburton 2009). The content of the subconscious mind has to be removed, it has to be cleaned and purified of unwanted desires and emotions, which can best be achieved through religious – and sometimes psychological – practice.

13 Dr John, Kottayam, 7 March 2014.

14 Ahamkara is one of the different mental faculties alongside discriminating intelligence and mind. Usually translated as self-identification or ego-consciousness, Dr John used the term it to denote selfishness or egotism. In the context of *dalit* [lower caste] ritual healing in Garhwal, the term *hamkar* that derives from the Sanskrit term ahamkara "literally, 'I-ness,' which is associated with egoism, self-interest, and identification with the body" (Sax, Weinhold and Schweitzer 2010) refers to a malevolent spirit or ghost.

15 Cf the discussion of love marriages in "Depression and the medicalization of suicide", Chapter 3).

16 Dr John, Kottayam, 10 March 2014.

17 Dr John, Kottayam, 15 March 2011.

18 Actually, ethnographic evidence shows that kaivisham healing specialists are not interested in what comes out, and often they do not see it. But for patients, the content of the vomit is of high importance.

19 Dr John, Kottayam, 2 April 2010.

20 Dr John, Kottayam, 15 March 2011. Sometimes Dr John used the term "hysteria" when referring to physical symptoms related to depression while at other times he spoke of "somatoform disorder".

21 Dr John, Kottayam, 17 March 2011.

22 Laws in India allow Christian priests to take the responsibility for criminals released on bail.

23 Father Kurien, Kottayam, 26 March 2010.

24 Father Kurien, Kottayam, 26 March 2010.

25 Father Kurien, Kottayam, 19 March 2011.
26 Father Kurien, Kottayam, 27 January 2012.
27 Father Kurien, Kottayam, 27 January 2012.
28 Father Kurien, Kottayam, 27 January 2012.
29 Father Kurien, Kottayam, 26 March 2010. Exorcism requires a fully ordained priest with explicit authorization from the bishop. However, all Catholic priests can make deliverance prayers (a form of prayer against evil spirits without full-scale ritual exorcism). The employment of exorcism has increased in the last ten years or so. There is a sense of urgency among those participating in this movement who have identified a lack of training in exorcism. In 1999, requirements for exorcists were propagated following a series of murders with Satanist overtones. In the same year, an international association of exorcists was founded in Italy, and in alternate years, it sponsored an international conference and an Italian conference for training in spiritual practices. Towards the goal of appointing more exorcists, a training course was launched at the European University of Rome. In 2013, the course attracted 163 participants from 25 countries. A psychiatrist and a psychologist are required by Catholic regulations to consult an exorcist. One of their main tasks is to rule out mental illness prior to recognizing a problem of demonic influence (Csordas 2013). Dr Kurien was well aware of these developments and regulations. Apart from Dr John, he had no other psychiatrist or psychologist with whom he collaborated on diagnosing and treating mental illness. "Who does it here in Kerala?" he asked rhetorically, pointing towards the antagonistic attitude of most professionals against exorcism. Father Kurien told me that in most cases when people come and say, "I am possessed by an evil spirit," after he examines them it turns out that this is not the case. In turn, those who are in fact attacked or possessed often do not formulate it in this way.
30 Father Kurien often used the term "thing" to designate the spirit in her.
31 I did not record this session (audio or video), so for the account of this part of the deliverance, I rely on later discussions with Father Kurien and Anita and their recollections of the session.
32 Dr Rasheed, Kottakkal, 25 January 2013.
33 For a critique of this view see Engler (2003) who argues that Vedic aspects of the texts are too central to be considered inauthentic or marginal.
34 The Nambudiri healers of Poonkudil Mana, a traditional healing centre that combines Ayurveda and mantravadam are generally excluded from the designation "quacks" because they have a *parampara* [tradition].

Glossary[1]

abhicharam a form of occult violence
abhyanga oil bath, massage
abodham unconscious
achara good behaviour
acharya preceptor, teacher
adhi mental stress, mental pain, grief, anguish
adhijonmada mental illness following a loss, reactive depression
adravya drugless
agada tantra toxicology
agantu external
agantu unmada mental illness caused by external agents
agni digestive fire, metabolism
ahamkara ego, self-identification, selfishness
aharam diet
anjanam medicated eyewash
anganwadi lay health worker
anubhava experiential evidence.
anuthailam a classic *yogam* [compound]
apasmara convulsion, epilepsy
aparadha offence, crime
aristham fermented decoction
artha sense objects
avahana removal of spirits
avarana obstruction
ashrama religious centre
ashvagandha *Withania somnifera*, Indian ginseng
asthti bone, cartilage
atman inner self, soul
avastha inner state
avipathi churnam a powder used as a purgative to induce a bowel cleaning motion
ayat Qu'ranic verse
badha spirit, spirit affliction

badha ozhippikkal spirit removal
balam strength
bali sacrifice, offering
bhakti devotion
bharam heaviness
bhasma ash
bhringrai *Eclipta alba*
bhuta being, spirit, ghost, demon, past tense
bhuta chikitsa treatment of *bhutas*
bhuta unmada mental illness related to *bhutas*
bhutavidya knowledge of *bhutas*, Ayurvedic psychiatry
biriyani a fried rice dish
bodham consciousness
bodham illa unconscious
brahmi *Bacopa moneri*
brahmarakshas spirit of a dead Brahmin
branthan mad
branthan jail prison for the mad
buddhi intellect, intuitive intelligence
chesta psychomotor activity
chiktsa treatment
chintu worrying
chitotvega anxiety
chudu heat, anger, grief, romantic or sexual passion
churnam powder
dhyanam Christian healing retreats
dhinacharya daily regimes
daivavyapasraya chikitsa spiritual therapy
dargah a shrine built over the grave of a revered religious figure
deshyam anger or irritation
deva deity
dhara warm oil pouring over the forehead
dharma duty, norm, righteous path, often related to one's fate
dhat semen loss
dhat syndrome semen loss understood as a culture-bound syndrome
dhairya courage
dhatu tissue
dhi short form of *buddhi*
dhuma smoke, fumes
dhumapanam medical smoking
dhupanam fumigation
dosha humour, principle
dosham problem, affliction, fault
dosha unmada mental illness due to an imbalance of the *doshas*
drakshadi churnam an Ayurveda compound

dravyaguna Ayurvedic pharmacology
dukham grief
dur mantravadam black magic
dyanam Christian healing retreats
elassu amulet, talisman
ellam manasika all mental disorders
erichil rising gas or heat in the stomach
gandharva celestial musician
garavisha magic poisoning
gatodvegam hypochondriasis
gavya cow
ghrtam medicated ghee
gokshura *Tribulus terrestris*
graha grasping entity, possession, psychosis
graha chikitsa treatment of *graha*
graha unmada mental illness related to *graha*
gulika hand rolled pill
guna property, quality
gurukula traditional school
hamkara a malevolent spirit
hina sattva deficient *sattva*; a predisposition for mental illness
hingu *Asafoetida, Ferula asafoetida*
homam fire sacrifice
house surgency internship
indriya sense
Inquilab zindabad !
Long live the revolution!
ishtam liking
jatamansi *Nardostachys jatamasni*
jiva soul
jnana knowledge
jyothisham astrology
jyotishi astrologer
jyotishmati *Celastrus paniculatus*
kaivisham magic poisoning, type of sorcery or occult violence
kama erotic love, desire
Kama Deva god of erotic love, desire
kanji soup of broken rice
kantaka shani a difficult phase in his life due to the influence of Saturn
kapha phlegm, stabilizing principle
kaphonmada Ayurvedic disease category denoting a phlegmatic, despondent state often correlated with severe depression
karma actions in this life or in past lives
kashaya vasti enema with fermented decoction
kashayam fermented decoction

kavu small shrine
kaya chikitsa general medicine
kathakali classical Sanskrit theatre
katti knot
kizhi massage with warm herbal poultices
kriyas death ceremonies
krodha anger
kshinam weakness, tiredness
kudotram type of sorcery or occult violence
kuracc a bit
kuracc depression undayirunnu there was a bit of depression
kuttam guilt
kuttabodham guilt consciousness
lakshana characteristics, symptoms
lehyam an Ayurvedic medical preparation
mahapanchagavya ghrtam a medicated ghee, made of the five products of the cow
mahachandanadi thailam an Ayurvedic oil
majja marrow
mamsa muscles
manas mind, emotion
manasamitram vatakam an Ayurvedic *yogam* used mainly for mental health problems and restlessness
manasika mental, psychiatry
manasikarogyasupathri mental hospital
manasikarogyakendram mental health centre
manasika asukham lack of mental well-being
manasika bhavas mental states
manasika doctors doctors of the mind
manasika OPD psychiatric outpatient clinic
manasika rogam mental illness, mental disease, mental disorder
manasika tension mental tension
manasika vibranthi mental difficulties
manasikam mental
manasikaprakrti mental constitution
manasu heart, mind
mano vigyan avum mano rogam literally "knowledge of the mind and mental illness", often synonymous with Ayurvedic psychiatry or manasika
manobalam will power, mental power, mental strength
manodurbalam lack of *manobalam*
manovahashrotas specific channels that carry thoughts, ideas, and emotions
manovikaras abnormal emotional conditions, overflowing emotions or passions
mantra syllable, word or verse
mantravadam magic, sorcery

mantravadi Hindu healer
marma vital point
marumakkatayam matrilineal joint family practices of residence, descent and inheritance
marunnum mantravum medicine and *mantras*
mattam change
medas fat
medhya mind booster
medhya rasayana mind rejuvenating
mishra integrated
mujahid post-1950s Islamic reformers and proponents of rationality, science, education and progress
murukku tightness, twisted, stiff, hot, constipated
musliyar Muslim priest
nadu marunnu folk medicine in Kerala
naga snake spirit
nakshatra birth star
namaz Muslim daily prayers
nara nerve
nasyam nasal drops to eliminate *kapha* from the head
nellika thalam head application of Indian gooseberry
nenchil kettu knot on the chest
nenjinn bharam heaviness in the chest
nenju chest
nenju edippu racing pulse
nenjinn vedana chest pain
neyy ghee, clarified butter
nidana etiology
nija internal
nilavilakku a religious lamp
ojakshaya depletion of the vital essence of the metabolic process
ojas vital essence
orkkam sleep
orkkam illa lack of sleep
paisachu ghost
pancha five
panchagavya ghrtam a ghee made of the five products of the cow
panchakarma literally the five treatments, consisting classically of the purifying procedures vomiting, enema, purgation, nasal purification and blood letting, and certain pre- and additional procedures
panikkar astrologer
parampara hereditary, lineage
parampara dosha intergenerational fault
para a measurement of weight, about 10 kg
pathashala traditional school

pathyam Ayurvedic diet recommendations
pathyahara unhealthy food habits
peti fear
perippu tingling, numbness
petichu scared
petikkuka to scare or shock
pharma wallahs pharmaceutical sellers in the pharmacies
picchu oil application on the head
pitre ancestor
pippali *Piper longum*
pitta bile, heal, transforming principle
pittonmada a state characterized by excessive emotions or passions
pokachile a burning sensation
prabhava specific effect
prajna wisdom or intelligence
prajnaparadha offence against wisdom, moral trangsgression
prakrti constitution, matter, nature, healthy state
prana breath, life force
pranayama breathing exercises, part of Asthanga yoga
prashnangal difficulties
prashnam problem-oriented horoscope
pravara sattva strong sattva
pravaram, madhyam or hina strong, medium or weak, respectively
preta spirit of a dead person
preta badham affliction by the spirit of a soul who died a of bad death or of suicide
puja prayer, ritual of reverence
punyaham a cleaning ritual
purusha consciousness without content or quality
rajas activity
rajasika predominance of *rajas*
raktavahashrotas blood carrying channels
rasa lymph, plasma, taste, emotion
rakta blood, haemoglobin
rasayana rejuvenation aiming at nourishing the tissues
rasam a vegetable soup with a tamarind juice base
rogam disease
saar a respectful form of addressing a doctor or superior
samadhi higher consciousness
samana dosha pacifying
sambandham customary institution that framed sexual relations between men and women in matrilineal communities
samnipadunmada mental illness due to the vitiation of all three *doshas*
sampoorna manasikarogyam mental health for all
samprapti pathogenesis, the course of the disease

samsayarogam the illness of doubt
sankadam sadness
sannipadonmada mental illness involving the vitiation of all three *doshas*
sarpam serpent spirit, deity
sarpa dosham affliction related to the serpent deity
sarpa kavu snake shrine
sarpagandha *Rauwolfia serpentina*
sattvabalam mental strength
sattvavajaya Ayurvedic psychotherapy, controlling or disciplining the mind
sattva purity
sattvika predominance of *sattva*
shaithan satan
shalya chikitsa surgery
shankhpushpa *Convolvulus pluricaulis*
shankhupushpa *Clitoria ternate*
shantam a balanced mental and emotional state, peace
shanti priest
sharira body
shastra the classical texts
shastric scholastic
shila habits, temperaments
shirodhara pouring medicated oil onto the forehead
shiroshodanam head purification
shodana purifying
shrotas channels
shukra semen and reproductive tissues
shunyata emptiness
shrungataka simanta marma a vital point
smrti memory
sneham care, affection, grease, unctuousness
snehapanam drinking of medicated ghee in large quantities
snehavasti enema with oil or ghee
suddha pure
sukham health, well-being
sukham illa I am not well
surat chapter of the Qu'ran
svedana steam therapy
thakkidu protective amulet
takrapanam the drinking of large quantities of buttermilk to make the body dry and rough
tala vedana headache
talapodichil medicated mudpack for the head made with Indian gooseberry and other ingredients
taluk sub-district
tamas ignorance

tamasika predominance of *tamas*
tapas literally heat; also meditation, austerity, discipline
tashibiya Islamic prayer beads
tenshan tension
thailavasti oil enema
thailikk bharam heaviness in the head
thakradhara pouring medicated buttermilk on the forehead
thala chudu heat in the head
thalam oil application on the head
thangal Muslim healer
thairippu tingling or numbness in the head
thechippoo a flower used for *puja*
tikshna penetrating
tridosha three *doshas*
tullal possession
ulvaliyuka introvert
unmada madness, mental illness
upayangal drugless remedial practice
ustad Muslim scholar
vacha *Acorus calamus*
vaidya traditional Ayurvedic practitioner
vamana therapeutic vomiting
vashyam sweets given to seduce a woman
vasti enema
vastu architecture
vata wind, moving principle
vatonmada a state characterized by unsteadiness of thought and emotions and psychotic features
vatta crazy
vayu wind
vazhipadu offering
vedana ache, pain
vega emotion, motion
velichappadu Hindu oracle
veshamam sadness
virya potency
viharam daily activities
vijnana specific knowledge
vikara abnormal condition
vilwadi gulika a classic Ayurveda compound
vipak post-metabolic effect
virechanam purging
vishada, vishadam depression, confusion, melancholia
vishada avastha a state of depression, confusion or melancholia
vishada rogam depression, depressive disorder

vishada yogam yoke of *vishadam*
utkanta anxiety
vishonmada mental affliction due to toxins
vishvasam faith or belief
vishvasa chikitsa faith or religious treatment
vyadhi disease
yogam union, compound
yukti logical inference or reason; rationality
yuktivyapasraya chikitsa rational treatment

Note

1 Whenever English terms were used in Malayalam speech, I set them in italics. I have used Malayalam terms so frequently because translations are not necessarily direct or straightforward. The translations in the glossary and throughout the text are therefore rough to serve a first approximation. Malayalam is the language spoken by the inhabitants of Kerala.

References

Abraham, D. (2009). *A Comparative Study on an Ayurvedic Compound (J J Tablet) Against SSRI Groups of Antidepressant Drug in Moderate Depression.* Kottakkal: Vaidyaratnam P.S. Varier Ayurveda College Kottakkal.

Adams, V. (2002). Randomized Controlled Crime: Postcolonial Sciences in Alternative Medicine Research. *Social Studies of Science*, 32(5–6), 659–690.

Addlakha, R. (2008). *Deconstructing Mental Illness. An Ethnography of Psychiatry, Women, and the Family.* New Delhi: Kali for Women.

Agrawal, P. & Saibaba, P. (2001). TRIPS and India's Pharmaceuticals Industry. *Economic and Political Weekly*, 36(39), 3787–3790.

Ahmed, S. (2007). The Happiness Turn. *New Formations*, 63, 7–15.

Alter, J. S. (1999). Heaps of Health, Metaphysical Fitness. Ayurveda and the Ontology of Good Health in Medical Anthropology. *Current Anthropology*, 40 Supplement, 43–66.

Amorth, G. (1999). *An Exorcist Tells His Story.* San Francisco: Ignatius Press.

Anwar, K. S. (2004). *A Study on Kaphonmada in Relation with Depressive Disorders.* Kottakkal: Vaidyaratnam P.S. Varier Ayurveda College Kottakkal.

Appadurai, A. (1986). *The Social Lives of Things. Commodities in Cultural Perspective.* Cambridge, UK: Cambridge University Press.

Appadurai, A. (1996). Introduction. Commodities and the Politics of Value. In A. Appadurai (Ed.), *The Social Life of Things. Commodities in Cultural Perspective* (pp. 3–63). Cambridge, MA: Cambridge University Press.

Appadurai, A. & Breckenridge, C. L. (1988). Why Public Culture? *Public Culture*, 1(1), 5–9.

Applbaum, K. (2006). *Educating for Global Mental Health. The Adoption of SSRIs in Japan.* In A. Petryna, A. Lakoff & A. Kleinman (Eds.), *Global Pharmaceuticals. Ethics, Markets, Practices* (pp. 85–110). Durham & London: Duke University Press.

Arunima, G. (2003). *There Comes Papa: Colonialism and the Transformation of Matriliny in Kerala, Malabar, c. 1850–1940.* New Delhi: Orient BlackSwan.

Ayurveda Medical Association of India. (2013). *Suggestions for Additions in Health Policy.* Retrieved from www.ayurveda-amai.org/suggestions-for-additions-in-health-policy/, 5 April 2014.

Baer, R. D. & Bustillo, M. (1993). Susto and Mal de Ojo among Florida Farmworkers: Emic and Etic Perspectives. *Medical Anthropology Quarterly*, 7(1), 90–100.

Balanchandran, E. (1998). Kerala. A Consumption Society in Distress. *Economic and Political Weekly*, 33(42–43), 2700.

Banerjee, M. (2002). Power, Culture, and Medicine: Ayurvedic Pharmaceuticals in the Modern Market. *Contributions to Indian Sociology*, 36(3), 435–467.

Banerjee, M. (2008). Ayurveda in Modern India: Standardization and Pharmaceuticalization. In D. Wujastyk & F. S. Smith (Eds.), *Global and Modern Ayurveda. Pluralism and Paradigms*. Albany: State University of New York Press.

Basu, H. (2014). Davā and Duā. Negotiating Psychiatry and Ritual Healing of Madness. In H. Naraindas, J. Quack & W. S. Sax (Eds.), *Asymmetrical Conversations. Contestations, Circumventions, and the Blurring of Therapeutic Boundaries* (pp. 162–199). New York, Oxford: Beghahn Books.

BBC News. (2010). Kerala's Love Affair with Alcohol. Retrieved from http://news.bbc.co.uk/2/hi/south_asia/8557215.stm, 8 April 2014.

Bemme, D. & D'Souza, N. A. (2014). Global Mental Health and Its Discontents: An Inquiry into the Making of Global and Local Scale. *Transcult Psychiatry*, 51(6), 850–874.

Benyamin (2008). *Goat Days*. New Delhi: Penguin Books.

Bhabha, H. (1984). Of Mimicry and Man. The Ambivalence of Colonial Discourse. *October*, 28, 125–133.

Bhattacharyya, D. (1986). *Pagalami. Ethnopsychiatric Knowledge in Bengal*. Syracuse, NY: Maxwell School of Citizenship and Public Affairs.

Bhatia, S.C., Madabushi, J., Kolli, V., Bhatia, S. K. & Madaan, V. (2013). The Bhagavad Gita and Contemporary Psychotherapies. *Indian Journal of Psychiatry* 55(6), 315–321.

Bhugra, D. & Mastrogianni, A. (2004). Globalisation and Mental Disorders. Overview with Relation to Depression. *British Journal of Psychiatry* (184), 10–20.

Biehl, J. (2006). Pharmaceutical Governance. In A. Petryna, A. Lakoff & A. Kleinman (Eds.), *Global Pharmaceuticals. Ethics, Markets, Practices* (pp. 206–239). Durham & London: Duke University Press.

Blum, L. M. & Stracuzzi, N. F. (2004). Gender in the Prozac Nation Popular Discourse and Productive Femininity. *Gender & Society*, 18(3), 269–286.

Bode, M. (2002). Indian Indigenous Pharmaceuticals. Tradition, Modernity and Nature. In W. Ernst (Ed.), *Plural Medicine, Tradition and Modernity, 1800–2000*. London and New York: Routledge.

Bode, M. (2006). Taking Traditional Knowledge to the Market: The Commoditization of Indian Medicine. *Anthropology & Medicine*, 13(3), 225–236.

Bode, M. (2015). Assembling Cyavanaprash, Ayurveda's Best-selling Medicine. *Anthropology & Medicine, 22*(1), 23–33. doi:10.1080/13648470.2015.1005285

Bode, M. & Payyappallimanna, U. (2013). Evidence Based Traditional Medicine: For Whom and to What End? *e-journal of Indian Medicine*, 6, 1–20.

Brass, P. (1972). The Politics of Ayurvedic Education. A Case Study of Revivalism and Modernization in India. In S. Hoeber Rudolph & L. I. Rudolph (Eds.), *Education and Politics in India. Studies in Organization, Society, and Policy* (pp. 342–549). Cambridge, MA: Harvard University Press.

Breggin, P. (2001). *The Anti-Depressant Fact Book: What Your Doctor Won't Tell You About Prozac, Zoloft, Paxil, Celexa, and Luvox*. Cambridge, MA: Perseus Books.

Briggs, C. & Hallin, D. C. (2007). Biocommunicability. The Neoliberal Subject and its Contradictions in News Coverage of Health Issues. *Social Text 93*, 25(4), 43–66.

Brives, C. (2013). Identifying Ontologies in a Clinical Trial. *Social Studies of Science*, 43(3), 397–416.

Bromet, E.*et al*. (2011). Cross-national epidemiology of DSM-IV major depressive episode. *BMC Med, 9*, 90. doi:10.1186/1741-7015-9-90.

Brosius, C. (2010). *India's Middle Class. New Forms of Urban Leisure, Consumption and Prosperity*. New Delhi: Routledge.

Callan, A. (2012). *Patients and Agents. Mental Illness, Modernity and Islam in Sylhet, Bangladesh*. New York, Oxford: Berghahn.

Callon, M. & Latour, B. (1981). Unscrewing the Big Leviathan. How Actors Macro-Structure Reality and How Sociologists Help Them to Do So. In K. Knorr-Cetina & A. V. Cicourel (Eds.), *Advances in Social Theory and Methodology* (pp. 277–303). London: Routledge and Kegan Paul.

Cameron, M. (2008). Modern Desires, Knowledge Control, and Physician Resistance: Regulating Ayurvedic Medicine in Nepal. *Asian Medicine*, 4, 86–112.

Chakrabarty, V. (2013). *Indian Architectural Theory. Contemporary Uses of Vastu Vidya*. Richmond: Curzon Press.

Chandra, S. (Producer). (2011). Status of Indian Medicine and Folk Healing. [Report, 9 May 2016] Retrieved from http://reporttraditionalindianmedicine.blogspot.com/2011/10/status-of-indian-medicine-and-folk.htm , 15 June 2016.

Chopra, A. (n.d.) Asymmetrical Translations in Contemporary Ayurvedic Nosology.

Choudhury, S. & Kirmayer, L. J. (2009). Cultural Neuroscience And Psychopathology: Prospects For Cultural Psychiatry. *Progress in Brain Research*, 178, 263–283.

Choudhury, S. & Slaby, J. (Eds.). (2012). *Critical Neuroscience. A Handbook of the Social and Cultural Contexts of Neuroscience*. Wiley: Blackwell.

Chua, J. L. (2009). *The Productivity of Death. The Social and Political Life of Suicide in Kerala, South India*. Stanford: Stanford University.

Chua, J. L. (2011). Making Time for the Children. Self-Temporalization and the Cultivation of the Antisuicidal Subject in South India. *Cultural Anthropology*, 26, 112–137.

Chua, J. L. (2013). Reaching Out to the People. The Cultural Production of Mental Health Professionalism in the South Indian Public Sphere. *Ethos*, 41(4), 341–359.

Chua, J. L. (2014). *In Pursuit of the Good Life: Aspiration and Suicide in Globalizing South India*Berkeley, Los Angeles, London: University of California Press.

Clarke, A. E., Shim, J. K., Mamo, L., Fosket, J. R. & Fishman, J. R. (2010). Biomedicalization. Technoscientific Transformations of Health, llness, and U.S. Biomedicine. In A. E. Clarke, L. Mamo, J. R. Fosket, J. R. Fishman & J. K. Shim (Eds.), *Biomedicalization. Technoscience, Helth, and Illness in the U.S.* (pp. 47–87). Durham and London: Duke University Press.

Cleetus, B. (2007). Subaltern Medicine and Social Mobility: The Experience of Ezhavas in Kerala. *Indian Anthropologist, 37*(1), 142–172.

Cohen, D. & Jacobs, D. H. (2007). Randomized Controlled Trials of Antidepressants. Clinically and Scientifically Irrelevant. *Debates in Neuroscience*, 1, 44–54.

Cohen, D., McCubbin, M., Collin, J. & Pérodeau, G. (2001). Medications as Social Phenomena. *Health*, 5(4), 441–469.

Cohen, L. (1995). The Epistemological Carnival: Meditations on Disciplinary Intentionality and Ayurveda. In D. Bates (Ed.), *Knowledge and the Scholarly Medical Traditions* (pp. 320–344). Cambridge, UK: Cambridge University Press.

Cohen, L. (1998). *Alzhymer's, the Bad Family, and Other Modern Things*. Berkeley, Los Angeles, London: University of California Press.

Csordas, T. J. (1997). *The Sacred Self. A Cultural Phenomenology of Charismatic Healing*. Berkeley, Los Angeles, London: University of California Press.

Csordas, T. J. (2013). The Contemporary Resurgence of Exorcism as a Catholic Healing Practice. Paper presented at Encounters and Engagements: Creating New Agendas for Medical Anthropology, Tarragona, 13 June 2013.

Cussins, C. (1996). Ontological Choreography: Agency through Objectification in Infertility Clinics. *Social Studies of Science*, 26(3), 575–610.

Daniel, V. E. (1984). *Fluid Signs. Being a Person the Tamil Way*. Berkeley: University of California Press.

de Laet, M. & Mol, A. (2000). The Zimbabwe Bush Pump. Mechanics of a Fluid Technology. *Social Studies of Science*, 30(2), 225–263.

Deleuze, G. & Guattari, F. (1987). *A Thousand Plateaus. Capitalism and Schizophrenia*. Minneapolis, London: University of Minnesota Press.

Department of AYUSH, Government of Kerala (2016). Kerala AYUSH Health Policy 2016 (Report). Retrieved from www.meditv.in/ayush.pdf

Desjarlais, R., Eisenberg, L., Good, B. & Kleinman, A. (1995). *World Mental Health: Problems and Priorities in Low-income Countries*. New York: Oxford University Press.

Devika, J. (2007). *En-Gendering Individuals. The Language of Re-Forming in Early Twentieth Century Keralam*. New Delhi: Orient Longman.

Dumont, L. (1980). *Homo Hierarchicus. The Caste System and Its Implications*. Chicago & London: University of Chicago Press.

Eapen, M. (2002). Mental Health of Women in Kerala. *Samyukta*, 2(2), 25–35.

Eapen, M. & Kodoth, P. (2003). Family Structure, Women's Education and Work. Re-Examining the "High Status" of Women in Kerala. In S. Mukhopadhyay & R. Sudarshan (Eds.), *Tracking Gender Equity under the Economic Reforms. Ontinuity and Change in South Asia* (pp. 227–267). New Delhi: Kali for Women.

Ecks, S. (2004). Bodily Sovereignty as Political Sovereignty. "Self-Care" in Kolkata, India. *Anthropology & Medicine*, 11(1), 75–89.

Ecks, S. (2005). Pharmaceutical Citizenship: Antidepressant Marketing and the Promise of Demarginalization in India. *Anthropology & Medicine*, 12(3), 239–254.

Ecks, S. (2008). Three Propositions for an Evidence-Based Medical Anthropology. *Journal of the Royal Anthropological Institute*, S77–S92.

Ecks, S. (2011). Polyspherical Pharmaceuticals: Global Psychiatry, Capitalism, and Space. In J. H. Jenkins (Ed.), *Pharmaceutical Self: the Global Shaping of Experience in an Age of Psychopharmacology* (pp. 97–116). Santa Fe, NM: School for Advanced Research Press.

Ecks, S. (2013). *Eating Drugs. Psychopharmaceutical Pluralism in South Asia*. New York & London: New York University Press.

Ecks, S. & Basu, S. (2009). The Unlicensed Lives of Antidepressants in India. Generic Drugs, Unqualified Practitioners, and Floating Prescriptions. *Transcultural Psychiatry*, 46(1), 86–106.

Ecks, S. & Basu, S. (2011). How Wide is the Treatment Gap for Antidepressants in India? Ethnographic Insights on Marketing Strategies. *Journal of Health Studies*, 2, 68–80.

Ecks, S. & Sax, W. S. (2005). The Ills of Marginality: New Perspectives on Health in South Asia. *Anthropoly & Medicine*, 12(3), 199–210.

Eisenberg, Leon (1977). Disease and Illness. Distinctions between Professional and Popular Ideas of Sickness. *Culture, Medicine & Psychiatry* 1(1), 9–23.

Elliott, C. (2004). Introduction. Prozac as a Way of Life. In C. Elliott & T. Chambers (Eds.), *Prozac as a Way of Life* (pp. 1–18). Chapel Hill and London: University of North Carolina Press.

Engel, G. L. (1977). The Need for a New Medical Model: A Challenge for Biomedicine. *Science* 196, 129–136.

Engler, S. (2003). "Science" vs. "Religion" in Classical Ayurveda. *Numen*, 50.

Ernst, W. (2007). Madness and Colonial Spaces – British India, c. 1800–1947. In J. Moran, L. Topps & J. Andrews (Eds.), *Madness, Architecture and the Built Environment. Psychiatric Spaces in Historical Context* (pp. 215–238). London, UK: Routledge.

Exotic India (Producer). (2016, 23 June 2016). Stresscom Ashvagandha Capsules. Retrieved from www.exoticindiaart.com/product/ayurveda/stresscom-ashvagandha-capsules-for-stress-strain-fatigue-combats-price-per-strip-of-10-capsules-AMH06/ , 15 August 2016.

Fabrega, H. J. (2009). *History of Mental Illness in India: A Cultural Psychiatry Retrospective*. Delhi: Motilal Basarsidass Publishers.

Farmer, P. (1990). Sending Sickness: Sorcery, Politics, and Changing Concepts of AIDS in Rural Haiti. *Medical Anthropology Quarterly*, 4(1), 6–27.

Fernando, S. (1991). *Mental Health, Race and Culture*London: Palgrave Macmillan.

Foucault, M. (1973). *The Birth of the Clinic. An Archeaology of Medical Perception*. London: Tavistock Publications

Foucault, M. (1982). The Subject and Power. In H. L. Dreyfus & P. Rabinow (Eds.), *Michel Foucault: Beyond Structuralism and Hermeneutics* (pp. 208–226). Chicago: University of Chicago Press.

Foucault, M. (1988). *The Care of the Self*. New York: Vintage Books.

Frances, A. (2013). *Saving Normal: An Insider's Revolt Against Out-Of-Control Psychiatric Diagnosis, DSM-5, Big Pharma, and the Medicalization of Ordinary Life*. New York: HarperCollins Publishers.

Frank, R. & Stollberg, G. (2004). Conceptualising Hybridisation: On the Diffusion of Asian Medical Knowledge to Germany. *International Sociology*, 19, 71–88.

Friedman, L., Furberg, C. D., DeMets, D. L., Reboussin, D. M. & GrangerC. B. (1998). *Fundamentals of Clinical Trials*, Heidelberg et al: Springer.

Fuller, C. J. (1976a). Kerala Christians and the Caste System. *Man, New Series*, 11(1), 53–70.

Fuller, C. J. (1976b). *The Nayars Today*. New York: Cambridge University Press.

Ganguly, R. (2012). *Staging "Open-Minded Science": Culture and Evidence in Contemporary Ayurvedic Laboratory Research in India*. Minnesota: University of Minnesota.

Ganguly, R. (2014). Sense and Evidence. *Asian Medicine*, 9(1–2), 102–140.

Gaudillère, J.-P. (2014). Herbalized Ayurveda? *Asian Medicine*, 9(1–2), 171–205.

Gaudillière, J.-P. (2015). Marketing Loops. Clinical Research, Consumption of Antidepressants and the Reorganization of Promotion at Geigy in the 1960s and 1970s. In J.-P. Gaudillère & U. Thoms (Eds.), *The Development of Scientific Marketing*. London & New York: Routledge.

Geertz, C. (1974). From the Natives' Point of View. On the Nature of Anthropological Understanding. *Bulletin of the American Academy of Arts and Sciences*, 28, 26–45.

Geetha, C. (2014). Malayali Sthreekalude Manas [The Mind of a Malayali Woman]. *Arogya Masika*, 1 June.

Giguère, N. (2009). Dosa, Satvabalam, Genes, and Pūjā. A God for Everything. An Ethnographic Study of a Government Ayurvedic Mental Hospital. In B. Sébastia (Ed.), *Restoring Mental Health in India: Pluralistic Therapies and Concepts* (pp. 48–70). Delhi: Oxford University Press.

Goffman, E. (1963). *Stigma. Notes on the Management of Spoiled Identity*. London: Penguin.

Good, B. (1977). The Heart of What's the Matter. *Culture, Medicine and Psychiatry*, 1, 25–38.

Good, B. (1994). *Medicine, Rationality, and Experience: An Anthropological Perspective*. Cambridge et al: Cambridge University Press.

Good, B., Good, M.-J. D. & Moradi, R. (1985). The Interpretation of Iranian Depressive Illness and Dysphoric Affect. In A. Kleinman & B. Good (Eds.), *Culture and*

Depression. Studies in the Anthropology and Cross-Cultural Psychiatry of Affect and Disorder (pp. 369–428). Berkeley, Los Angeles, London: University of California Press.

Goodale, M. & Merry, S. E. (2007). *The Practice of Human Rights*. Cambridge: Cambridge University Press.

Gough, K. (1959). The Nayars and the Definition of Marriage. *Journal of American Folklore*, 71, 23–34.

Granado, S., Manderson, L., Obrist, B. & Tanner, M. (2011). Appropriating "Malaria": Local Responses to Malaria Treatment and Prevention in Abidjan, Cote d'Ivoire. *Med Anthropol*, 30(1), 102–121.

Gulati, L. & Rajan, S. I. (1991). *Population Aspects of Aging in Kerala. Their Economic and Social Context*. Thiruvananthapuram, India: Center for Development Studies.

Gulati, L. & Rajan, S. I. (1993). *In the Absence of their Men. The Impact of Male Migration on Women*. New Delhi: Sage Publications.

Gupta, M. (2007). Does Evidence-based Medicine Apply to Psychiatry? *Theoretical Medicine and Bioethics*, 28(2), 103–120.

Hacking, I. (1995). *Rewriting the Soul. Multiple Personality and the Sciences of Memory*. Princeton, NJ: Princeton University Press.

Hacking, I. (2002). *Historical Ontology*. Cambridge, MA: Harvard University Press.

Hacking, I. (2007). Kinds of People. Moving Targets. *Proceedings of the British Academy*, 151, 285–318.

Hahn, H.-P. (2004). Global Goods and the Process of Appropriation. In P. Probst & G. Spittler (Eds.), *Between Resistance and Expansion. Explorations of Local Vitality in Africa* (pp. 213–231). Münster: LIT Verlag.

Halliburton, M. (1998). Suicide: A Paradox of Development in Kerala. *Economic and Political Weekly, 33*(36/37), 2341–2345.

Halliburton, M. (2004). Finding a Fit: Psychiatric Pluralism in South India and its Implications for WHO Studies of Mental Disorder. *Transcultural Psychiatry*, 41(1), 80–98.

Halliburton, M. (2005). "Just some spirits": the erosion of spirit possession and the rise of "tension" in South India. *Medical Anthropoly*, 24(2), 111–144.

Halliburton, M. (2009). *Mudpacks & Prozac. Experiencing Ayurvedic, Biomedical & Religious Healing*. Walnut Creek, CA: Left Coast Press.

Halliburton, M. (2011). Resistance or Inaction? Protecting Ayurvedic Medical Knowledge and Problems of Agency. *American Ethnologist*, 38(1), 86–101.

Hamilton, M. (1989). Frequency of Symptoms in Melancholia (Depressive Illness). *British Journal of Psychiatry*, 154, 201–206.

Hapke, H. M. (2013). Theorizing Patriarchy: Development Paradoxes and the Geography of Gender in South Asia. *Gender, Technology, and Development*, 17(1), 1–29.

Harilal, M. S. (2009). "Commercialising Traditional Medicine". Ayurvedic Manufacturing in Kerala. *Economic and Political Weekly*, 44(16), 44–51.

Hartnack, C. (2001). *Psychoanalysis in Colonial India*. Delhi: Oxford University Press.

Healy, D. (1997). *The Antidepressant Era*. Boston:Harvard University Press.

Healy, D. (2004). *Let Them Eat Prozac*. New York: New York University Press.

Healy, D. (2006). The New Medical Oikumene. In A. Petryna, A. Lakoff & A. Kleinman (Eds.), *Global Pharmaceuticals. Ethics, Markets, Practices* (pp. 61–84). Durham & London: Duke University Press.

Healy, D. (2015). Serotonin and Depression. The Marketing of a Myth. *British Medical Journal*, 1771.

Heaton, M. M. (2013). *Black Skin, White Coats. Nigerian Psychiatrists, Decolonization, and the Globalization*Athens: Ohio University Press.
Holbraad, M. (2009). Ontography and Alterity: Defining Anthropological Truth. *Social Analysis*, 53(2), 80–93.
Horwitz, A. V. (2010). How an Age of Anxiety Became an Age of Depression. *Milbank Quartery*, 88(1): 112–138.
Horwitz, A. V. & Wakefield, J. C. (2007). *The Loss of Sadness. How Psychiatry Transformed Normal Sorrow into Depressive Disorder*. New York: Oxford University Press.
Illich, I. (1975). The Medicalization of Life. *Journal of Medical Ethics*, 1, 73–77.
Indu, P.V. (2014). Varthikkitile vishada rogam [Depression In Old Age]. *Arogya Masika*, 1 April.
Insel, T. R. (2014). The NIMH Research Domain Criteria (RDoC) Project: precision medicine for psychiatry. *American Journal of Psychiatry*, 171(4), 395–397.
Isaac, Mohan, Kapur, R. L., Chandrasekhar, C. R., Kapur, M.& Pathasarathy, R.(1982). Mental Health Delivery Through Rural Primary Care: Development and Evaluation of a Training Programme. *Indian Journal of Psychiatry*, 24(2), 131–138.
Jackson, S. W. (1986). *Melancholia and Depression: From Hippocratic Times to Modern Times*. New Haven: Yale University Press.
Jadhav, S. (2000). The Cultural Construction of Western Depression. In V. Skultans & J. Cox (Eds.), *Anthropological Approaches to Psychological Medicine. Crossing Bridges* (pp. 41–65). London and Philadelphia: Jessica Kinsley Publishers.
Jadhav, S. & Littlewood, R. (1995). Defeat Depression Campaign: Attitudes to Depression. *Psychiatric Bulletin*, 19(4), 259–260.
Jain, S. & Jadhav, S. (2008). A Cultural Critique of Community Psychiatry in India. *Int J Health Serv*, 38(3), 561–584.
Jain, S. & Jadhav, S. (2009). Pills That Swallow Policy: Clinical Ethnography of a Community Mental Health Program in Northern India. *Transcult Psychiatry*, 46(1), 60–85.
Jansen, E. & Lang, C. (2012). Transforming the Self and Healing the Body Through the Use of Testimonies in a Divine Retreat Center, Kerala. *Journal of Religion and Health*, 51(2), 542–551.
Jayaprakash, R. (2009) Manasika rogatinde thettudharana [Misconceptions about Mental Illness]. *Arogya Masika*, 1 June.
Jeffrey, C. (2010). *Timepass. Youth, Class, and the Politics of Waiting in India*. Stanford, CA: Stanford University Press.
Jeffrey, R. (1992). *Politics, Women and Well-Being. How Kerala Became "a Model"*. Houndsmills, UK: Macmillan Press.
Jeffrey, R. (1997). Malayalam: "The Day-to-Day Social Life of the People". *Economic and Political Weekly*, 32(1–2), 18–21.
Jeffrey, R. (2004). Legacies of Matriliny: The Place of Women and the "Kerala Model". *Pacific Affairs*, 77(4), 647–664.
Jenkins, J. H. (1988). Ethnopsychiatric Interpretations of Schizophrenic Illness: The Problem of Nervios within Mexican-American Families. *Culture, Medicine, and Psychiatry*, 12(3), 303–331.
Jenkins, J. H. (2011). Psychopharmaceutical Self and Imaginary in the Social Field of Psychiatric Treatment. In J. H. Jenkins (Ed.), *Pharmaceutical Self. The Global Shaping of Experience in an Age of Psychopharmacology* (pp. 17–40). Santa Fe, NM: School for Advanced Research Press.

John, C. J. (2009). Chikitsayedukkunnathinu Munpu [Before Seeking Treatment]. *Arogya Masika*, 1 June.

John, C. J. (2010). Vishadathal Chuttappedunna Keralam (Depression Engulfs Kerala). *Arogya Masika*, 1 April.

John, C. J. (2014). Kanneeru Kutikkunna Sthreekal [Women Who Drink Tears]. *Arogya Masika*, 1 April.

Kakar, S. (1982). *Shamans, Mystics, and Doctors. A Psychological Inquiry Into India and Its Healing Traditions*. Chicago: University of Chicago Press.

Kallivayalil, R. A. (2012). The Importance of Psychiatry in Undergraduate Medical Education in India. *Indian Journal of Psychiatry*, 54(3), 208–216.

Kapur, R. L. (2004) The Story of Community Mental Health in India. In S. P. Agarwal, D. S. Goel, R. L. Ichhpujani, R. N. Salhan & S. Shrivastava (Eds.). *Mental Health. An Indian Perspective 1946–2003* (pp. 92–100). New Delhi: Elsevier for Directorate General of Health Services, Ministry of Health and Family Welfare.

Kerala University of Health Sciences. (2012). Regulations, Curriculum and Syllabus of Postgraduate Course (MD/MS) in Ayurveda, Thrissur. Available at: http://14.139.185.154/files/syllabus/2010_11/PGAy/mdayur.pdf

Kirmayer, L. J. (1988). Mind and Body as Metaphors. Hidden Values in Biomedicine. In M. Lock & D. Gordon (Eds.), *Biomedicine Examined* (pp. 57–93). Dordrecht, Boston, London: Kluwer Academic Publishers.

Kirmayer, L. J. (2002). Psychopharmacology in a Globalizing World: The Use of Antidepressants in Japan. *Transcultural Psychiatry*, 39(3).

Kirmayer, L. J. & Gold, I. (2011). Re-Socializing Psychiatry. In S. Choudhury & J. Slaby (Eds.), *Critical Neuroscience: A Handbook of the Social and Cultural Contexts of Neuroscience*. Oxford, UK: Wiley-Blackwell.

Kirmayer, L. J. & Minas, H. (2000). The Future of Cultural Psychiatry: An International Perspective. *Canadian Journal of Psychiatry*, 45(5), 438–446.

Kirmayer, L. J. & Pedersen, D. (2014). Toward a New Architecture for Global Mental Health. *Transcult Psychiatry*, 51(6), 759–776.

Kishore, A. N. R., Shaji, K. S. & Praveenlal, K. (2010). Revalidation: Are we Meeting Training Needs? Training and its Influence on the Practice of Child Psychiatry and Psychotherapy. *Indian Journal of Psychological Medicine*, 32(1), 3–6.

Kitanaka, J. (2012). *Depression in Japan. Psychiatric Cures for a Society in Distress*. Princeton and Oxford: Princeton University Press.

Kleinman, A. (1977). Depression, Somatization and the "New Cross-Cultural Psychiatry". *Social Science & Medicine*, 11(1), 3–10.

Kleinman, A. (1980). *Patients and Healers in the Context of Culture*. Berkeley, CA: University of California Press.

Kleinman, A. (1982). Neurasthenia and Depression: A Study of Somatization and Culture in China. *Culture, Medicine, and Psychiatry*, 6(2), 117–190.

Kleinman, A. (1986). *Social Origins of Distress and Diseases. Depression, Neurasthenia and Pain in Modern China*. New Haven: Yale University Press.

Kleinman, A., Das, V. & Lock, M. (1997). Introduction. In A. Kleinman, V. Das & M. Lock (Eds.), *Social Suffering* (pp. ix–xxvii). Berkeley, Los Angeles, London: University of California Press.

Kleinman, A. & Good, B. (1985). Meanings, Relationships, Social Affects. Historical and Anthropological Perspectives on Depression. In A. Kleinman & B. Good (Eds.), *Culture and Depression. Studies in the Anthropology and Cross-Cultural Psychiatry of Affect and Disorder* (pp. 1–42). Berkeley, Los Angeles, London: University of California Press.

Kline, N. S. (1954). Use of Rauwolfia Serpentina Benth in Neuropsychiatric Conditions. *Annals of the New York Academy of Sciences*, 59, 107–132.

Kodoth, P. & Eapen, M. (2005). Looking Beyond Gender Parity. Gender Inequities of Some Dimensions of Well-Being in Kerala. *Economic and Political Weekly*, 40(30), 3278–3286.

Kramer, P. (1993). *Listening to Prozac. A Psychiatrist Explores Antidepressant Drugs and the Remaking of the Self*. Princeton: Princeton University Press.

Krishnakumar, P. (2010). Vishadam Kuttikalil [Depression in Children]. *Arogya Masika*, 1 April.

Krishnakumar, R. (2000). State of Despair. Retrieved from www.hinduonnet.com/fline/fl1708/17080970.htm , 2 January 2016.

Kumar, A. (2006). *Sattwa, Rajas & Tamas Factors among Patients with Depression*. (MPhil). Bangalore: National Institute of Mental Health and Neurosciences.

Kumar, A. (2010). Adravya chikitsa [Treatment Without Drugs]. *Arogya Masika*, 1 April.

Lakoff, A. (2005). Diagnostic Liquidity: Mental Illness and the Global Trade in DNA. *Theory and Society*, 34(1), 63–92.

Lamb, S. (2000). *White Saris and Sweet Mangoes. Aging, Gender, and Body in North India*. Berkeley, Los Angeles, London: University of California Press.

Lambert, H. (2006). Accounting for EBM. Notions of Evidence in Medicine. *Social Science & Medicine*, 62, 2633–2645.

Lang, C. (2014). Trick or Treat? Muslim Thangals, Psychologisation and Pragmatic Realism in Northern Kerala, India. *Transcult Psychiatry*, 51(6), 904–923.

Lang, C. & Jansen, E. (2013). Appropriating Depression: Biomedicalizing Ayurvedic Psychiatry in Kerala, India. *Medical Anthropology*, 32(1), 25–45.

Langford, J. M. (1999). Medical Mimesis. Healing Signs of a Cosmopolitcan "Quack". *American Ethnologist*, 26(1), 24–46.

Langford, J. M. (2002). *Fluent Bodies. Ayurvedic Remedies for Postcolonial Imbalance*. Durham and London: Duke University Press.

Langwick, S. A. (2007). Devils, Parasites, and Fierce Needles: Healing and the Politics of Translation in Southern. *Science, Technology & Human Values*, 32(1), 88–117.

Langwick, S. A. (2011). *Bodies, Politics, and African Healing. The Matter of Maladies in Tanzania*. Bloomington and Indianapolis: Indiana University Press.

Latour, B. (1986). Visualization and Cognition: Thinking with Eyes and Hands. *Knowledge and Society: Studies in the Sociology of Culture Past and Present*, 6, 1–40.

Latour, B. (1991). *We Have Never Been Modern*. Cambridge, MA: Harvard University Press.

Latour, B. (2010). *On the Modern Cult of Factish Gods*. Durham: Duke University Press.

Latour, B. & Callon, M. (1981). Unscrewing the Big Leviathan. How Actors Macro-Structure Reality and How Sociologists Help Them to Do So. In K. Knorr-Cetina & A. V. Cicourel (Eds.), *Advances in Social Theory and Methodology. Toward an Integration of Micro- and Macro-Sociologies* (pp. 277–303). London and New York: Routledge.

Latour, B. & Woolgar, S. (1979). *Laboratory Life. The Construction of Scientific Facts*. Beverly Hills: Sage Publications.

Leslie, C. (1976). The Ambiguities of Medical Revivalism in Modern India. In C. Leslie (Ed.), *Asian Medical Systems. A Comparative Study* (pp. 355–367). Berkeley, Los Angeles, London: University of California Press.

Leslie, C. (1992). Interpretation of Illness. Syncretism in Modern Āyurveda. In C. Leslie & A. Young (Eds.), *Paths to Asian Medical Knowledge* (pp. 177–208). Berkeley, Los Angeles, London: University of California Press.

Light, D. (2010). Bearing the Risks of Prescription Drugs. In D. Light (Ed.), *The Risks of Prescription Drugs* (pp. 1–39). New York: Columbia University Press.

Lindberg, A. (2005). *Modernization and Effeminization in India. Kerala Cashew Workers since 1930*. Copenhagen: NIAS Press.

Littlewood, R. & Dein, S. (Eds.). (2000). *Cultural Psychiatry & Medical Anthropology. An Introduction and Reader*. New Brunswick, New Jersey: Athlone Press.

Lovell, A. (2014). The World Health Organization and the Contested Beginnings of Psychiatric Epidemiology as an International Discipline: One Rope, Many Strands. *International Journal of Epidemiology*, i6–i18.

Luhrmann, T. (2000). *Of Two Minds. An Anthropologist Looks at American Psychiatry*. New York: Vintage Books.

Luhrmann, T. (2012). Beyond the Brain. Retrieved from http://wilsonquarterly.com/quarterly/summer-2012-american-vistas/beyond-the-brain/ , 6 July 2016.

Lukose, R. A. (2009). *Liberalization's Children: Gender, Youth, and Consumer Citizenship in Globalizing India*. Durham and London: Duke University Press.

Lynch, O. M. (Ed.) (1990). *Divine Passions. The Social Construction of Emotion in India*. Berkeley, Los Angeles, Oxford: University of California Press.

Marcus, G. (1995). Ethnography in/of the World System: The Emergence of Multi-Sited Ethnography. *Annual Review of Anthropology*, 24, 95–117.

Marriott, M. (1976). Hindu Transactions: Diversity Without Dualism. In B. Kapferer (Ed.), *Transaction and Meaning: Directions in the Anthropology of Exchange and Symbolic Behaviour* (pp. 109–142). Philadelphia: Institute for the Study of Human Issues.

Marriott, M. & Inden, R. (1977). Toward an Ethnosociology of South Asian Caste Systems. In K. David (Ed.), *The New Wind. Changing Identities in South Asia* (pp. 227–238). The Hague, Paris: Mouton Publishers.

Mathew, E. T. (1997). *Employment and Unemployment in Kerala. Some Neglected Aspects*. New Delhi: Sage Publications.

Metzl, J. M. (2003). *Prozac on the Couch: Prescribing Gender in the Era of Wonder Drugs*. Durham, NC: Duke University Press.

Meulenbeld, G. J. (1987). Reflections on the Basic Concepts of Indian Pharmacology. In G. J. Meulenbeld & D. Wujastyk (Eds.), *Studies on Indian Medical History*. Groningen: Egbert Fortsten.

Mevekari, H. (2003). *The Role of Dhupana and Dhumapana in the Management of Kaphaja Unmada*. Kottakkal: Vaidyaratnam P.S. Varier Ayurveda College Kottakkal.

Mills, C. (2014). *Decolonizing Global Mental Health: The Psychiatrization of the Majority World*. Hove and New York: Routledge.

Mines, M. (1994). *Public Faces, Private Voices. Community and Individuality in South India*. Berkeley: University of California Press.

Ministry of Health & Family Welfare. (2014). *New Pathways, New Hopes. National Mental Health Policy of India*. Retrieved from www.nhp.gov.in/sites/default/files/pdf/national mental health policy of india 2014.pdf , 6 January 2015.

Ministry of Health & Family Welfare, Government of Kerala (2013). *Kerala 2013*. Retrieved from http://dhs.kerala.gov.in/docs/draftpolicy.pdf , 3 January 2016.

Mitra, A. & Singh, P. (2007). Human Capital Attainment and Gender Empowerment. The Kerala Paradox. *Social Science Quarterly*, 88(5), 1227–1242.

Mohandas, E. (2009). Samanilla nashtapetathe jivikkum [Live Without Losing Balance]. *Arogya Masika*, 1 June.

Mol, A. (2002). *The Body Multiple. Ontology in Medical Practice*. Durham and London: Duke University Press.

Mol, A. (2010). Actor-Network Theory. Sensitive Terms and Enduring Tensions. *Kölner Zeitschrift für Soziologie und Sozialpsychologie*, 50(1), 253–269.

Moncrieff, J. (2008). The Creation of the Concept of an Antidepressant: An Historical Analysis. *Social Science & Medicine*, 66, 2346–2355.

Moncrieff, J. (2014). The Medicalization of "Ups and Downs". The Marketing of the New Bipolar Disorder. *Transcultural Psychiatry*, 51(4), 581–598.

Montagne, M. (1996). The Pharmakon Phenomenon. Cultural Conceptions of Drugs and Drug Use. In P. Davis (Ed.), *Contested Ground. Public Purpose and Private Interest in the Regulation of Prescription Drugs* (pp. 253–294). New York, NY: Oxford University Press.

Moynihan, R., Heath, I. & Henry, D. (2002). Selling Sickness. The Pharmaceutical Industry and Disease Mongering. *British Medical Journal*, 324(7342), 886–891.

Mukhopadhyay, C. C. & Seymour, S. (Eds.). (1994). *Women, Education, and Family Structure in India*. San Francisco: Westview Press.

Mukhopadhyay, S., Basu, J. & Rajan, S. I. (2007). Mental Health, Gender Ideology, and Women's Status in Kerala. In S. Mukhopadhyay (Ed.), *The Enigma of the Kerala Woman. A Failed Promise of Literacy* (pp. 71–101). New Delhi: Social Science Press.

Murray, C. J. L. & Lopez, A. D. (Eds.). (1996). *The Global Burden of Disease. A comprehensive assessment of mortality and disability from diseases, injuries, and risk factors in 1990 and projected to 2020*. Geneva: World Health Organization

Murthy, Srinivasa & Wig, Narendra N. (1983). The WHO Collaborative Study on Strategies for Extending Mental Health Care IV: A Training Approach to Enhancing the Availability of Mental Health Manpower in a Developing Country. *American Journal of Psychiatry* 140(11), 1486–1490.

Münster, D. (2012). Farmers' Suicides and the State in India: Conceptual and ethnographic notes from Wayanad, Kerala. *Contributions to Indian Sociology*, 46(1+2, special issue on suicide in South Asia), 181–208.

Nair, A. B., Kumari, A. & Sandeep, P. T. (2014). Vishadam-Puthiya Veshathil [Depression in New Attire]. *Vanitha*, 1 December 2014.

Naraindas, H. (2006). On Spineless Babies and Folic Acid: Evidence and Efficacy in Biomedicine and Ayurvedic Medicine. *Social Science & Medicine*, 62(11), 2658–2669.

Naraindas, H. (2014a). Nosopolitics. Epistemic Manging and the Creolization of Contemporary Ayurveda. In M. Dinges (Ed.), *Medical Pluralism and Homeopathy in India and Germany (1810–2010)* (pp. 105–136). Stuttgart: Franz Steiner Verlag.

Naraindas, H. (2014b). On 'Shastric' Yogams and Polyherbals. *Asian Medicine*, 9(1–2), 12–48.

Naraindas, H., Quack, J. & Sax, W. S. (2014). Introduction. Entangled Epistemes. In H. Naraindas, J. Quack & W. S. Sax (Eds.), *Asymmetrical Conversations. Contestations, Circumventions, and the Blurring of Therapeutic Boundaries* (pp. 1–25). New York, Oxford: Berghahn.

NDTV (Producer). (2015). Actor Deepika Padukone: Depression Interview with NDTV, 1 April 2015. Retrieved from www.youtube.com/watch?v=vQBNYRBpY7c , 15 December 2015.

Nichter, M. (1981). Idioms of Distress. Alternatives in the Expression of Psychosocial Distress. A Case Study from South India. *Culture, Medicine, and Psychiatry*, 5, 379–408.

Nichter, M. (1983). Paying For What Ails You. Sociocultural Issues Influencing The Ways And Means Of Therapy Payment In South India. *Social Science & Medicine*, 17(14), 957–965.

Nichter, M. (2010). Idioms of Distress Revisited. *Culture, Medicine, and Psychiatry*, 34(2), 401–416.

Nisula, T. (2006). In the Presence of Biomedicine: Ayurveda, Medical Integration and Health Seeking in Mysore, South India. *Anthropology & Medicine*, 13(3), 207–224.

Nunley, M. (1996). Why Psychiatrists in India Prescribe So Many Drugs. *Culture, Medicine, and Psychiatry*, 20(2), 165–197.

Obeyesekere, G. (1977). The Theory and Practice of Psychological Medicine in the Ayurvedic Tradition. *Culture, Medicine, and Psychiatry*, 1, 155–181.

Obeyesekere, G. (1985). Depression, Buddhism, and the Work of Culture in Sri Lanka. In A. Kleinman & B. Good (Eds.), *Culture and Depression. Studies in the Anthropology and Cross-Cultural Psychiatry of Affect and Disorder* (pp. 134–152). Berkeley, Los Angeles, London: University of California Press.

Obeyesekere, G. (1990). *The Work of Culture. Symbolic Transformations in Psychoanalysis and Anthropology*. Chicago: University of Chicago Press.

Obeyesekere, G. (1992). Science, Experimentation and Clinical Practice in Ayurveda. In C. Leslie & A. Young (Eds.), *Paths to Asian Medical Knowledge*. Berkeley: University of California Press.

Ong, A. & Collier, S. J. (Eds.) (2008). *Global Assemblages. Technology, Politics, and Ethics as Anthropological Problems*. Oxford: Blackwell Publishers.

Orr, J. (2010). Biopsychiatry and the Informatic of Diagnosis. Governing Mentalities. In A. E. Clarke, L. Mamo, J. R. Fosket, J. R. Fishman & J. K. Shim (Eds.). *Biomedicalization. Technoscience, Health, and Illness in the U.S.* (pp. 353–379). Durham and London: Duke University Press.

Osella, C. (2012). Desires under Reform: Contemporary Reconfigurations of Family, Marriage, Love and Gendering in a transnational South Indian Matrilineal Muslim Community. *Culture and Religion*, 13(2), 241–264.

Osella, C. & Osella, F. (2006). *Men and Masculinities in South India*. London, New York, Delhi: Anthem Press.

Osella, C. & Osella, F. (2008). Food, Memory, Community: Kerala as both 'Indian Ocean' Zone and as Agricultural Homeland. *South Asia Journal of South Asian Studies*, 31(1), 170–198.

Osella, F. & Osella, C. (1996). Articulation of Physical and Social Bodies in Kerala. *Contributions to Indian Sociology*, 30(1), 37–68.

Osella, F. & Osella, C. (1999). From Transience to Immanence: Consumption, Life-Cycle and Social Mobility in Kerala, South India. *Modern Asian Studies*, 33(4), 989–1020.

Osella, P. & Osella, C. (2000). *Social Mobility in Kerala. Modernity and Identity in Conflict*. London, Sterling, Virginia: Pluto Press.

Osella, P. & Osella, C. (2008). Islamism and Social Reform in Kerala, South India. *Modern Asian Studies*, 42(2–3), 317–346.

Patel, V. (2003). *Where There Is No Psychiatrist. A Mental Health Care Manual*. Glasgow, UK: The Royal College of Psychiatrists.

Petryna, A., Lakoff, A. & Kleinman, A. (Eds.). (2006). *Global Pharmaceuticals. Ethics, Markets, Practices*. Durham & London: Duke University Press.

Pigg, S. L. (1996). The Credible and the Credulous: The Question of "Villagers' Beliefs" in Nepal. *Cultural Anthropology*, 11(1), 160–210.

Pilania, M., Bairwa, M., Kumar, N., Khanna, P. & Kurana, H. (2013). Elderly Depression in India: An Emergent Public Health Challenge. *Australasian Medical Journal*, 6(3), 107–111.

Pinto, S. (2004). Development without Institutions. Ersatz Medicine and the Politics of Everyday Life in Rural North India. *Cultural Anthropology*, 19(3), 337–364.

Pinto, S. (2012). The Limits of Diagnosis: Sex, Law, and Psychiatry in a Case of Contested Marriage. *Ethos*, 40(2), 119–141.

Pinto, S. (2014). *Daughters of Parvati. Women and Madness in Contemporary India.* Philadelphia: University of Pennsylvania Press.

Pollock, S. (1985). The Theory of Practice and the Practice of Theory in Indian Intellectual History. *Journal of the American Oriental Society*, 105(3), 499–519.

Pordié, L. (2014). Pervious Drugs. *Asian Medicine*, 9(1–2), 49–76.

Pordié, L. & Gaudillière, J.-P. (2014). Introduction: Industrial Ayurveda. *Asian Medicine*, 9(1–2), 1–11.

Prakash, G. (1999). *Another Reason: Science and the Imagination of Modern India.* Princeton, NJ: Princeton University Press.

Prince, R. H. (1960). The Brain Fag Syndrome in Nigerian Students. *Journal of Mental Science*, 106, 559–570.

Quack, J. (2012). Ignorance and Utilization: Mental Health Care Outside the Purview of the Indian State. *Anthropology & Medicine*, 19(3), 277–290.

Quack, J. (2013). "What do I know?" Scholastic Fallacies and Pragmatic Religiosity in Mental Health-Seeking Behaviour in India. *Mental Health, Religion & Culture*, 16(4), 403–418.

Quack, J. (2014). Porous Dividuals? Complying to a Healing Temple (Balaji) and a Psychiatric Out-Patient Department (OPD). In H. Naraindas, J. Quack & W. S. Sax (Eds.), *Asymmetrical Conversations. Contestations, Circumventions, and the Blurring of Therapeutic Boundaries* (pp. 56–84). New York, Oxford: Berghahn.

Raghunadhan, A. (2001). Concept of Drugs Advised in Mental Diseases. In C. R. G. Agnives (Ed.), *Concept of Mind* (pp. 165–169). Kottakkal: Sankalpa, Department of Samhitas & Siddhantas, Vaidyaratnam P.S. Varier Ayurveda College Kottakkal.

Raguram, R., Weiss, M. G., Keval, H. & Channabasavanna, S. M. (2001). Cultural dimensions of clinical depression in Bangalore, India. *Anthropology & Medicine*, 8(1).

Raikhel, E. & Bemme, D. (2016). Postsocialism, the Psy-ences and Mental Health. *Transcultural Psychiatry*, 53(2), 151–175.

Rajan, I. S. & Zachariah, K. C. (2010). Remittances to Kerala. Impact on the Economy. Retrieved from www.mei.edu/content/remittances-kerala-impact-economy, 14 March 2014.

Ramanujan, A. K. (1989). Is There an Indian Way of Thinking? An Informal Essay. *Contributions to Indian Sociology*, 23(1), 41–58.

Ramdas, S. & Rameshkumar, P. P. (2014). Sthreekalile Vishadam: Rithubhedangalanusarichulla Mattangal[Female Depression through the Seasons]. *Arogya Masika*, 1 April.

Reddy, M.S. (2012) Psychotherapy. Insights from Bhagavad Gita. *Indian Journal of Psychological Medicine*, 34, 100–104.

Rhodes, L. A. (1980). Movement Among Healers in Sri Lanka. A Case Study of a SInhalese Patient. *Culture, Medicine, and Psychiatry*, 4, 71–92.

Robertson, R. (1995). Glocalization: Time-space and Homogeneity-heterogeneity. In M. Featherstone, S. Lash & R. Robertson (Eds.), *Global Modernities* (pp. 25–44). London: Sage Publications.

Rose, N. (1996). *Inventing Our Selves: Psychology, Power, and Personhood* . Cambridge, UK: Cambridge University Press.

Rose, N. (1999). *Powers of Freedom. Reframing Political Thought.* Cambridge, UK: Cambridge University Press.

Rose, N. (2003). Neurochemical Selves. *Society*, 46–59.

Rose, N. (2006). Disorders without Borders? The Expanding Scope of Psychiatric Practice. *BioSocieties*, 1(4), 465–484.

Rose, N. (2016). Reading the Human Brain How the Mind Became Legible. *Body & Society*. doi:10.1177/1357034X15623363

Röttger-Rössler, B. & Markovitsch, H., J. (Eds.). (2009). *Emotions as Bio-Cultural Processes*. . New York: Springer.

Roy, A. (2014). Vishadam Veshaprachannamayi [Depression in Disguise]. *Arogyam Masika*, 1 April.

Roy, A. (2016). Tagore's Triumph over Depression. *The Statesman*. 6 June 2016.

Saradamoni, K. (1999). *Matriliny Transformed. Family, Law, and Ideology in Twentieth Century Tranvancore*. New Delhi: Sage Publications.

Sax, W. S. (2009). *God of Justice. Ritual Healing and Social Justice in the Central Himalayas*. New York: Oxford University Press.

Sax, W. (2014). Ritual Healing and Mental Health in India. *Transcult Psychiatry*, 51(6), 829–849.

Sax, W. S. & Bhaskaran Nair, H. K. (2014). A Healing Practice in Kerala. In H. Naraindas, J. Quack & W. S. Sax (Eds.), *Asymmetrical Conversations. Contestations, Circumventions, and the Blurring of Therapeutic Boundaries* (pp. 200–236). New York, Oxford: Berghahn.

Sax, W. S., Weinhold, J. & Schweitzer, J. (2010). Ritual Healing East and West. A Comparison of Ritual Healing in the Garhwal Himalayas and "Family Constellation" in Germany. *Journal of Ritual Studies*, 24(1), 61–77.

Sébastia, B. (2009). Introduction. Restoring Mental Health in India. Pluralistic Therapies and Concepts. In B. Sébastia (Ed.), *Restoring Mental Health in India. Pluralistic Therapies and Concepts* (pp. 1–26). Delhi: Oxford University Press.

Seligman, R.,& Brown, R. A. (2009). Anthropology and Cultural Neuroscience: Creating Productive Intersections in Parallel Fields. *Progress in Brain Research*, 178, 31–42.

Sharma, A. K., Agrawal, A., Agrawal, U. & Dubey, G. P. (1990). Influence of Mentat on Memory and Mental Fatigue in Cases of Anxiety Neurosis and Depression. *Indian Journal of Cancer and Biological Research*, 3(1), 27.

Shorter, E. (1997). *A History of Psychiatry: From the Era of the Asylum to the Age of Prozac*. New York et al: John Wiley & Sons.

Shorter, E. (2013). *How Everyone Became Depressed. The Rise and Fall of the Nervous Breakdown*. New York: Oxford University Press.

Shukla, K. P. (1980). *Traditional Healers in Community Health*. Varanasi: Gomati Krishna Publications.

Shureshkumar, P.N. (2009). Utkantayum neurosisum [Anxiety and Neurosis]. *Arogya Masika*, 1 June.

Sieler, R. (2015). *Lethal Spots, Vital Secrets. Medicine and Martial Arts in South India*. New York: Oxford University Press.

Sismondo, S. (2009). Ghosts in the Machine. Publication Planning in the Medical Science. *Social Studies of Science*, 39(2), 171–198.

Slaby, J. (2010). Steps Towards a Critical Neuroscience. *Phenomenology and the Cognitive Sciences*, 9, 397–416.

Smith, F. M. (2006). *The Self Possessed. Deity and Spirit Possession in South Asian Literature and Civilization*. New York, Chichester, West Sussex: Columbia University Press.

Smith, F. M. (2011). Sattvāvajaya, Psychology, and Ritual Possession in India. *Asian Medicine*, 6, 22–32.

Sousa, A. J. (2011). *Pragmatic Ethics, Sensible Care. Psychiatry and Schizophrenia in North India.* (Doctor of Philosophy). Chicago, IL: University of Chicago.

Sreekumar, S. (2007). The Land of the "Gender Paradox"? Getting Past the Commonsense of Contemporary Kerala. *Inter-Asia Cultural Studies*, 8(1), 34–54.

Sujatha, V. (2011). Innovation Within and Between Traditions. *Science, Technology & Society*, 16(2), 191–213.

Summerfield, D. (2008). How Scientifically Valid is the Knowledge Base of Global Mental Health? *British Medical Journal*, 336, 992–994.

Sundaran, K. (1993). *Manoroga Chikitsa Ayurvedathil (Treatment of Mental Diseases in Ayurveda)* (B. Appat, Trans.). Kottakkal: Arya Vaidya Sala.

Swayamprava, S.(2009). *An Analytical Study on the Concept of Garaviṣa and its Contemporary Relevance.* Kottakkal: P.S. Varier Ayurveda College.

Tarabout, G. (1999). "Psycho-Religious Therapy" in Kerala as a Form of Interaction between Local Traditions and (perceived) Scientific Discourse. In M. Charrin (Ed.), *Managing Distress. Possession and Therapeutic Cults in South Asia* (pp. 133–154). Delhi: Manohar.

Tarabout, G. (2003). Magical Violence and Non-Violence. Witchcraft in Kerala. In D. Vidal, G. Tarabout & E. Meyer (Eds.), *Violence/Non-Violence. Some Hindu Perspectives.* Delhi: Manohar.

Taylor, C. (2001). Two Theories of Modernity. In D. P. Gaonkar (Ed.), *Alternative Modernities* (pp. 172–196). Durham, NC: Duke University Press.

The Economist. (2013). Rum, Rum Everywhere. Retrieved from www.economist.com/blogs/banyan/2013/03/drinking-kerala , 2 March 2015.

The Hindu. (2012). Kerala Lags behind in Mental Health Indices. Retrieved from www.thehindu.com/todays-paper/tp-national/tp-kerala/kerala-lags-behind-in-mental-health-indices/article3883759.ece , 14 December 2012.

Tousignant, M. (1984). Pena in the Ecuadorian Sierra: A Psychoanthropological Analysis of Sadness. *Culture, Medicine, and Psychiatry*, 8, 381–398.

Trawick, M. (1987). The Ayurvedic Physician as Scientist. *Social Science & Medicine*, 24(12), 1031–1050.

Turkle, S. (2011). *Alone Together. Why We Expect More From Technology and Less From Each Other.* New York: Basic Books.

van der Geest, S., Whyte, S. R. & Hardon, A. (1996). The Anthropology of Pharmaceuticals: A Biographical Approach. *Annual Review of Anthropology*, 25, 153–178.

Varma, S. (2012). Where There are only Doctors: Counselors as Psychiatrists in Indian-Administered Kashmir. *Ethos*, 40(4), 517–535.

Vatuk, S. J. (1990). "To Be a Burden on Others": Dependency Anxiety among the Elderly in India. In O. M. Lynch (Ed.), *Divine Passions: The Social Construction of Emotion in India* (pp. 64–90). Berkeley and Los Angeles: University of California Press.

Venkoba Rao, A. (1978) Bhagavad Gita and Psychotherapy. *Bhavan's Journal July 2 and 16*, 19–23, 35–38.

Visvanathan, S. (1993). *The Christians of Kerala: History, Belief and Ritual among the Yakoba.* New Delhi: Oxford University Press.

Watters, E. (2010). *Crazy Like Us. The Globalization of the Western Mind.* New York, NY: Free Press.

Weiss, M.G. (1977) *Critical Study of Unmāda in the Early Sanskrit Medical Literature. An Analysis of Ayurvedic Psychiatry with Reference to Present-Day Diagnostic Concepts.* Pennsylvania: University of Pennsylvania.

Weiss, M. G. (2015). Classification of serious mental illness according to Ayurveda. *World Cultural Psychiatry Research Review*, 10(1), 16–26.

Weiss, M.G. (2001). Cultural Epidemiology. *Anthropology & Medicine*, 8(1), 5–29.

Weiss, M.G., Isaac, M., Parkar, S.R., Chowdhury, A.N. & Raguram, R. (2001) Global, National, and Local Approaches to Mental Health: Examples from India. *Tropical Medicine and International Health* 6(1), 4–23.

Weiss, M. G., Jadhav, S., Vounatsou, P. & Littlewood, R. (2001). Psychiatric Stigma across Cultures: Local Validation in Bangalore and London. *Anthropology & Medicine*, 8(1), 71–87.

Whyte, S. R., van der Geest, S. & Hardon, A. (2002). *Social Lives of Medicine*. Cambridge: Cambridge University Press.

Wig, N.N. (1983). DSM-III. A Perspective from the Third World. In R.L. Spitzer, J.B.W. Williams & A.E. Skodol (Eds.), *International Perspectives on DSM-III* (pp. 79–89). Washington DC: American Psychiatry Press.

Wig, N. N. & Awasthi, A. (2005). Origin and Growth of General Hospital Psychiatry. In S. P. Agarwal (Ed.), *Mental Health. An Indian Perspective 1946–2003*. New Delhi: Elsevier.

Wolfgram, M.S. (2009). *Ayurveda in the Age of Biomedicine. Discursive Asymmetries and Counter-Strategies*. Michigan: University of Michigan.

Wolfgram, M. S. (2010). Truth Claims and Disputes in Ayurveda Medical Science. *Journal of Linguistic Anthropology*, 20(1), 149–165.

World Health Organization. (1946). *Preamble to the Constitution of the World Health Organization as adopted by the International Health Conference*. Retrieved from www.who.int/governance/eb/who_constitution_en.pdf , 7 April 2016.

World Health Organization. (2001a). *General Guidelines for Methodologies on Research and Evaluation of Traditional Medicine*. Geneva: World Health Organization.

World Health Organization. (2001b). *The World Health Report 2001. Mental Health – New Understanding, New Hope*. Geneva: World Health Organization. Retrieved from http://www.who.int/whr/2001/en/whr01_en.pdf?ua=1, 2 November 2016.

World Health Organization. (2008). *mhGAP Mental Health Gap Action Program. Scaling Up Care for Mental, Neurological, and Substance Use Disorders*. Geneva: World Health Organization. Retrieved from http://apps.who.int/iris/bitstream/10665/43809/1/9789241596206_eng.pdf, 2 November 2016.

Wujastyk, D. (2008). The Evolution of Indian Government Policy on Ayurveda in the Twentieth Century. In D. Wustastyk & F. M. Smith (Eds.), *Global and Modern Ayurveda. Pluralism and Paradigms* (pp. 43–76). Albany: State University of New York Press.

Wujastyk, D. & Smith, F. M. (Eds.) (2008) *Global and Modern Ayurveda. Pluralism and Paradigms*. Albany: State University of New York Press.

Young, A. (1995). *The Harmony of Illusions. Inventing Post-Traumatic Stress Disorder*. Princeton, NJ: Princeton University Press.

Zachariah, K. C. (2001). Social, Economic and Demographic Consequences of Migration on Kerala. *International Migration*, 39(2), 43–71.

Zimmermann, F. (1979). Remarks on the Conception of the Body in Ayurvedic Medicine. *South Asian Digest of Regional Writing*, 8, 10–26.

Zimmermann, F. (1987). *The Jungle and the Aroma of Meats: An Ecological Theme in Hindu Medicine*. Delhi: Motilal Banarsidass.

Zimmermann, F. (2014). Medical Individualism and the Dividual Person. In H. Naraindas, J. Quack & W. S. Sax (Eds.), *Asymmetrical Conversations. Contestations, Circumventions, and the Blurring of Therapeutic Boundaries* (pp. 85–117). New York, Oxford: Berghahn Books.

Zita, J. (1998). *Body Talk. Philosophical Reflections on Sex and Gender*. New York: Columbia University Press.

Zysk, K. (1991). *Asceticism and Healing in Ancient India*. New York: Oxford University Press.

Index

For Product Safety Concerns and Information please contact our EU representative GPSR@taylorandfrancis.com Taylor & Francis Verlag GmbH, Kaufingerstraße 24, 80331 München, Germany

Batch number: 10726532

Printed by Printforce, the Netherlands